"These intricate, interwoven stories speak the truths women too often leave unsaid, the losses we keep to ourselves. They contrast the dichotomies medicine sometimes presents with the uncertain gray areas where so many of us have found ourselves—and even doctors are not immune, as *Held Together* gently proves. The wide breadth of experiences in these pages can help the rest of us make sense of our own lives. Many books tell us how to care for others, but far fewer show us how we might heal ourselves. Thankfully, there is such a book now."

—Amy Wilson, cohost of *What Fresh Hell: Laughing in the Face of Motherhood* and author of *Happy to Help*

"*Held Together* is a simply wonderful collection, beautifully written, of deep stories of women who have undergone personal loss and have come out on the other side. It is about pain, suffering, danger, endurance, survival, and transcendence. It is so experientially rich that I couldn't put this book down without wanting to know what would come next. Rebecca Thompson has caught life itself and shared it with us. Mothers, husbands, grandparents, doctors, and nurses should read it and will come away with something so very rare—hard-earned wisdom for the art of living!"

—Arthur Kleinman, MD, Harvard University Professor of Psychiatry, Anthropology, and Global Health and Social Medicine and author of *The Soul of Care*

"This book does not seem like a book. It seems like a quilt that weaves together stories to create a treasure, and reading it is a healing. The women within these pages share the impact of deep loss, fear, self-doubt, and surprises both agonizing and wondrous. As I read, I was *with* these women, sitting before them like the receptive and open pages of a journal, absorbing their truths. I hung on every word."

—Wendy N. Davis, PhD, PMH-C, President and CEO of Postpartum Support International

"This tapestry of intimate stories is a testament to the common humanity found after loss and the beauty found in connection. Thrumming with sorrow and hope, *Held Together* will comfort those facing challenges on their path to creating families—the families they are born into and the ones they choose."

—Mimi Zieman, MD, author of *Tap Dancing on Everest* and coauthor of *Managing Contraception*

"Rebecca Thompson shares stories that exemplify what mental strength looks like during the darkest days, shedding light on topics that are rarely discussed and showing us that we aren't alone in our pain."

—Amy Morin, LCSW, author of *13 Things Mentally Strong People Don't Do*

"Immersive, compassionate, and vulnerable, *Held Together* invites us to walk with Dr. Thompson as she navigates her own journey to parenthood and the beautiful, messy, uplifting stories of the families she cares for along the way."

—Lori Gottlieb, MFT, *New York Times* bestselling author of *Maybe You Should Talk to Someone*

"In this timely and touching memoir, Rebecca Thompson captures the heartfelt stories of an incredibly diverse group of women. She approaches these women and their families as the thoughtful and experienced physician that she is, recording intimate and sensitive accounts that add critical understanding about complex periods of human development. *Held Together* is at once powerful and tender—essential reading not only for mothers but for anyone concerned with building a constructive future in a troubled era."

—Robin Karr-Morse, MEd, LPC, Family Therapist, Founding Director of the Children's Trust Fund of Oregon, and coauthor of *Ghosts From the Nursery* and *Scared Sick*

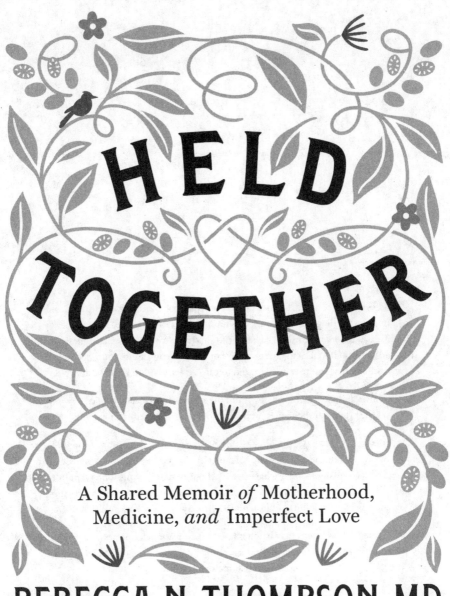

HELD TOGETHER

A Shared Memoir *of* Motherhood,
Medicine, *and* Imperfect Love

REBECCA N. THOMPSON, MD

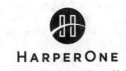

HarperOne

An Imprint of HarperCollinsPublishers

HELD TOGETHER. Copyright © 2025 by Rebecca N. Thompson. All rights reserved. Printed in the United States of America. No part of this book may be used or reproduced in any manner whatsoever without written permission except in the case of brief quotations embodied in critical articles and reviews. For information, address HarperCollins Publishers, 195 Broadway, New York, NY 10007.

HarperCollins books may be purchased for educational, business, or sales promotional use. For information, please email the Special Markets Department at SPsales@harpercollins.com.

FIRST EDITION

Designed by Yvonne Chan
Art throughout by Dana Tanamachi

Library of Congress Cataloging-in-Publication Data has been applied for.

ISBN 978-0-06-333901-9

25 26 27 28 29 LBC 5 4 3 2 1

This project is dedicated with love

To all of our families, born and built and chosen

To everyone whose story is reflected within these pages,
for sharing a piece of your patient, generous, miraculous self

To the women, the mothers, and the people we are—
and to those we're still becoming

CONTENTS

HELD TOGETHER

Soyez comme l'oiseau, posé pour un instant
Sur des rameaux trop frêles,
Qui sent ployer la branche et qui chante pourtant,
Sachant qu'il a des ailes

Be like the bird who
Halting in her flight
On a limb too slight
Feels it give way beneath her
Yet sings
Knowing she has wings

Les chants du crépuscule
Songs of Twilight

Victor Hugo

AN INVITATION

Seventeen years ago, when I endured a string of life-threatening pregnancy losses and rare medical conditions, being a physician didn't protect me from feeling isolated and overwhelmed. What I longed for was a community of women—or even one encouraging story—to reassure me that I wasn't the only person finding the path to motherhood so complicated.

But talking about my struggles seemed unimaginable. Watching friends and colleagues host baby showers and celebrate their children's milestones, I balanced precariously along the edges of their lives. I guarded my sadness like a shameful secret, terrified of being seen as a failure or, worse, being treated as an object of pity. As the months wore on, I recognized that my silence wasn't easing the burden. Instead, it was preventing me from healing, both by hindering the forward movement that I needed to heal myself and by inhibiting my ability to serve as the attentive, compassionate doctor that I aspired to be to help others heal.

So I began to reveal my story, tentatively at first. As I did, other women eagerly offered their own stories in return: Stories about becoming a mother, about growing up as a daughter, about being part of a family. Stories that were deeply felt and self-defining, laced with wonder and anguish and persistence and grace. Stories full of moments they had never shared before, even with their closest friends. Stories about holding their lives together just as everything seemed to be falling apart.

Though few would have chosen their difficulties, every one of them believed that they wouldn't be who they were if their lives had been simpler, and they were grateful for the wisdom they'd gained. They didn't accept the intolerable assertion we too often foist on the grieving—that everything happens for a reason—but they were making meaning out of everything that had happened. The stories they told were uplifting and joyful, even in the face of great loss. The clear-eyed optimism they embodied, resolute and never naive, led the way down a tangle of paths that diverged from what they had expected and veered instead into what they had experienced. I was in awe of the strength and beauty of these ordinary women in extraordinary circumstances.

As I took in the stories of the women all around me, I realized that they were the community I had been longing for. These women changed how I understood my own narrative. Their eloquence reminded me of the power of words and the catharsis in feeling heard. Their trust gave me permission to reach out to others even while I was still finding my way. During a long stretch of time overshadowed by uncertainty, it was their resilience that steadied me, allowing me to imagine a more hopeful future. When I asked each of them if I might retell their stories alongside my own to support other women and families, they generously agreed.

And so *Held Together* invites you to walk alongside us as the details of our lives unfold: Infertility, multiples, abortion, surrogacy. Pregnancy losses, death of a child, death of a spouse. Genetic disorders, mental illnesses, physical and emotional abuse. Poverty, legal struggles, family conflict, career change. Coping with life-altering diseases in our children and in ourselves. Confronting turning points in national and global history. Watching scientific breakthroughs occur in real time. Finding faith and questioning it. Rejecting assumptions about womanhood while experiencing gender as more fluid than binary. Devoting long hours to delivering babies and caring for new mothers while pregnant. Motherless mothering. Adoption, international and domestic, successful and failed. Foster parenthood. Stepparenthood. Teen parenthood. Putting off parenthood for so long that it almost doesn't happen. Ambivalence about whether to become a mother—or wanting to be a mother desperately and ultimately redefining what motherhood could come to mean.

As we embarked on this work together, I began to understand just how far collaboration might take us. What I had first seen as small moments were actually the heart of something much bigger. Where our stories intersected, they came alive. Where grief and joy converged, where oppression and resistance coexisted, we were exploring uncomfortable ideas, and this comforted us deeply. Rejecting the notion that valid narratives required resolutions clearly achieved and adversity neatly conquered, we embraced doubt. We admitted that our stories were messy and complicated—and that we were a long way from knowing how they might end. We relished coherence, dissonance, redemption, and imperfection alike. We welcomed vulnerability and humility. We liberated ourselves and built connections with those around us by sharing our stories, again and again, and we heard our voices grow more self-assured and more resonant each time.

Held Together opens with my own story—because how can I ask others to bare their most intimate thoughts until I am ready to do the same?—then connects to the lives of women who have shaped me through the obstacles and triumphs that have woven our stories together. One close friend struggles to bond with her exceptionally unsoothable newborn as I mourn multiple pregnancy losses. Another recounts her experience of surviving a devastating cancer as I wait to learn my prognosis after pregnancy complications requiring chemotherapy. My patients teach me how to accept the pain and absurdity of the human condition with humor and dignity, even when our days are endlessly different from what we expected. My colleagues' doubts about their choices emerge as we lament the impossibility of ever finding true balance in motherhood and medicine.

All of the people whose stories we share in this project identify as mothers and as women. But they are also so much more. They are physicians, nurses, engineers, biologists. They are architects, artists, activists, teachers. They are homemakers, hired maids, office workers, massage therapists. They are partnered and single, widowed and divorced, gay and straight, city dwellers and homesteaders. They and their families represent a wide range of racial, cultural, religious, and socioeconomic backgrounds. Some have had limited opportunities for formal education while some hold multiple advanced degrees. They have lived all over the United States and have immigrated here from other countries. Their pregnancies took place from their mid-teens to their mid-forties, and their children range from newborns to fiftysomethings who are mothers of young adults themselves. They grew up financially secure and destitute, coddled and neglected, bold and afraid, innocent and tough. They have become, every one of them, courageous and outspoken women who are committed to using their stories to help support others.

They know—we know—that our words can create worlds. We are made of the stories we tell ourselves, the stories we tell each other, and even the stories we hold too tightly, fearing the power they contain in the waiting to be told. Loosening our grip on our most closely held stories can bring us together in ways that nothing else can. In every conversation, we have the opportunity to listen more carefully, to engage more thoughtfully, to give of ourselves more generously, and to ask questions that transform our personal relationships into dynamic and resilient communities. Above all, the wide-ranging perspectives of *Held Together* ask us to consider our common humanity. We are all just people, shepherding each other's memories. We are creating life, raising children, and building families, even as we search for reassurance that we are not unique in our struggles. We are all patients, and we are all healers, navigating tenuous boundaries between wellness and disease. We are realizing that burdens are sometimes gifts. We are living in the liminal spaces of these fragile, beautiful moments.

Collaborating with such an amazing group of women to write *Held Together* has changed how I see my role as a physician as well. In the listening, in the telling, in the bearing witness and the being witnessed, this project has become my practice of medicine. I am honored to call the women whose voices fill these pages my patients, my colleagues, and my dearest friends—some, in fact, are all three, and half of them are medical professionals themselves—and we have cultivated years upon years of sustaining and intertwined relationships. I have learned more from them about compassion than from all my days in hospitals and in classrooms. From them, I have come to understand what true healing requires.

Physical recovery is not enough. The passage of time is not enough. Success in unrelated aspects of life is certainly never enough. More than one woman has told me, over hours of coffee shop conversations and lingering backroad strolls and tearful clinic revelations, that it was only in sharing the story of these pivotal moments that she has been able to move beyond them. To reimagine them in a way that replaces grief and regret with growth and purpose. To revisit her past—and herself—and come out stronger.

Held Together now welcomes you into this place of healing, into this refuge built from the stories that surround us and that will shelter each one of us if we are brave enough to seek them. We are holding each other together in love, offering the same to all who would join us. We are lifting our voices even as we feel the ground give way beneath us. Our foundations may not always be strong, but *we* are.

We hope that you will find yourself among us and know that you are not alone.

NOTES ON THE CREATION
OF THIS BOOK

Held Together **began** as a series of ordinary conversations—conversations between patient and doctor, between longtime friends, between passing strangers. But I quickly realized that our individual connections could be the start of something much more far-reaching and inclusive. As I listened to the stories of the women in my community, so many of them resonated profoundly with the challenges I'd encountered as a mother, as a physician, and as a person. I knew that I wanted to find a way to preserve our words and our experiences and to offer them back so others could benefit from them too.

And so we have kept these conversations going, with intention. Through early-morning and late-night calls across time zones, we have whispered while children slept. On muddy winter walks, we have talked while wind and rain swirled around us. In noisy sandwich shops, we have sought out quiet corners and leaned close. We have recorded every conversation and revisited topics over many meetings. With time, and with each woman's permission, I have sifted through hours upon hours of our interviews, reviewed notes and letters and journal entries from her past and present, and delved into our shared observations of surprising connections that reveal universal themes.

Using these oral and written histories as my foundation, I have worked directly and collaboratively with these incredible women to retell their stories, always striving to capture their most authentic voices by weaving together the pieces of their lives they've so graciously shared with me. As I've done so, I have tried my best to portray the unique experiences of individuals while overlaying a unifying tone that ensures the cohesion of the project as a whole. I hope that reading each of these stories feels like accompanying a close friend through a time of need—and like being accompanied as you find your own way.

While all the people represented here identify as women, this space welcomes all readers of any identity and stands by the right of each person to define who they are. Some of the collaborators have requested that names, familiar places, or personal details be changed, and I have honored that. Some have preferred that their real names be used and identifying information be included, and I have supported that too. Any errors or oversights are my own.

Every account in these pages is true—though not every detail will be accurate. This distinction matters. If a woman mentioned wearing a gray sweater as she recalled an event, I didn't ask her to bring me the sweater, provide a photograph, or find someone else who could vouch for her wardrobe on that day. The sweater was gray to her. And so her telling was worthy of belief.

Memory, like love, is imperfect, but it is all we have. These are the events as we recall them. These are our truest selves, as we wish to be remembered. We hope that our stories will inspire you to reconsider your own experiences, to feel a renewed curiosity about the lives of those around you, and to discover a deeper sense of community by sharing your own story, when you are ready to reach out.

Thank you so much for reading.

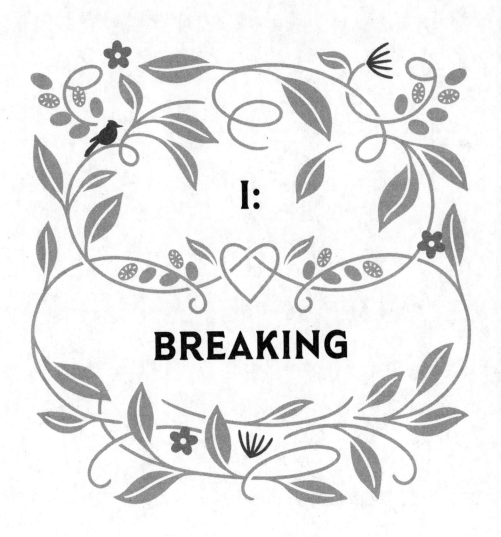

I:

BREAKING

CHAPTER 1

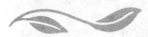

As I recovered from surgery, Ian and I dug in the dirt outside our bedroom window. I pushed the edge of my shovel into the crumbling soil, watching fragments of decaying leaves tumble and resurface as I broke through layers of sand, silt, clay, rock. I imagined the deposits beneath being carried here by the advancing floods and rumbling volcanoes that had shaped the slopes of our forested neighborhood when it was just an untamed expanse of land. My abdomen ached to remind me that I was no longer pregnant. The raw wounds on the surface of my skin stung as they healed into scars.

That morning, we were planting baby kiwis. Before digging, we had mapped out four holes nine feet apart in a perfect square, planning to drive a wooden post into the ground at each corner and plant one spindly start beside it, then run a series of crossbeams, creating an arbor for the vines to climb as they grew. We had placed three more saplings along the periphery of the yard. Smaller and hardier than the better-known fuzzy varieties, these kiwis would take several years to produce the first of their smooth green fruits and several more to deliver a full crop. We were prepared to wait.

We worked side by side to loosen the root balls of each plant in turn as I breathed in the fresh June air and loamy scent of earth. It was a relief to have a project to move my focus out of my head and into my hands, to be doing something that felt useful. Productive. Optimistic, even.

To say that the last several months had not gone as we'd hoped would be a huge understatement. In January, after being together for nearly seven years, Ian and I had decided we were ready to have a baby. We'd both always wanted to be parents, but we'd met during my first year of medical school and gotten married in the thick of my internship, a job that too often demanded that I log hundred-hour workweeks, consider five hours of sleep a luxury, and let a granola bar devoured during a stolen moment qualify as a meal. I was about to graduate from public health residency and take a faculty research job with predictable hours. I was solidly into my thirties. We could finally imagine parenthood fitting into our lives.

Still, we had stared at each other in disbelief when the home pregnancy test had turned positive just seconds after I'd dipped it into the cup. Busy finishing a big project at work, I had waited more than a week after my missed period to test. I'd had just one cycle since trading my birth control pills for prenatal vitamins. I knew that my mother had had two miscarriages before having me and that I was an only child in part because of the anguish those losses had caused my parents. I knew that Ian's parents had endured five years of unexplained infertility before conceiving him and his sister. I had never expected motherhood to come easily.

That afternoon, Ian and I went for a walk as we tried to take in what had just happened. We kept turning to each other and saying, "So, do you want to have a baby?" then giggling incredulously. "Guess we didn't need the two-pack of pregnancy tests," I joked. I nearly floated down the street, dazed with excitement and smug relief that the timing we had planned was working out perfectly. We weren't going to have to endure what our parents did to have a family. Our baby was due at the end of November.

When I started bleeding at a friend's birthday get-together the next evening, all the certainties I had felt the day before vanished. Standing up from the dinner table, I felt a strange gravity, a sinking sensation heavy and deep in my pelvis. In the bathroom, I confirmed it. Bright red blood had soaked through my underwear and into my—very fortunately—black pants. I crafted a makeshift pad out of layers of toilet paper and a plastic soap wrapper I'd scavenged from under the sink. I returned to the table and tried to signal to Ian that I wanted to leave. Although I knew that bleeding in early pregnancy is common and often harmless, I wasn't in any mood to make dinner party small talk.

Away from the gathering, I started to worry more. We were planning to drive from our home in Oregon to rural Washington the next morning to visit our friends Nick and Emily for the weekend. While Ian put some clothes into a duffel bag for us, I rested in bed and we discussed whether it would be safe for me to go to their small farm several hours outside the city. What if I was having a miscarriage and started hemorrhaging? What if I had an ectopic pregnancy, in which the embryo implants outside the uterus and can rupture the fallopian tube as it grows, causing catastrophic internal bleeding? Even if the bleeding stopped, was I going to be capable of socializing when all I wanted was to stay in bed, holding as still as possible? The rational doctoring part of me knew there was little I could do to influence the outcome of this pregnancy. But the instinctive mothering part of me couldn't accept that. When I finally turned out the light, my sleep was fitful and fragmented.

In the morning, I settled on mapping out hospitals and urgent care centers along our route and hoping for the best. I called my doctor's office, where the on-call physician tried to reassure me by reviewing the common benign causes of bleeding in early pregnancy that I already knew. She also recommended that I stop by for a blood draw. By measuring my levels of human chorionic gonadotropin—the same hormone detected in urine by home pregnancy tests—on

Saturday and again on Monday, she would be able to see if the forty-eight-hour change in hCG suggested a healthy pregnancy or a failing one. After a quick stop at the clinic lab, we were on our way.

As we headed north, I found comfort in the promise that I'd have more information soon. I told myself that I was overthinking the situation because I knew too much from my training. Rare complications were just that—rare. And Nick and Emily were old friends, trusted friends. We'd long traveled together, both literally and metaphorically, and we knew that if something went wrong during our visit they would be supportive and resourceful.

But the reason we were going to visit them also made the trip more complicated. They had a newborn. After being surprised by their son's arrival two months before his due date, they had been home with him for less than three weeks after an extended stay in the neonatal intensive care unit. Ian and I had been excited to meet him and to surprise them with our news. But now I wasn't sure how much I wanted to share—or if I'd be up for holding little Leo.

At their house, I quickly realized that I needn't have worried too much about holding the baby. Nick and Emily hovered around their impossibly tiny son, nervously learning to be new parents. Leo woke to eat every two hours, breastfeeding for at least thirty minutes and then taking a supplementary bottle of fortified preemie formula for another thirty. His brief windows of wakefulness were largely consumed by eating and diaper changes.

When he did fall asleep, Emily laid him down on the apnea monitor, a sensor placed under his mattress that sounded a jarring alarm any time it detected a decrease in his breathing movements. I understood her urge to protect him. I wished that I could protect the pea-sized ball of cells inside me, and I wasn't even sure it was still alive. I thought about how parenthood—or the possibility of parenthood—had transformed us all so suddenly into such tentative, timid creatures, unrecognizable as the adventurers we used to be. I watched in wonder as Leo's shadowy eyelashes fluttered with dreams.

But my heart sank when I stepped into their guest room. The decor was simple and elegant, with a rustic four-poster bed and an antique mahogany dresser. Everything else was unforgivingly white: the wall-to-wall carpet, the high-backed side chair, the hand-quilted bedspread, the sheets folded back to welcome us. In the shower, I watched shades of red and pink swirl around the drain. The hot water turned warm, then cool, then cooler still as I stalled, lifting my face into the stream, dreading the plush white towel that Emily had draped so thoughtfully across the rack beside me. I knew that Ian and I wouldn't be sharing any news with our friends that weekend.

By Monday morning, I was back at work, having stopped by the clinic for a second round of tests on my way in. When I hadn't heard any results by noon, I walked out to the parking lot to find some privacy while I waited for the call, since I wasn't able to concentrate on the medical journals I was supposed to be reviewing anyway. Now six weeks pregnant, I was still bleeding, and the cramping had gotten worse on the car ride back the night before.

I barely hesitated when my phone rang. I knew what my doctor was going to say. In her soft voice, she confirmed that my numbers had dropped by more than half. The embryo had likely died more than a week ago, or never fully implanted at all. She tried to comfort me with facts I already knew: At least twenty percent of clinically recognized pregnancies end in the first trimester, and many more end unnoticed, marked only by a heavy or delayed period. The decrease in hCG showed that my body was healing as it should. Most miscarriages are caused by genetically abnormal embryos that wouldn't have survived to become children. Most women who have early losses go on to get pregnant again, and one miscarriage doesn't decrease the chances of having a healthy baby next time. The miscarriage wasn't my fault. We could try again as soon as we were ready.

After she hung up, I sat on the yellow curb feeling numb. I knew that everything she had told me was true, and she had conveyed it with the same gentle words I would have used to reassure my own patients. Still, I agonized over what I could have done differently. I launched into worst-case scenarios. I shifted from believing that Ian and I had escaped the difficult path of our parents into realizing that our story could end up every bit as complicated as theirs. As a doctor, I understood that miscarriage was incredibly common, essentially a normal event in the landscape of reproductive life, and that mine was medically straightforward. The practical side of me was grateful. At least this wasn't something dangerous, like an ectopic pregnancy. The rest of me was devastated anyway.

In the days that followed, moving forward did seem like the best way to heal. I learned how to chart basal body temperature and cervical fluid consistency to predict my peak fertility, trying to walk the fine line between taking charge of my health and obsessing about tenths of a degree on the thermometer I held under my tongue each morning before getting out of bed. Nine days after all signs indicated that I'd ovulated—less than two weeks after I'd stopped bleeding from the miscarriage—Ian and I held our breath over the second pregnancy test from the two-pack as a faint positive emerged. I let myself imagine things going differently this time. But a rusty smear of blood two days later was enough to vanquish those wishful thoughts. I was right back where I had been last month.

On the phone with my doctor's office in the morning, I tried to schedule blood work to see if my hormones were rising appropriately. The medical assistant put me on hold, then came back to say that my doctor wanted me to wait a few more days, that spotting was common in early pregnancy. I thanked her and hung up, disappointed by her response. I was aware that I probably would have attributed the small bit of blood to implantation if this had been my first pregnancy, if I'd had healthy pregnancies before, or if I weren't a physician myself who understood all the ways that pregnancy could be complicated. But I couldn't shake the feeling that something was wrong.

The next day, when I developed a sharp pain on my right side, I called back. This time the message from my doctor, relayed less than patiently again through her medical assistant, was that I should try to relax. That I was just worrying because I'd had a miscarriage so recently and because I knew too much. That I should see how things went over the weekend—it was now almost noon on Friday—but that there was no need to come in yet.

On Sunday, to distract ourselves from the unfortunate fact that it was Mother's Day, Ian and I went for a hike. If my doctor was so confident everything was okay, then I just wanted to do ordinary things, and one of my favorite ordinary things was taking long walks with Ian through nearby Forest Park. With its five thousand acres of steeply wooded hills and seventy miles of paths, the park feels like a remarkably remote retreat in the heart of Portland. As we traversed its rambling trails that afternoon, the twinges of pain on my right side came and went. I loosened the waistband on my daypack and bent side to side and forward and back, nearly folding myself in half as I tried to adjust to the deepening pressure in my bloated abdomen. My discomfort was even more unsettling in its contrast to the solemn peace of the forest's centuries-old cedars. Nothing about this felt ordinary.

Monday morning, I called the clinic as soon as it opened. The medical assistant sighed, exasperated, when I asked again to schedule an appointment for a blood test. "Fine," she conceded tersely. "Why don't you come in this afternoon and see the nurse."

The nurse turned out to be a savvy nurse practitioner who had been in practice for nearly thirty years. She seemed concerned immediately as I described my symptoms. "I'm not finding any masses or swelling," she thought out loud as she pressed a gloved hand along my pelvis, inside and out, "and you don't seem to be in much pain. But just to be safe, let's check blood work and send you to radiology." I began to let down my guard a little. The fact that this attentive, experienced clinician hadn't turned up any alarming findings did reassure me. My doctor was probably right. I was just worrying unnecessarily because I knew too much about what could go wrong.

"I don't think you're overreacting," she said, perhaps noticing the mixture of relief and self-doubt in my expression. "But the odds are good that everything will be okay." She paused and smiled a little. "You know," she ventured, "I had some bleeding in my first pregnancy. But she's a teenager now. And her name is Maggie."

As Ian and I walked out of the clinic, now closing its doors for the night, she handed us an appointment card for an ultrasound at the hospital the next day.

CHAPTER 2

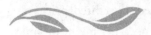

The next morning at nine o'clock, still buoyed by the nurse's encouraging assessment, Ian and I made our way to the sprawling hilltop hospital complex that hovered over the city's vast network of bridges and waterways. The radiologist who greeted us for the exam was wearing a fitted blue dress that accentuated her visibly pregnant figure. As she positioned the ultrasound probe, we watched streaks of light and shadow emerge on the screen, hinting at nothing that resembled a healthy embryo.

She confirmed that I had an ectopic pregnancy lodged in my fallopian tube rather than a viable baby who might go on to be named Maggie. I was grateful that she delivered the news in a straightforward, sympathetic, and respectful tone. But it hurt to hear it from someone who so clearly had what I'd just learned I was about to lose.

Slowly taking in the realization that my worries had been validated, Ian and I walked across the street to the emergency room, where the nurse who checked my blood pressure was also hugely pregnant in her oversized scrubs. I sat numbly in the curtained exam bay for an hour waiting to see a physician. When the on-call obstetrics and gynecology resident introduced herself as Devorah, I was relieved that she seemed kind and thoughtful and about my age—and that she didn't appear to be pregnant.

Devorah listened to my story carefully, then we reviewed my ultrasound results and hormone levels. She outlined the three primary options for managing an ectopic pregnancy: expectant, medical, and surgical. My mental haze didn't allow me to fully process the information she offered about the risks, benefits, and statistics of each method. But I understood that my hCG result from yesterday measured higher than permitted for the wait-and-see approach of expectant management. And having never undergone abdominal surgery, I was terrified of its invasiveness and intimidated by the idea of general anesthesia, even though I got the sense that swift intervention would be Devorah's preference. I was fixated on having the medication.

Devorah consulted with her supervising attending physician—who earned my trust instantly when he joined her at my bedside and asked to see the cycle chart I'd been keeping to confirm my dating—and they decided that I was a reasonable candidate for nonsurgical treatment. My ultrasound made the diagnosis clear. The embryo had no heartbeat and measured within the size range that typically responded to the dosing protocol. I lived very close to the hospital. I was otherwise healthy. And I was the most reliable and compliant patient possible.

But medical management presented its own risks. I would be given an injection of methotrexate, a form of chemotherapy that halts the development of rapidly dividing cells, to stop the pregnancy from growing and allow my body to resorb the tissue on its own. Methotrexate could also cause nausea, vomiting, stomach pain, lung lesions, mouth sores, hair loss, skin rashes, dizziness, anemia, immune suppression, organ damage, or lymphoma. Though the risk of encountering severe complications was low, we had to confirm that my liver and kidneys were up to the task of processing the harsh chemical before the doctors administered it. The nurse came back in to draw my blood. Her eyes were gentle, but her pregnant belly stared me down, reinforcing my failure.

Still wearing the flimsy cloth gown I'd been given on arrival, I was moved from the curtained alcove to a gurney in the hallway to await my results. Several hours dragged by as we watched doctors and nurses pass back and forth in varying states of calm and urgency. By the time my tests confirmed normal liver and kidney functions and blood counts, the staff had changed shifts. The new doctor reviewed my story and the lab results, then ordered the medication from the pharmacy. Each time he walked by us, he apologized for the exposed corridor and the long wait. Since methotrexate is such a biologically active drug, the powder has to be mixed with liquid immediately before use. The pharmacy was swamped. We had arrived on campus right after breakfast, but when I was finally given the long needle of neon yellow liquid in my backside and handed my discharge paperwork, it was night.

I spent the rest of that seventh week of pregnancy on medical leave, frozen on my living room couch and afraid to move lest I make a terrible situation even worse. Methotrexate wasn't an instant cure. If treatment succeeded, the cells of the embryo would stop dividing and my body would resorb them. If it failed, the embryo could continue to grow, pressing outward from within the fallopian tube, causing the narrow passageway to burst, and filling my pelvis and abdomen with blood. Even if the methotrexate arrested further development in the embryo, the weakened tube could tear open and begin to bleed.

The likelihood was high—on the order of nine out of ten—that the methotrexate would work. Although I now had the exact complication that I had been so relieved not to have during the prior cycle's miscarriage, at least the ectopic hadn't ruptured. Still, while I was waiting for it to resolve, the risk of catastrophe was real. I knew that hemorrhage from ectopic pregnancy was the leading cause of maternal death in the first trimester. I alternated between reading everything I could find about fertility after pregnancy loss and trying not to think about what was happening. Each time I managed to forget about the whole sad, scary, overwhelming thing for a few minutes, the constant dull ache in my abdomen would electrify into sudden, sharp flashes. Ian and I curled up under cozy blankets with our two tabby cats and watched endless hours of television, trying to find reruns and movies that were entertaining enough to distract me but not so funny that I couldn't resist laughing—which would cause the stabbing pain to return.

On Saturday morning, after three long days of tiptoeing around my fears and limitations, I woke at sunrise feeling restless. By six o'clock, I had resigned myself to the reality that I wasn't going back to sleep in my bed. I snuck out to the living room to try to get some more rest on the couch. After dozing off for a few minutes, I was awakened again by the strangely warm, weighty feeling of something expanding deep within my pelvis. I felt queasy and unbalanced when I stood up, and my discomfort only intensified in the bathroom. The bleeding got heavier as I felt something lurch forward inside me. The room spun erratically. As I slid to the floor, I knew that there was barely enough space for me to lie down in the narrow aisle between toilet and tub. Ian came in to check on me and found me staring at the ceiling in my green fleece robe. In a deliberate and measured voice, I told him that I thought the pregnancy had ruptured.

When the paramedics arrived less than five minutes later, I'd made it to the hallway beside the bathroom. They kneeled on either side of me, strapped an oxygen mask to my face, and started two large-bore intravenous lines before carrying me to the stretcher they'd parked outside our front door. With Ian in the passenger seat of the ambulance as lights and sirens announced our drive through the neighborhood, I wondered if whatever was happening really merited all this commotion, then, on the other extreme, if I should be more worried that my life was in imminent danger.

Safely delivered to the emergency department, I still felt dizzy and unsettled. By the time the on-call obstetrics and gynecology group came in to assess me, the pain in my side had decreased slightly. Two new residents and their supervising physician stood over me as I recounted my story again. They reviewed my vital signs, including a slightly elevated heart rate and borderline low blood pressure. They looked over my lab results, which revealed a mild anemia and a small dip in pregnancy hormone levels. Sounding tired and impatient, as if nearing the end of a long overnight shift, the supervising physician told me that she thought the ectopic was resolving, albeit slowly. As they left the room, I overheard her tell the residents that I was probably just dehydrated and anxious.

But I didn't feel dehydrated, and I didn't feel any better after two liters of IV fluid. I didn't even feel very anxious—at least not out of proportion to my concern about being dismissed while I was quite possibly experiencing a life-threatening pregnancy complication. In fact, I felt surprisingly calm. And I didn't agree with their assessment.

Ian and I walked out of the emergency department much as we had rolled in, confused and not particularly reassured. Again, I wavered between doubting my own instincts and being indignant about feeling unheard. When we realized that we had no car with us and that I was barefoot and wearing a bathrobe, we called our good friend and neighbor, who—in the midst of her own painful and complicated fertility struggles—drove over to pick us up. During the ride home, the jostling of rutted spring roads and school-zone speed bumps launched bright waves of pain through my abdomen as I tried to lie motionless on the back seat. When I breathed too deeply, a twinge sparked up to the tip of my shoulder—a sign that suggested internal bleeding irritating the underside of my diaphragm where the muscle separated abdomen from chest cavity. I was still worried that the pregnancy had ruptured.

On Monday, feeling no better but being decidedly relieved that the past forty-eight hours had been uneventful, I returned to the emergency department for my scheduled recheck. A too-slight decrease in my hCG level quickly revealed that I wouldn't be in that fortunate ninety percent of women whose ectopics are successfully treated with a single shot of methotrexate. After more discussions with new doctors and more waiting for the pharmacy to mix and send the medication, I received a second dose and an appointment for my next follow-up in three days.

On Thursday, Ian and I met with Devorah and yet another supervising physician. They confirmed with blood work and a repeat ultrasound that I also wasn't among the even larger group—now approaching ninety-five percent—of women whose ectopics are successfully treated with a second dose of methotrexate. Incredibly disappointed but knowing it was time to move forward, I tearfully agreed to surgery. Devorah advised us to go home and collect a few things for the hospital stay while she tried to secure an operating room for that afternoon.

She called less than forty-five minutes later. She had me on the schedule, was going to stay to perform the surgery herself even though it would start four hours after her shift ended, and had booked me a post-operative room in a medical wing of the hospital, far from the crying babies of the labor and delivery ward. Yet again, Devorah had listened to what I'd said and what I hadn't said. She'd understood what I needed. She was doing all she could to provide me with the care she would have wanted if our situations had been reversed. Calmed by my gratitude and resigned to the plan, I finally surrendered to her help completely.

The ceilings of the back corridors that I rolled through a few hours later, as we transitioned from the pre-op area to the operating rooms, were a drab grayish white. I had said goodbye to Ian at a set of wide double doors what seemed like miles ago. Now I shivered in a paper gown as we moved through a maze of hallways and rode a freight elevator—up or down, I don't know. Everything looked flat and sterile and unfamiliar. Even as a resident myself, I'd never visited this dimly utilitarian part of the hospital.

In the operating room, I fixed my gaze on the round lights that stared down at me like bug faces, with their compound eyes formed by dozens of tiny bulbs and the strange proboscises of their handles sheathed in disposable green plastic. One nurse checked my IV. Another repositioned my legs and draped warm blankets over them. The anesthesiologist asked me to count backward from one hundred as she covered my nose and mouth with a clear mask that smelled vaguely like lemons. The last number I remember saying was ninety-two.

When I woke up in the recovery room, Ian was beside me again and it was well past midnight. The surgery had gone much longer than expected. He told me that Devorah had called him shortly after starting, when she had realized that she was looking not at an uncomplicated tubal swelling that she could easily dissect but instead at a mess of ovary and tube and embryo, plastered together by congealed blood and scar tissue, dangerously close to my bladder. This unanticipated finding gave almost certain confirmation that the pregnancy had ruptured at least once and tamped down its own bleeding. Devorah's clinical judgment was telling her to remove the entire right ovary and fallopian tube to avoid any chance of leaving behind pregnancy tissue that could continue to grow and cause serious complications, but she hadn't obtained prior consent from me for this possibility. So she'd asked Ian what I would want. He'd assured her that I'd trust whatever she believed would allow me to move beyond this and try to get pregnant again safely.

I was grateful that my husband so implicitly understood what my priorities and preferences would be and that my doctor was so respectful in honoring them. I was equally grateful to be far from labor and delivery in this post-op room that Devorah had reserved, which happened to be in the oncology wing of the hospital. My presence here reminded me that I was fortunate not to have another condition that methotrexate chemotherapy is used for in pregnancy: the rare and horrifying molar pregnancy, in which the embryo itself doesn't develop but placental tissue can become cancerous and metastasize aggressively, necessitating a much more complex treatment regimen than we'd tried for the ectopic. Though I'd lost a significant portion of my reproductive tract, at least the situation wasn't life-threatening anymore. I found comfort in the knowledge that the surgery was curative, definitive, and done.

In my hospital room the next morning, the sun reflected harshly off an adjacent building and shone straight into my eyes as I woke. I tried to move gingerly under my starched white sheets without jarring the IV line, the thickly intrusive urinary catheter, or my exquisitely tender abdomen. Ian hunkered deeper into the blankets on the visitor couch beside the window ledge. We both rubbed the too-short sleep from our eyes when the senior obstetrician who'd assisted in my surgery came by to check on me.

She reviewed my chart and examined my bandaged wounds. Then she sat gently down on the bed beside me. "Well," she said with a wan smile, looking back and forth between Ian and me, "you must have used up all your pregnancy bad luck by now, so things should be easy for you from here on out." I think I nodded, but I can't remember if I believed her.

A month after my surgery, spring had turned to summer. The newly built kiwi arbor stood outside our bedroom window. While the spindly limbs hovered bare at the bottom of the posts, the structure was in place, ready to support their future fruits. We watered the roots and adjusted the green garden tape as the plants began to climb. I thought about how I was supposed to be almost twenty weeks pregnant, almost halfway to my due date, sensing eager potential and steady growth within myself.

Instead I felt broken.

The magnitude of everything I'd been through suddenly hit me as I stepped away from the arbor and slumped down on a decrepit bench that had long overstayed its welcome in our yard. This was my only life. There would be no do-overs, and I was missing pieces I would never get back. I felt damaged, defective, unrepairable, empty. What if this was the strongest I would ever be?

For the first time, I let the devastation of the past three months overwhelm me as my body convulsed with choking sobs. I was angry at myself for letting my primary care doctor convince me to wait longer to be seen in clinic. I felt guilty for losing several weeks to failed medical management. I took in the realization that my resistance to surgery had cost me an ovary and that it may have cost me my ability to give birth to a living child. No amount of patience or determination or medical knowledge could protect me from these bleak, unchangeable truths.

I felt all the more isolated because no one else knew we were going through these losses. At work, after weekly department conferences, I faded away with the excuse of some hastily imagined administrative task as other doctors gathered to chat about their pregnancies and young children. When my supervisor, trying to console me after I mumbled something vague about recovering from a surgery during my recent absence from the office, launched into a long and animated monologue about how her perspective on her own health had changed completely in becoming a mother, I slouched farther down in the chair beside her desk. I focused all my energy on not crying as she detailed the emergency cesarean birth of her daughter and her memories of selflessly shouting, "Do whatever you need to do to me! Just save the baby!"

We hadn't even told our family and friends that we were trying to get pregnant. Unlike at work, where I'd guarded my privacy deliberately to maintain professional boundaries, we hadn't made a conscious choice to withhold information from those closest to us. But the complications had mounted so swiftly and so relentlessly that I hadn't decided how or when to tell others I was pregnant before I suspected I wasn't pregnant anymore. I felt like I'd gone from noticing a drifting snowflake one moment to finding myself buried in an avalanche the next.

Consumed with getting through each immediate crisis, Ian and I barely had time to grasp what was happening, let alone consider how to seek support. Even among good friends, I was hesitant to reach out. The people who knew me best were used to my stories being filled with rugged optimism, obstacles overcome by perseverance, and challenges resolving into personal growth. Now, I felt weak and embarrassed, with every instinct imploring me to hide my uncertainty. Many of our friends had young children already, but none of them had been through a miscarriage that we knew of, let alone a complicated series of losses. I doubted that any of them could relate to what I was going through. So—regrettably—I didn't even let them try.

Because this unwillingness to reveal my story to others was my own choice, I knew it wasn't fair to resent their unintentional insensitivity. But I did anyway. When one of my closest friends from medical school complained to me over the phone about the third-trimester exhaustion in her healthy first pregnancy, I went silent. After her daughter was born and became an inconsolably colicky infant, I had no reserves of sympathy to offer my friend. Tess was struggling with the things I wished I could be struggling with. Her complaints seemed so trivial, so enviable. So normal.

Observing each other's lives across the deep divide of our separate pains, Tess and I let our friendship dim as we each turned inward. We drifted apart. We pushed ahead. I hoped we might reconnect on the other side of these hours even if we couldn't imagine how or when the other side would come. I hoped we might still recognize each other.

Tess ~ Love Letters

Elena writes me love letters. She sneaks one under my pillow in the morning and tiptoes away, giggling, thinking I'm still asleep. She hides one in her backpack, where I find it when I reach in to pull out her sweater. She leaves one on the counter, where I discover it while I'm gathering up the breakfast dishes after she's left for school. In our quiet kitchen, the paper feels weightless in my hands. I hold it for a moment, trace its smooth surface, run my finger along its neatly folded crease, before I open it to read. Later, when I pick her up outside her second-grade classroom, Elena runs toward me, beaming, with arms open wide. We embrace, kneeling together on the sidewalk as other families swirl around us. At bedtime, I hold her tight on my lap, and we sit still and silent for several long minutes that feel like a lifetime. We are the whole world to each other, providing a comfort and a calm deeper than either of us has ever known.

I think we're making up for lost time.

Before I became a mother, I believed that one of the most rewarding experiences a woman could have would be to bring a child into the world and to love that child unconditionally. I'd spent hours daydreaming about a mysterious baby who would have my sharp Scandinavian cheekbones and my husband Khenan's dark and smooth Jamaican skin, whose eyes would be whatever color is halfway between clear ocean blue and the warmest brown imaginable.

When I was thirty-five weeks pregnant with Elena, just before I went on maternity leave from my clinical practice as a child psychiatrist, the mother of a longtime patient brought me a gift. It was a precious infant blanket, pink and fluffy, with two matching burp cloths and a card that read *Treasure your new baby. This will be one of the most wonderful times of your life.* I brought the blanket home, took it out of its shiny silver box, and set it gently in the crib I had prepared for my daughter, envisioning the day I would meet her.

Giving birth was one of the happiest moments I've experienced. Elena was beautiful—small and delicate, with intense hazel eyes and a shadow of dark hair. She had surprised us by being born on a sweltering August day a month before her due date, but she seemed healthy and strong. When the hospital discharged her after three days of monitoring, I was glowing as I carried our baby out the door.

But as we settled in at home, our routine quickly became complicated. Breastfeeding was nothing like the peaceful bonding experience I had anticipated. I had imagined my newborn nuzzled up against me and gazing up with a milky, half-lidded smile. Although Elena did doze off constantly at my breast, it wasn't because she was full and content. She could barely stay awake long enough to take in any nourishment.

To encourage her to nurse more vigorously, I started pumping and feeding the extra milk back to her through a tube taped next to my nipple. The endless cycle repeated every two hours: Plug in the machine and position the cones. Pump the milk in whirring rhythm. Transfer it carefully to the supplementer. Try to angle Elena's tiny mouth to drink from my breast and the tube at the same time. Feed her for as long as I could keep her awake. Wash the gear with a narrow bottle brush, trying to rinse each delicate accessory thoroughly without dropping anything down the drain. By the time we were done, it was almost time to start over again. I was exhausted, and the extra milk didn't seem to have any effect on my baby. *Things will get better soon,* I thought to myself. *The first few weeks must be the hardest.*

The crying began when Elena was three weeks old. But crying doesn't truly describe what she was doing. I had never heard such a sound. She sounded tortured, in agony, as her screams echoed out our windows, escalating in volume until I was sure our neighbors for miles around thought we were terrible parents. Restless and inconsolable, Elena turned tomato red with eyes squeezed to slits. She looked like she would stop breathing at any moment. My stomach churned to watch her suffering.

Her wailing would start by midmorning and continue through the night, until she and Khenan and I were utterly spent. The moments that she did stop were almost eerie. Loud screeches suddenly ceased when her little body collapsed in sleep. On one particularly rough day, I calculated that she had slept for six hours in the past twenty-four—which left eighteen hours of crying.

When she was awake, she couldn't coordinate her brain and her mouth and her limbs to breastfeed effectively. She arched her back and shrieked, pulling away as I tried to cradle her head. As I leaned off-kilter in our padded blue rocker, my arms grew tired and my nipples grew sore. The back-and-forth motions of the chair made monotonous clunking noises, like a weary horse. Elena's room was painted a bright and flawless white with a warm peach accent wall, but I remember everything as a dull, heavy gray through those long autumn hours.

We had been weighing Elena every few days, and her doctor reassured us that—tiny as she was, barely in the fifth percentile—she was gaining weight appropriately. A thorough medical evaluation was completely unremarkable. I wondered if there was something in my milk that was bothering her. The idea came to me like a ray of light, that this could hold the explanation for—and maybe the solution to—her misery. So I read about elimination diets. I stopped eating dairy products and tried every substitute for regular milk and cheese and yogurt. I read food labels diligently, searching out hidden ingredients. There was not a single knife that had touched butter that grazed anything on my plate. I waited a week, but nothing got better.

Her doctor said maybe it was soy. I cut out soy. Another week, and nothing. I learned that broccoli could make babies gassy and decided it must be the broccoli. Within a few days, I had stopped eating any vegetables. Then I read that in the true elimination diet, the least allergenic foods are rice and chicken. So I ate only white rice and plain grilled chicken for weeks and weeks. It was barely palatable, and I was hungry all the time. Still, Elena's screaming was relentless.

We offered her formula after each breastfeeding session. We stopped breastfeeding entirely and switched to formula mixed with pumped milk. We switched to soy formula. We switched to partially hydrolyzed low-allergen formula, which features the cow's milk proteins already broken into pieces to make digestion easier. We switched to elemental formula made of pure amino acids, which is reserved for only the sickest babies who can tolerate nothing else—but which smells like rotting potatoes and costs six times as much as regular formula. Nothing changed.

Khenan and I ignored everything in our lives that wasn't essential. We rested in fifteen-minute shifts, during those tiny windows between feedings and diaper changes when Elena was sometimes sleeping herself. It didn't occur to us as first-time parents to take turns taking care of her so we could carve out longer stretches of sleep individually— and I couldn't bear to sleep when my baby was crying.

Khenan was a doting husband and devoted father, doing just as much as I was to try to care for our family. Because we did everything together, I never felt alone. We were stumbling through, discouraged and depleted, but we wanted to be strong for each other. We were both barely hanging on by the time Elena was one month old—before we had even expected her to be born. I was humbled by the depth of my helplessness and vulnerability.

Khenan's mother and both of my parents came to support us. We swaddled, swung, shushed, and side-patted Elena's tiny body. We gave her binkies and blankets and hats, walks and baths and mobiles. My mother rocked and rocked and rocked her so tirelessly that I thought she'd wear a hole through the bedroom floor. But even five adults could not find a way to stop the crying.

No one had an explanation, but everyone had a theory.

My mother: "It must be something in your breastmilk." But the only things I had eaten for the past three weeks were chicken and rice.

My father: "There must be something *really* wrong with that child." I didn't appreciate his follow-up suggestion that she might be dying from a rare stomach tumor.

Our neighbor: "You must not be swaddling her properly." She came over to show me her methods and seemed genuinely surprised when everything she did only made Elena scream louder.

Khenan's coworker: "Sometimes babies have unresolved birth trauma and are picking up on their parents' unhappiness." But

Khenan and I were incredibly happy—or we had been, before the crying had started.

My psychiatry colleague: "She must be upset when she looks at you and realizes that you don't look alike." I was deeply offended by his interpretation of my biracial child's inner life.

Elena's pediatrician: "I'm not really sure." At least she was honest.

Though they all had different ideas about the root of the problem, everyone agreed that Elena had colic. And everyone said it would stop by the time she was three to four months old. So I searched for resources about colic. I found books that made promises about learning to baby whisper, finding no-cry sleep solutions, having the happiest baby on the block, knowing what to expect, and becoming baby wise. I read them all, and more. Where was the chapter that would tell me why this was happening and what I could do to help my baby? Sometimes I searched the pages as Elena wailed in the bassinet beside me. Sometimes I fell asleep with half-open texts strewn around me on the bed, only to be startled awake a few minutes later by her piercing cry.

There was no book for me. I found only one that came close to describing what we were going through. It had been written by a mother whose son had had severe colic for the first several months of his life. When I read her stories about how horrible things used to be for their family, I felt a little bit of encouragement. There was at least one other person on the face of the earth who had been through this and survived. But the good outcome of her story almost made me angry. Her child had grown into a happy toddler and then a delightful preschooler, and he seemed completely normal now. I wasn't that optimistic. I couldn't imagine where we'd be in five years. And none of the tips she suggested for soothing a colicky baby had any effect on Elena. Still, I started a countdown. I could endure anything for a few months.

I called my supervisor to let him know that I wouldn't be able to come back to work at eight weeks postpartum as planned. In fact, very little was going as planned. I felt like I'd been hit by a train, and

I couldn't imagine keeping my eyes open long enough to get through half a workday, let alone having the sound judgment needed to practice as a physician. I felt like a fraud as a child psychiatrist. I was supposed to be an expert in human behavior, but I couldn't even handle my own infant. The delicate pink blanket from my patient had long been put back in its silver gift box and stowed away on a high closet shelf. Its naive beauty posed too sharp a contrast against our reality for me to tolerate seeing it in Elena's bedroom.

The four-month mark came and went, and nothing was getting better. Some days I was bitter, but most days I was bewildered and afraid. I numbly wondered what I would do if Elena's screaming never stopped. We began to visit developmental pediatricians, infant psychologists, and pediatric neurologists, seeking an explanation for her behavior. She still resisted being fed and her weight had begun to drop off the growth curve. We started her on a trial of antacid medication, cautiously went back to breastfeeding, and pursued evaluation after evaluation, searching for a medical diagnosis that we could name and thereby—we hoped—fix. Sometimes I wished desperately for the reassurance that would come with being able to put a label on our experience. Sometimes it made me feel better that the experts were just as baffled as Khenan and I were. Although the specialists seemed reluctant to diagnose Elena officially with failure to thrive, clearly none of us were thriving.

Six months in, with no improvement in sight, I went back to work. I felt guilty about being apart from my daughter, then even guiltier about the overwhelming relief I felt sitting in my quiet office while Khenan's mother looked after Elena. I wanted to want to be home with her. But I didn't. While some of my friends struggled with leaving their babies to go to work each day, I struggled with leaving work in the evenings to come home to what I knew awaited me.

I felt deeply embarrassed by my inability to console my child. I avoided public places and social events. I was incredibly disappointed to miss my childhood best friend's wedding, knowing she thought that I didn't value our friendship anymore or that I was too wrapped up in my work to take time off. But the truth is that I knew Elena would scream for six hours straight on the cross-country flight and continue through the ceremony and reception. I was terrified to let anyone see us this way.

When friends would tell me they were pregnant, I cringed. I wanted to warn them that this was going to be the worst thing that ever happened to them. But I said nothing. Every other mother seemed to agree that having a new baby was difficult but wonderful, one of the hardest but also one of the best times of their lives. Watching other women enjoying their pregnancies and young children, I felt alienated from what I imagined everyone else was experiencing as I grieved our lost moments. I was constantly aware of how incongruent motherhood was with the joy of connection I had expected. Elena never looked at me. She never smiled. She never stopped screaming and flailing her arms while she was awake.

My friends were sympathetic, but they didn't understand the depth of my anguish. Most of them tried to be supportive. But, deep within their own challenges or their own joys, they had a hard time relating to my plight. I worried that friends who were struggling with pregnancy complications and infertility would think I should be more grateful to have the baby I'd always wanted. One of my closest friends from medical school had only recently confided in me that she'd gone through multiple pregnancy losses over the year before I had Elena. Looking back, I remembered that when we'd talked one evening during my third trimester—when, I now knew, my friend was still recovering from a surgery to address complications from one of those losses—I had complained about how exhausted I felt hauling myself up the stairs after a long day of work and had heard her go silent. ·

From my perspective now as Elena's mother, I couldn't believe how insensitive I had been. To me, miscarriage was a medical condition to be memorized for clinical rotations and board exams. I had no idea what my friend was going through. I began to appreciate that the range of experiences women navigate in the process of becoming mothers is phenomenally vast. As challenging as life was at that moment for us, Elena and I were safely on the other side of pregnancy and birth. I regretted that I didn't feel grateful. I wished I could start over, trade places with anyone, even my friend who was struggling to have a child. The conflict was agonizing. My guilt escalated. I began to understand that motherhood was laden with grief. That motherhood could bring grief even to those who did not yet look like mothers to the world. That I was far from the only one in pain.

As I spent my days walking circles around the block with Elena squirming fitfully against my chest, intrusive worries clouded my mind. Had I made a serious mistake to have a child? The thought confused me. I loved my daughter so much even as I struggled to remind myself what was lovable about her. Still, in those rare hours of reprieve when she stopped screaming, I would find myself collapsed in tears beside her crib, feeling hopeless, wanting to help her but not knowing how. I wondered if my experience was actually universal but there was something wrong with me because I couldn't handle it.

Just after Elena's first birthday, we were filling out a tax form when we came upon the question *Have you been through a natural disaster?* Khenan looked at me as if to say, *Should I mark "Yes"?*

We just stared at each other for a long moment before we started to laugh, hesitantly and incredulously. There'd been no major floods or hurricanes near our coastal South Carolina home that year. Life had gradually fallen into more predictable patterns over the past few months. Elena's constant screaming had finally stopped. We had made it to the other side. We couldn't even remember how or when the transition happened. Khenan thought it was because we were too devastated to notice. I suspected it was because we never trusted that anything that got better would stay that way.

At Elena's twelve-month checkup, I asked her doctor what I should think about next. I was looking for reminders of which developmental milestones to monitor—but she smiled and said, "Your next child." Khenan and I had always wanted two children, but I had to admit that I could barely imagine starting over. If our next child were as needy as Elena, how would I be able to handle them both? If that baby were easy, what if I couldn't help loving our second child more? What would adding a new person to our family do to the relationship that Elena and I were finally beginning to enjoy?

I still worried about Elena. In her increasing periods of quiet, there was something about her that seemed weathered and worn, always on edge and wary of the world. Khenan and I were convinced she had autism, since—calmer though she had become—she still wasn't bonding with us or making much eye contact. She didn't even babble. She seemed disengaged.

At fourteen months, we took her for another series of evaluations. A psychoanalyst we consulted suggested an attachment disorder. As much as this label resonated with the concerns we had as we struggled to connect with our daughter, it also felt like an insult. As a child psychiatrist, I was acutely aware that the diagnosis of an attachment disorder signifies exposure to trauma, abuse, or neglect that has interfered with the ability to form a normal bond with a primary caregiver. Elena had certainly never been abused or neglected. Was the colic itself her trauma? I was her primary caregiver. I had spent more than a year doing everything in my power to foster attachment and to love this child, and I had failed for reasons beyond both my understanding and my control.

Eventually, our team of specialists confirmed that neither autism nor attachment disorder was an accurate descriptor but that Elena had language delays, placing her in the range of an eight-month-old in verbal skills. With nearly continual crying, there had been no space for speech to develop. Still, her doctors noticed what she was doing well. They showed us the ways she was communicating without speech, watched her pointing from one corner of the room to the other as she glanced back at us hopefully.

"Yes, she's delayed," they acknowledged. "But look what she *can* do!" Gradually, I began to see the good in my child through other people's eyes. I began to appreciate her again. I had been so mired in what wasn't working that I hadn't been able to recognize her gifts. For the first time in more than a year, I felt like there was hope for us.

Speech emerged slowly. One of her few words at nineteen months was *Wuh-muh! Wuh-muh!* As Khenan and I splashed her into the water at the community pool, she would giggle and shout, begging us to dunk her *one more* time. We did this over and over, passing her back and forth between us. The water was incredibly soothing, bringing out a level of trust and connection that we never felt on land. Steam rose up around us under the domed tent that shrouded the outdoor pool year-round, and rows of glowing track lights made me feel like we were cradled by an incubator as the sky outside the shelter darkened. Since Elena had never tolerated skin-to-skin contact as a baby, these hours pressed together felt like some sort of a beginning. For the first time, she was smiling and looking at us with pleasure. We could sense our love being returned. We were finally starting to bond.

As we wrapped ourselves in thick bath towels after a swim one evening, memories of the comforts of swimming during my own childhood washed over me. Growing up in Miami, I had spent entire summers at our city pool. Those were blissful days of mornings regimented by swim practice drills followed by lazy afternoons of playing water volleyball in the shallow end and sharing licorice sticks from the vending machines. I can still smell the strawberry shampoo we passed around in the locker room as we lathered up and clapped soap bubbles in our hands. We took turns sleeping over at each other's houses, where we fell asleep with faces nuzzled in friends' half-dry hair, drinking in the lingering scent of chlorine mixed with berries. Swimming made everything right with the world, if just for those moments.

By the time Elena turned two, I was pregnant with her sister. One afternoon, while cleaning to make room for the baby's arrival, I came across a few old photos that had been gathering dust in a desk drawer.

The first showed five-week-old Elena at her baptism, cheeks blazing scarlet against her starched white gown as she wailed and I squinted into the camera, trying to muster a smile. This summarized her first nine months pretty well. Another showed Elena at ten months, sitting on Khenan's lap and looking quiet but not quite happy, her eyes glazed over with a vacant stare. This was a fair representation of her second nine months. A third showed Elena as a newborn, nestled up against a favorite auntie and trying to chew on her sweater. A fourth showed our family smiling in the pool. I studied these last two pictures for just a beat longer before putting them all into a keepsake box, savoring the reminder that there had been happy moments through it all and that the connections were starting to outweigh the voids in our lives.

Our second daughter, Cecilia, now five, turned out to be a calm, soothable child, who reassured me of what I logically knew but had trouble believing: Elena's temperament wasn't caused by bad mothering. Shortly after Cecilia was born, I finally pulled that delicate pink blanket out of the silver box. Soon she was snoozing peacefully beneath it. In the next room, Elena snuggled with her ratty old tan throw, a simple, unadorned bit of unraveling crocheted yarn that she has now fallen asleep under for more than seven years. She still weaves her toes between the soft acrylic loops every night, while her long fingers stretch the fabric up to her chin. She's almost too tall to fit under it. Over the years, I've repaired it at least a half dozen times.

Although Elena, who just turned eight, is still sensitive and sometimes challenging, I cannot imagine a more loving, more closely bonded child. She is generous and kind and wise beyond her years. I watch her make new friends effortlessly at the park. She hugs me and cries a little when she tells me how much she misses me when she's at school. I have finally become a special person to her.

Today, it's hard to believe that there were times when I didn't know if I'd ever be meaningful to this child. I revel in both my daughters' attachments when only Mommy will do, and I can even have patience when everyone needs Mommy at the same time, and everyone needs just a little more Mommy than everyone else.

As close as Elena and I are, I can't say that the feelings associated with those early days are gone. Colic continues to seem too tame a word to describe our experience, but I've accepted that we'll probably never come to a better explanation. Still, there's a deeper wound that carries over, a subtle but dangerous effect of our past that can undermine the strength of our current relationship. When we are pushed to our limits, I default to some of the same patterns from her infancy. My mind begins to spin: *What if I can't ever calm her down? What if she'll live with this unhappiness forever?* When Cecilia is upset, I feel sorry for her but confident that my interventions will help. But when Elena is upset, I find myself back in those dark places that I thought we'd never escape.

Building our attachment has taken years. It has been a halting process, a constant balancing of gains and losses. Sometimes, during the too-rare moments I take to myself these days, I swim laps in our community pool. As I float on my back and look up at the ceiling, I'm transported to the peace of steamy evenings under the same glowing lights, when we first started to connect as a family of three in the water together. My arms trace circles in a soothing slap and glide and my breathing falls into easy rhythms. I think about how comfortable Khenan has always been in the water too, going back to his childhood outside Kingston, when he started making two-kilometer open water swims at eight years old, the same age I was when I spent my summers at city pools along the Gold Coast of Florida, the same age that Elena is now. I realize that, for every member of our family, water is a source of serenity and safety. Water brings out our bravest and truest nature. I realize that Elena is still an amazing swimmer.

Every time I go back and reflect on our story, it heals me a little bit. Some of the emotion fades. This healing has made remembering the feelings, and capturing their immediacy in the writing or the telling of our story, a little bit harder—but living with the memories immeasurably easier. I remember a seasoned psychiatrist that I studied with years ago talking about recovery from trauma. He referred to studies showing that the higher the quality of a survivor's narrative—the more detailed and nuanced the story she tells herself about her experiences—the less severe her suffering as she tries to move forward. His words, which had seemed abstract enough to me as a trainee to be nearly useless, now give me hope. Telling our stories might save us all.

The pain associated with Elena's infancy is still so fresh in my mind, but the details are gone. I've blocked out the most difficult memories, and we don't have many records of those early years. What I do have are love letters, stacks of notes and drawings saved in boxes alongside those rare few photos of her babyhood. From the time Elena could hold a pencil, when she was not quite three, she has marked our time together this way.

At first Elena's letters were just shapes: stick figures of Mommy and Elena, with a heart enveloping us. Then her letters became words, delightfully misspelled: *u me we luv.* Soon she moved on to bigger ideas: *thank you mom fur helping me feal beter.* Now her letters have topic sentences, supporting details, and conclusions, and they come in both English and Spanish. All her letters are heartfelt, so some reveal her frustrations too. Once she scrawled an angry signature across her sister's face on our family portrait and left it on my desk. But she also engraved a huge, puffy heart encircling all four of us, to represent her love for our family, on that same defaced photo. Elena has never shied away from emotions, however complicated or conflicting, and I love that about her.

I do worry about sharing the story of our struggles with Elena as she gets older. I wonder about what memories were imprinted on her from infancy, about what will come of the mixture of inconsolable distress and offerings of maternal comfort that was her constant for so long. I wonder what will carry forward in her. I never want Elena to doubt my love, or to think I've been selfish for hoping for better times for all of us. Part of me hesitates to reveal our history for fear of tarnishing the incredible bond that she and I share now.

But more than anything, I want to be honest.

I want to unearth these dark moments that formed the beginning of our complex love story, to allow healing and growth out of pain. I want to add this difficult but important chapter—one that was written long before Elena took pen to paper. I want to capture these memories to make sense of something that seemed senseless at the time, to discover the beauty, and sometimes even the humor, in what would otherwise be insufferable. I want to remember that our family's path, cobbled together though it may be with laughter and tears, frustration and pride, is the foundation for our love letters.

So this is my love letter to Elena.

May you always understand how much we have endured without giving up on each other. Believe me when I say that if I could lift the burden of those painful hours from either of us, I would. But I thank you for so profoundly deepening my capacity to feel empathy for others who are hurting.

May you come to appreciate how hard-earned our love has been, and how deep our commitment, even when the days and nights were long and we both grew despondent. We have built our bond together, through years of physical and emotional work, sometimes excruciating and sometimes exhilarating. I will never take it for granted.

May you seek and discover and create your own loves in this life. May you remember that sometimes the people you love the most will not be able to show or tell you how they feel and that sometimes you won't be able to express the depth of your love even to someone you care boundlessly about. May you have patience with yourself when this happens, especially if you have children of your own someday.

May you find your way to who you want to become, unhindered by my expectations. May you continue to grow as the capable and compassionate person I've had the privilege to witness you becoming. When you struggle, may you find the grace to believe that you are strong enough to tolerate the unbearable, even in the face of uncertainty.

May you never feel alone in the world. May you always know how much I love you. May our love always be a story that we're still in the process of telling.

II:

RECONNECTING

CHAPTER 3

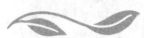

After the ectopic, I wanted to try to get pregnant again immediately, and I was scared of ever trying again. Fortunately, the decision
was partly made for me. What scant medical literature I could find
estimated that the liver took, on average, one hundred sixteen days to
clear the body of methotrexate. For my peace of mind, I needed all
traces of chemotherapy to be gone before we tried again, which gave
me four cycles—the rest of the summer and the first bit of fall—to
heal and grieve and prepare myself for whatever might come next.

Deciding to wait was much easier than the waiting that followed.
In June, I finished residency. In July, I started my research position at
the university. In August, I busied myself studying for medical board
exams. Through the summer, I swam and ran and biked and hiked,
setting a goal to exercise every day without fail. I was determined to
channel sadness into strength.

But nothing could distract me from the obvious void. Everywhere
I looked, women were snuggling babies in carriers and lifting toddlers
into race-car grocery carts. Each week brought new pregnancy and birth
announcements from friends and coworkers. Each month stretched out
to feel like a year. We still hadn't told anyone else what had been happening. I was frozen in time while the rest of the world moved on.

In October, when the positive result flashed bright and quick on the plastic strip, I felt a tangled mix of relief, dismay, excitement, and dread. I'd ovulated two weeks late—the first time my cycle had been irregular since I was a teenager. Because I'd been charting, I was sure of my dates. I worried that the delay indicated that something was wrong with this embryo, or with my hormone levels, or with my sleep or nutrition or stress level as I'd juggled starting a new job with preparing for the biggest exam of my career—which I'd sat for that morning. I suddenly wished we had waited one more cycle. I felt like this pregnancy was doomed already.

Calculating the six-and-a-half-week mark, when we might be able to detect a heartbeat, I called and made an appointment with Devorah. I felt almost giddy imagining how delighted she'd be to see my name on her schedule for a prenatal visit, after all our prior interactions had revolved around discouraging news and unwanted outcomes. I tried to push off my doubts as I counted down eighteen days until the appointment.

In the clinic on that crisp fall morning, Devorah was every bit as happy for us as I'd hoped she'd be. She had brought the bedside ultrasound in with her, knowing that I'd have a difficult time chatting casually before trying to see the pregnancy. The image appeared on the screen right away, a white line of embryo and nearby circle of yolk sac. Everything looked about the right size, and everything was in the right place. I breathed my relief out heavily, reverently. It wasn't another ectopic. She moved the ultrasound wand gently to get a better view.

"I'm so sorry," she said.

It took me a moment to notice that she had stopped smiling. Then I realized that the tiny white line wasn't pulsating as it should. The embryo was still.

My first surge of grief wasn't for the impending miscarriage itself.

It was for the loss of the joyful conclusion to our story that I'd already imagined, already calculated. This baby was supposed to be due the last week of June, which was also the last week of Devorah's residency. This baby was supposed to arrive into the world caught by the hands of this colleague, this peer, this friend who would understand how desired and how hard-won this pregnancy had been as she attended us during labor. This baby was supposed to bring our experience full circle—mine, Ian's, Devorah's, the child's—and deliver the validation of a happy ending to us all.

Although we understood that the pregnancy probably wouldn't succeed, we agreed to watchful waiting. Ian and I both needed time to accept what was going on, and maybe Devorah did too. At a formal ultrasound one week later, the same picture persisted: a solitary embryo with no heartbeat, and with no further growth. Again at two weeks. And at three.

At our next appointment, Devorah met us in the waiting room and walked us to a small counseling alcove with a round wooden table and four padded chairs. I didn't suspect that this room was the setting for many lighthearted conversations.

As soon as we sat down, I told her that I was ready to move on. Though my body hadn't recognized it yet, this embryo was clearly not viable. She offered me misoprostol, a medication that would end the pregnancy and encourage my body to bleed it out on its own, or a dilation and curettage, which would remove the pregnancy using a surgical procedure. Contrary to my feelings with the ectopic, and I think surprising her a little, I interrupted her to insist on the D&C.

"I want the tissue to go to pathology," I said. "I think it's a molar pregnancy."

Molar pregnancy: a bizarre genetic misstep in which placental tissue from an abnormal embryo can become malignant and metastasize aggressively as it transforms into a disease called choriocarcinoma. Molar pregnancy: one of the rarest, most feared, and least understood of early pregnancy complications. Molar pregnancy: the very condition I had been relieved not to have back while I'd been recovering from the ectopic surgery on the oncology ward.

"Oh, Becca." So much history swirled between us as Devorah paused, regarding me with exasperation, kindness, pity, and longing to reassure. "There is no way you have a molar pregnancy."

Even as she tried to convince me that having a molar pregnancy now would be too much bad luck for one person, my mind shifted to the evidence in support of my theory. Over the past three weeks, each time I had seen the yolk sac on the ultrasound, it had looked strangely calcified, which I knew could correlate with chromosomal anomalies. I was also troubled by the hCG levels that my recent blood work had shown. With a healthy embryo undergoing normal development, these levels typically double every forty-eight hours for the first few weeks. As development gets further along, doubling times should slow. Or, more grimly, when an embryo is faltering, levels should decrease. I was worried that mine were rising too quickly in the setting of no interval growth or heartbeat, with values well above the median for eight, nine, ten weeks into pregnancy. Devorah, citing the textbook standard of two-day doubling, suggested that they seemed to be rising too slowly.

I had grown accustomed to medical staff dismissing my concerns. But Devorah's tone was different. She didn't agree with me, and she didn't believe me—but she didn't criticize me either. Though she made no effort to hide the fact that she found my logic dubious and my conclusions improbable, she listened patiently while I explained my perspective. She respected my voracious reading of the obstetrics literature about first-trimester complications and monitoring, and never let on if she had reservations about my detailed scrutiny of my own medical data. She understood why I needed the information we'd get from sending the pregnancy tissue to the pathology department for laboratory analysis.

Because of her willingness to validate my observations and to consider my questions, I trusted her so deeply that when we realized no anesthesiologist was available to assist her in performing the procedure, I told her I'd be fine with local numbing medication and ibuprofen. I wasn't afraid of the physical pain or of being awake as she worked. It was enough for me to feel safe in her care, and a part of me wanted to be fully present to what was happening, with nothing to filter or obscure the experience. We scheduled the D&C for the next afternoon.

Exactly one week before the due date of my first pregnancy, I found myself on a cold metal procedure table listening to the lurching vibrations of a suction machine, acutely aware that I could have instead been in a very different wing of the hospital listening to the cries and coos of my newborn. Five days after that, when I might have been at home, surrounded by friends and family to celebrate the beginning of the winter holiday season with my baby, I was instead sitting in a movie theater parking lot answering a phone call from Devorah, whose incredulous voice told me that the pathology lab's results were back.

My instincts and interpretations had been right. It was a molar pregnancy.

Because the mutations involved in this disorder meant that any left-behind cells could metastasize, I would now undergo a minimum of six months of follow-up to confirm that my pregnancy hormones resolved to undetectable levels and stayed there. Suddenly, I had to invert all my expectations. Instead of being encouraged by the rising hormone levels of a healthy pregnancy, I hoped for dropping numbers when I got my blood drawn each week. Instead of charting to identify fertile days, we were consigned to many cycles of careful contraception.

Being on hold with these broken dreams felt worse than trying but failing, and I hated the flood of memories triggered by each visit to the hospital lab. But getting pregnant would complicate my monitoring and put my health in danger. A new pregnancy would make hormone levels rise again, overshadowing any smaller increase that could signal persistence of the molar pregnancy.

After the D&C, we decided it was time to tell our families what had been happening. My hormones were dropping reassuringly, which felt like a distant cousin of good news. Somehow, almost imperceptibly, the balance was shifting. Explaining what we were going through finally seemed simpler than withholding it.

Since settling in Oregon had brought us far from our childhood homes, we broke the news to our families over a series of phone calls. We provided the barest minimum of details, not wanting to overwhelm anyone. Yes, we'd been trying to get pregnant. Yes, we had actually succeeded. Three times, in fact. But no, there would be no baby in the near future. We described the procedures I'd undergone, trying to reassure our parents that all the interventions—daunting as they sounded to would-be grandmas and grandpas digesting them in one great bolus of dismay—had gone smoothly. We told a few close friends the same.

Even revealing this much was exhausting. As we moved through December and into January, I felt disconnected from this season of celebrating fresh starts. I wondered somberly if projecting hope for the future would be a sign of resilience or just another form of denial.

Two weeks into the new year, we watched the due date for the ectopic come and go—on Ian's thirtieth birthday. We carried on. We went to work. We planned scuba expeditions and backcountry ski trips that we wouldn't have been able to take if I'd been pregnant or if we'd had a newborn. In between these welcome distractions, I hunkered down against the winter chill while the scrawny spindles in the kiwi arbor withstood a harsh frost outside our bedroom window.

CHAPTER 4

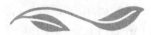

One night in February, we were out to dinner with Shreya and Kyle, old friends we hadn't seen much over the past couple of years. Sitting with them while the server brought a parade of sushi to our quiet corner table, we chatted about work, exchanged news about mutual friends, and reminisced about the mornings we used to spend together at the local rock climbing gym.

As I poked at a plate of salmon and tuna nigiri with my chopsticks, the same thought kept distracting me from our conversation: *This really isn't worth it.* This lavish meal of raw fish that would have been forbidden in pregnancy—this bittersweet privilege that I felt guilty not to be more grateful for—was yet another reminder that I would have willingly forgone the exotic dives, the snow camping, and every restaurant offering in town to become a mother.

Still, I was making the effort. After a long stretch of declining far more invitations than I accepted, just getting out for the evening was a step. Part of me relished the familiar comfort of sitting with friends who knew us well enough to pick up right where we'd left off. But part of me remained guarded, detached, inhibited by so much that had happened since we'd last been together, unsure of where to begin.

Then Shreya started talking about international adoption. Like us, Shreya and Kyle had decided to wait until she'd completed more of her medical training before starting a family. Now, in her final year of medical school, they were deep into the process of figuring it out.

On their side of the table, Ian and Kyle had moved into a discussion of lightweight gear for overseas travel when Shreya asked me if we were thinking about having kids too. Despite the obvious progression of this conversation, I hadn't anticipated her question. We'd never talked about our plans for parenthood beyond timelines. I stammered something about *Yes, probably, not right now but maybe soon*, before trailing off awkwardly.

There was a beat of silence before I ventured a question of my own.

"Did you always know you'd adopt? Or did you consider having biological children?"

"We can't." She shrugged.

Good friends that we were, her frank reply surprised me. Shreya and Kyle were, in some ways, intensely private people. Yet she spoke openly as she went on to describe a complicated series of events they'd been through long before we'd met. Her history was full of physical pain, emotional anguish, invasive procedures, and toxic medical regimens. But she didn't seem to see any of these challenges as shortcomings, as her fault. She was so self-assured.

Our stories blended seamlessly as we continued to talk, sentences weaving together with an ease that felt not like interruption but completion. Shreya listened as I began to explain the monitoring I was undergoing and how we'd know if I needed methotrexate again. She asked relevant, thoughtful questions about my diagnosis and complications. She offered insights about what I might expect emotionally based on her own experiences navigating a convoluted path to motherhood.

Parts of her story reminded me of the time I'd spent on the oncology ward recovering from surgery for the ectopic pregnancy, and I realized that my gratitude until now had been more abstract than I'd admitted. I knew things could get worse, but reality had felt distressing enough that my imagination stopped in the moment, allowing denial to defend me a little too well. In the dim light of that restaurant, I was struck by a visceral sense of how much more complicated our story could have become—how easily the miscarriage could have turned to hemorrhage, the ectopic rupture could have been catastrophic, the molar pregnancy could still progress into a malignant choriocarcinoma.

As I sat with Shreya, telling my story suddenly seemed like something that might heal me rather than just force me to keep revisiting my grief. Before that night, we'd mentioned our pregnancies to a few other close friends, hastily glossing over details to say that they hadn't worked out, that we weren't pregnant anymore, that we were taking a break for a while. But this was the first time I had articulated the experience of going through such rare and dangerous complications to someone whose own story made her capable of truly understanding mine.

Shreya had endured worse and come out stronger. She was living with intention, seeking the best options available to her without lamenting what could have been or envying what others had. But she was neither naive nor blindly optimistic. Every part of her story affirmed that she accepted things as they were. Now I understood: she was a realist who chose hope.

After that night, I knew that if Ian and I wanted to become parents we would find a way to become parents. By the end of April, I had painted the small bedroom beside ours a bright and cheerful yellow. On the wall, I had placed three framed batik prints—a tiger, a lion, and a bear—that used to hang above my own crib. On a narrow wooden bookshelf, I had arranged a dozen children's classics and a pair of tiny red sandals.

I wondered what Shreya and Kyle were doing to prepare.

Shreya ~ Contrasts

India is a land of contrasts. Encircling an expanse of more than one million square miles, its borders traverse the snowy peaks of the Himalayan range in the north, windswept desert plains in the west, silver-sand beaches in the south, and damp jungles of mangrove swamp along the eastern coast. In the capital territory of Delhi, skyscrapers tower over the ruins of palaces, tombs, and medieval forts that have almost returned to the earth.

India is a land of diversity. Its more than one billion inhabitants communicate in twenty-two official languages and more than sixteen hundred local dialects. Though three-quarters of the population practice Hinduism, the religions of Islam, Christianity, Buddhism, Sikhism, and Jainism are also observed by many. The country's flag displays three horizontal bands: a saffron stripe symbolizing strength and courage, a green stripe invoking fertility and growth, and a white stripe between them—punctuated by the navy blue spoked wheel of the Dharma Chakra—representing hope for peace, enlightenment, and truth for all.

India is a land of extremes. Its past and its present alike are marked by poverty and privilege, by devastation and magnificence, by war and tranquility, by tradition and innovation. It is where my family's story begins, no matter how I mark the beginning.

My father had just arrived in Pune, a sprawling city in his home state of Maharashtra, when he started acting strange. Helping his cousins prepare for an upcoming Hindu festival by setting up for the puja—the ceremonial worship ritual before the feast—he had trouble balancing or lifting anything. He couldn't name the statues of deities he'd known since childhood. He complained of a worsening headache and went to lie down.

In Kansas, on vacation from my biophysics master's program in Massachusetts and eager to celebrate the winter holidays together, I was with my mother at my childhood home when she received the call. Her voice sounded worried and confused. I didn't understand everything she was saying, her fluent English interspersed with whispered Marathi and medical terminology informed by her training as an obstetrician-gynecologist. The next morning, she began the thirty-two-hour journey to collect my father, leaving me behind to await my sister's return.

Once we were all reunited at home, instead of the festivities we'd planned, our family visited neurologists and surgeons, then learned from a brain biopsy that my father had an aggressive and inoperable form of cancer called glioblastoma multiforme. For three months, I flew back and forth between Boston and Wichita every few weeks, watching his function decline at each visit. It was heartbreaking to witness my father's independence slipping away just as I, at twenty-five, was beginning to establish my own. In March, he was hospitalized for pneumonia, transferred to intensive care, and intubated. He never came off the ventilator.

After my father's funeral, my mind was worn down by the events of the winter. My body was equally depleted. I'd been having trouble sleeping, making no time for exercise, and eating whatever was convenient, with little regard for my own well-being. The spotty vaginal bleeding I'd noticed had now dragged on for at least six weeks. Attributing it to the stresses of caring for my father and the pressure of having resumed my studies immediately after his death, I expected it to resolve once I got back into my usual routines.

But by April, the bleeding had only increased. Beginning to wonder if this might be related to the abnormal Pap smear I'd had a few months before my dad got sick, I scheduled an appointment at the student health center between a statistics lecture and an optics lab one afternoon.

The primary care physician who examined me said that she felt something on my cervix but wasn't too concerned, suggesting I return tomorrow to see the gynecologist. My mom told me that it was probably a harmless polyp, like the ones she removed all the time in her own practice. But when the gynecologist examined me the next day, she didn't reassure me so easily, referring me instead to the gynecologic oncology specialty group at the teaching hospital.

Now my mother and I were both worried. In two days, I had gone from almost dismissing some irregular bleeding to realizing that the doctors I'd consulted thought I had cancer. The endometrial biopsy with the oncologist was a horrible experience. I wasn't sure which was worse: the vulnerability of having seven residents and fellows stand over me observing the procedure as I lay flat on my back in stirrups or the sensation that—not having been offered strong enough pain medications—I was being stabbed repeatedly in my pelvis.

The biopsy did show cancer. My mother stayed by my side for the follow-up procedure that removed a sizable chunk of my cervix to clarify the diagnosis. The next morning, the oncologist met us in her office to explain the results. The cancerous cells were coming from the lining of my uterus. She recommended a complete hysterectomy.

I clutched my mother's hand and started bawling. The doctor's words made no sense. I was distraught, but I felt physically fine. I felt healthy. Her suggestion of illness felt like the only thing making me sick, her insistence at interventions defining me as a patient. Every impulse compelled me to stand up and walk out of the clinic so I could make the whole thing stop.

Through my sobs, I asked her what would happen if I did nothing.

"You'll die," she said quietly. Then she told me she wanted to schedule the surgery as soon as possible. As the three of us sat together in the silence that followed, I felt like all my babies had just died too, before even having a chance to be born.

Over the next few days, my mother called her colleagues and asked what they would do if I were their daughter. Several of them mentioned a new high-dose oral progesterone protocol that had seen some success with these types of tumors, without requiring a hysterectomy. After consulting with several other cancer centers around the country for second opinions, I decided to return home to Kansas to try this treatment, where my mom could continue to help me navigate procedures and evaluations that were so closely related to her area of expertise. Through three rounds of treatment and monitoring over eight months—through flying back and forth to Boston to finish the last few requirements for my graduate degree, through traveling to India with my mom and sister to spread my dad's ashes by a river near his ancestral home—every result came back normal, reassuring us all that the cancer had been eradicated.

That fall, when a mutual friend introduced me to Kyle, he struck me as that rare combination of kind and quiet with an open mind and an adventuresome spirit. Within a month of our first date, I had told him everything—the story of my dad, my diagnosis, my treatment, my uncertainty. He took it all in, nodding and listening. Amazingly, he wasn't scared away. I felt so optimistic about this new relationship, about how smoothly my treatments were going, about the possibility of reclaiming my life.

Then, in the spring, I developed terrible pelvic pain. A preliminary ultrasound at my gynecologist's office showed masses on both my ovaries. She recommended we repeat the imaging in a month to be sure these weren't simple cysts related to hormonal fluctuations. Skeptical though I felt, I was willing to entertain any possibility that left room for hope.

When I told Kyle, he seemed surprisingly unfazed. But I wanted to give him an out. I truly had no idea what might lie ahead.

"You know, if you don't want to be here, I'll understand," I told him when we were alone in the elevator of his apartment one day.

He hardly paused. "No. I want to be here. You need me and I want to be here."

That was the extent of our conversation. I knew I could trust him. We continued on.

The cysts looked bigger and more complex on the next ultrasound. The following week, the surgeon removed my entire left ovary and a large portion of my right, and the pathologist confirmed that both masses were malignant. Incredibly, the report also showed that these were new primaries, not related to the endometrial cancer. My oncologist recommended we remove my uterus, my fallopian tubes, and the rest of my right ovary immediately.

I felt like I was back in that original appointment when I'd first been told I had cancer. I started begging for options. Were there any nonsurgical treatments? Could she just remove more of the area around the cyst? Could we harvest my eggs? *No, no,* and a gentle but firm *no.* Fertility medicine was in its infancy, and finding a clinic to do this wouldn't be straightforward because assisted reproductive procedures were illegal for unmarried women in many parts of the United States. I didn't have time to wait. Given how suddenly these tumors had sprung up, they might fill my entire abdominal cavity if we delayed for even the two menstrual cycles that egg collection would take, and the ovarian-stimulation protocol could accelerate tumor growth. We scheduled the surgery for the following week.

When I woke up from the anesthesia, I was vainly grateful to find a low horizontal incision along my bikini line rather than a long vertical slice from my belly button down. A catheter snaked up into my bladder. The nurse kept waking me to take blood samples and check my vital signs. My mother and my sister and Kyle took turns sitting with me or napping on the tiny built-in couch by the window in the hospital room.

By the time my doctor came in to check on me a few hours later, I was completely spent. Still in a haze of painkillers, I felt like I'd been hit by a truck as I listened to her explain that they'd sampled my lymph nodes, stripped away a large portion of the lining of my abdominal cavity where it touched my small intestines, stomach, and diaphragm, and removed all my reproductive organs. It had been a huge undertaking, and it had gone as well as it could have.

When she paused, I broke down crying again. I had been silently questioning my fate for too long, and now it all came out in a choked sob.

"Why does God hate me so much?" I whispered, more to myself than to her.

She put her arm around me gently.

"I think your body just didn't like those organs. I think you're going to be okay now."

Somehow, her words were exactly what I needed to hear in that moment. I wiped my tears and smiled a little, for what seemed like the first time in months.

Once I'd had some time to heal from the surgery, about six weeks later, I started chemotherapy. Still wanting my mother by my side, I traveled to Kansas for treatment every three weeks. In contrast to my denial when I was first diagnosed, my anger now fortified my resolve. I had been told I could have three to six treatments. I insisted on all six. I kept working—I needed to, to pay the bills and to maintain my health insurance—and my supervisors were truly understanding, even when fatigue forced me to leave by late morning some days and a blood clot scare landed me briefly back in the hospital.

Losing my hair was kind of devastating and kind of a relief. I had been hoping for so long that it wouldn't fall out to definitively announce my status as a cancer patient. Seeing my eyebrows fade away and my underarms go baby smooth was bizarrely upsetting. My scalp was tender, as if I could feel each wavy black hair release from its follicle before it fell to the shower floor and swirled around the drain. But when I finally shaved my head, it was freeing. I was cool for the summer. And I needed less than ten minutes to get ready in the morning.

The port on my chest was the physical intrusion that bothered me most. Placed just below my collarbone and giving direct access to the large blood vessels near my heart, it would certainly make my treatment easier. Instead of constant needling of sensitive arm veins, blood samples could be collected here. Instead of eroding delicate local tissues, harsh medications could be delivered to where they would most safely and efficiently circulate throughout my body. But every time I saw it or felt it, I started to cry. Without it, I wouldn't have been left with any obvious marks from my disease. With it, a thick and lumpy scar would mar the once-smooth honey-colored skin just above my breast, indelible and visible any time I wore a bathing suit or a strappy top. I hated being reminded of how damaged I felt. I just wanted to look like everybody else.

I just wanted to *be* like everybody else. My friends were planning weddings and honeymoons while I was scheduling chemotherapy and doctors' appointments. But I wasn't exactly jealous. I was sad and angry that I had to spend my time doing something so different from what everyone else was doing. It felt so unfair that, while my friends were looking forward to starting families, I was coming to terms with the removal of my entire reproductive system. And I always seemed to be the youngest patient in the waiting room, in the clinic, in the oncology practice. When I was admitted to the hospital once to treat a sudden fever, the on-call physician, exploring possible sources of infectious disease, asked me if I had any younger siblings at home instead of if I had any kids. At first this strange question made me laugh. But as soon as he left, I broke down in tears. I had lost my fertility before some people thought I even looked old enough to have children.

Shortly after I finished the six months of treatment, my hair started growing back. I felt a little twinge of hope each time I moved through a new hairstyle, from pixie to short bob to long, soft ringlets. I felt relieved as winter gave way to spring and as I watched the body I remembered reemerging—but I sure didn't relish shaving my legs again. By the beginning of summer, almost two years after Kyle and I had begun dating, my doctors finally started using the word *cured*. Finally, we began to sense the relief in feeling truly optimistic for the first time since we'd been together, and to appreciate the clarity of purpose that brought us. We got married in a small family ceremony a few months later.

With the memory of my father's final weeks still just as present as the impact of my own illness, I also started volunteering at a local hospice facility. From my first shift, I loved being around my patients and their families, offering care that honored lives that were coming to a close rather than trying to prolong lives at any cost. I wished we had used hospice when my father had died. Hospice held no guarantee of perfect closure, but it bestowed a special kind of dignity and value on life. Being part of it made me feel like medicine was the ultimate humanity. Shortly after we got married, I told Kyle that I wanted to be a doctor. When I was offered admission to medical school in Texas after three years of night school premedical coursework and the grueling application process, I felt excited and liberated and undaunted. I was eager to do something big and meaningful with my life.

Medicine is a discipline inclined toward dichotomies, reliant on drawing boundaries between sick and well, physical and emotional, patient and physician. But I knew what it was to live in all these spaces—and between them. I understood that medicine was a land of contrasts but that many of them were artificial. I was thrilled to bring what I had learned from my own experience of illness into my training to benefit others. I was also relieved that no one in medical school would know my history. My hair had grown back. I didn't look sick. And I was beyond grateful for the fresh start.

Exploring different specialties, I considered the fine line between feeling a personal connection to my profession and triggering too many painful memories. I discovered that I loved uncovering complicated diagnoses. I was intrigued by medical technology and innovation. I needed to find a field that would position me as a problem solver, a doctor's consultant, an expert who had specialized knowledge to share. Then I discovered the role of the clinical pathologist.

During my rotation with the pathologist who would become my most influential mentor in medical school, I could immediately appreciate the constant intellectual stimulation she found in her work. I saw how her day moved in rhythms of intense concentration punctuated by breaks to review results with her colleagues, much like my former days in the lab. I loved that her work was active and cerebral and didn't require extensive charting or detailed consideration of social dynamics. And I remembered how the definitive diagnosis granted by the pathologist after my first surgery had guided the treatment that had ultimately saved my life.

As I began my final year of medical school, Kyle and I decided that—given the reality that nothing was going to get any easier once I moved into my pathology residency—we were ready to start a family. As soon as we started talking about adoption, we knew we would adopt from India. Having lost my ability at such a young age to carry a pregnancy, I relished the possibility of having a child who might look like me, who might manifest that visible link. Even more, I wanted to give my mom the opportunity to pass down traditions from our family's cultural heritage and Hindu religion to her first grandbaby.

The Indian adoption system held its own appeal—though for a distinctly unappealing reason. Unlike the open adoptions common in the United States, adoptions in India are almost always shrouded in secrecy because many of the children available are born outside marriage, a start in life that carries nearly insurmountable social stigma. The oppression of women that has led to shame around adoptions troubled me deeply, but the simplicity that a closed adoption might offer us as adoptive parents was, admittedly, attractive. I didn't know anyone who'd been involved in an open adoption, as a parent or an adoptee, and I couldn't envision how I might navigate the complex relationships it would create.

Kyle jumped into the research eagerly. He said that, since his ancestry was mostly Scottish and he had no personal connection to India, doing more of the work through this process would give him a special connection to our child's origins. I loved his enthusiasm. Watching him take this on reassured me that he was fully invested in our future family and the big decisions we were making. He identified a nearby agency that had been certified in accordance with the Hague Convention, the international agreement that guards the safety of children and families participating in intercountry adoptions. Within weeks, we were undergoing background checks, scheduling finger-printing sessions, and collecting all the documents and photographs and recommendation letters that would go into our dossier to demon-strate, both to our country and to our child's country of origin, that we could provide a reliable and loving forever home. We underwent a seven-visit home study from the social worker as she investigated every aspect of our life—from how we approached finances in our marriage, to what challenges and losses we'd faced together, to what our own childhoods were like, to where we planned to store our most poisonous cleaning chemicals—but her kind and patient presence felt surprisingly noninvasive. Her diligence reinforced the gravity of what we were undertaking.

Having specified no gender preference for our child, we were aware that we would likely be matched with a girl. I understood from my childhood visits that India has a strong social and cultural pref-erence toward boys, and even baby girls whose parents are married are at risk of being abandoned. Confirming sex through ultrasound has been forbidden since 1994—a disproportionate number of girls are aborted when this information is available to families—but many doctors still follow an unwritten code to tell expectant parents what they want to know. A girl, likely to marry and require her parents to offer the groom's family a dowry and to pay for lavish wedding festiv-ities, might be indicated with the offering of a pink candy or a frown. A boy, likely to get a job, provide for his parents, and contribute to his family's financial security, might be signaled with blue sweets or a smile.

I didn't see a girl as less desirable at all. I pictured making a lifetime of mother-daughter memories in our home: adorning her hair with barrettes, hanging frilly curtains in her bedroom, painting fingernails together before going out to buy dresses. I found it odd and humorous that my mind gravitated toward these stereotypical trappings of femininity, since I had never done these things with my own mother and sister, and I didn't spend much time shopping or wear nail polish myself.

Though the process felt interminable, everything was going smoothly. I'd recently secured a spot in my first choice of residency programs, so we could stay where we were settled in Texas and Kyle could keep his job. We were grateful that the permanent visa granted by my Overseas Citizenship of India status would make our adoption easier too. The year before we began the process, OCI card holders had been afforded parity with Indian citizens abroad in adopting Indian children, and agencies had a strong preference for matching children with people of Indian descent.

Still, when we got a referral just six weeks after our home study was completed, we were astonished—and even more so to learn that the child was a boy. As I held the single picture the agency had sent of a beautiful nine-month-old, belly button poking out from his too-tight undershirt as he pulled himself up on a whitewashed crib railing, I had a hard time believing that I was looking at my son.

My son. Suddenly he was real. His huge brown eyes stared up at me from the photograph. My heart felt sad and warm at the same time. What circumstances had brought him to an orphanage? What had his life been like so far? Was he being well taken care of? Did anybody hold him? Read to him? Comfort him at night when he couldn't sleep? Did anybody love him? I knew immediately that I wanted this child to be part of our family—that I wanted him to make us into a family.

We had a son, but we knew almost nothing about him. Kyle and I reviewed the records our agency representative had gotten from the orphanage. We learned that the baby had been born in Mumbai, where his young, unmarried mother lived. His first language was Marathi, the same local language my parents had grown up speaking and had spoken to me as a baby. While he had no known congenital anomalies, infectious diseases, or developmental delays, we were told nothing else about his medical history or his milestones. *No data*, *No data*, *No data* scrolled down pages of printed reports in the brackets corresponding to every other category.

We didn't even know when we'd get to bring him home. The adoption had to be approved through the Indian court system, which could be a slow and halting process. Every time we received more paperwork to fill out, we'd complete it within a couple of days and send it back to our agency, then wait a month or more to hear back from the Indian government that it had been accepted.

As we considered what to name him, we knew we wanted something easy to spell and easy to say that also had ties to India. We were passing around his picture over dinner one night with friends when one of them said, "Maybe you could call him something simple and sweet, like Vic." She hadn't realized it, but Vic was perfect—classically American, but connected to the common Indian boys' name Vikram, meaning *valor* in Sanskrit. Within days we were thinking of him as Vic.

In May, nine long months after we'd received the referral, it was finally time to bring our son home. Twenty-eight hours, three flights, and one teeth-clenching taxi ride later, we arrived at the hotel in Mumbai feeling exactly as miserable as expected after traveling more than eight thousand miles. My mother, who was accompanying us on the trip, stepped up to the desk to speak with the clerk, drawing on the Marathi of her own childhood to secure us two blissfully air-conditioned rooms.

After a deep but fitful sleep, our first full day in India was devoted to finalizing reams of paperwork and reviewing the prearranged schedule for our two-week visit, all under the guidance of our local social worker. She confirmed that we would travel to the orphanage the next morning. I barely slept at all that second night, full of anticipation and still tossing and turning when sunlight began to illuminate our room. A strange blend of jitters and numbness carried me through the very ordinary motions of washing my face, brushing my teeth, and putting on my clothes.

One by one, I placed the gifts we had brought for Vic's caregivers—watches, chocolates, lotions, lip balms—into a loose-weave fabric sack. I shifted the bag nervously from one shoulder to the other as I waited for Kyle to gather up his things. I wanted time to slow down so I could savor these last moments of preparation. I wanted time to speed up so we could hold our son. I wished I could be magically transported to my child that instant without missing any bit of this momentous day.

Soon we were in our hired van, with a driver who smiled as he sped along the dusty roads and blared his horn at passing motorbikes. As we traveled farther from the city center, the buildings became smaller, squatter, and more run-down, soon giving way to the tin-roofed cacophony of shantytowns, while the number of wandering roadside cows increased. Cracked earth and scraggly aloe plants heralded the beginning of the hot season, adding to the landscape's sense of desolation. The monsoons wouldn't start for another month.

Suddenly, coming around a corner, we recognized the structure we'd seen in pictures our social worker had shared. The orphanage rose three stories tall, directly in front of us. With its yellowish-tan concrete walls and covered balconies sheltering rows of uneven railings, only small murals of trees and butterflies beside the door distinguished it from the surrounding apartments and office spaces.

After paying our driver, we climbed out of the van to see an older man standing at the entrance, waiting to greet us. He was smartly dressed in the business attire typical of warm Southeast Asian climates: a collared short-sleeved polyester shirt, straight-legged pants, and open-toed sandals. His hair was slicked back and graying a little, and I had the thought that he looked like my dad might have at this age if he had lived as long.

He guided us to the second floor, to an open lobby area along the outer edge of the building. The adjacent hallway was strangely quiet, lined as it was with closed, windowless doors. Though we knew that about thirty children lived at the orphanage, we also understood that the staff was fiercely protective of the children's privacy. Our purpose that day was not to observe or to judge anything else, but solely to meet Vic.

Less than a minute later, a small woman stepped out from one of those doors to join us on the balcony. She was also dressed for the occasion, elegantly but functionally draped in the tunic and trousers of a deep red salwar kameez that matched the bindi in the center of her forehead. And she was holding a baby—*our* baby!

At first he was quiet, looking sweaty and disheveled in a colorful cotton jumper, as if he had just been woken up from a nap. His huge brown eyes glared warily at us, like the strangers that we were. As his caregiver walked him toward us, he started crying, then buried his face in her shoulder as he gripped her long black braid. He seemed terrified to let go of this soft and gentle woman who felt like home.

For the next thirty minutes, we sat together on the floor. Kyle, my mother, and I formed a semicircle, while Vic and his caregiver sat across from us as he pouted and clung to her. We tried to say sweet, reassuring things to him, but he didn't understand any of our words. We offered him a bottle of water, a small stuffed puppy, and salty American crackers. My mother whispered a singsong children's rhyme to him in Marathi, but even then he looked skeptical.

Finally, as I held out an Indian tea cookie, he stopped crying. His caregiver placed him beside me. He took the delicate tan sweet in his hand, turned it over quizzically, and stared up at me. His face softened. He looked back and forth between us, with more curiosity than suspicion, and I felt a glimmer of trust emerge.

The long day became evening. We performed a small puja, lighting a candle, saying a prayer, and dabbing the kumkuma powder of blessing on each of our foreheads. As Kyle gathered our things, I lifted my hand and Vic's, guiding him to wave a tired goodbye to the adults who had helped bring him to us.

Back in the van, I held Vic in my lap as we drove over the rutted road leading away from the orphanage. I was so happy to finally have my son and so sad to watch him watching the only home he'd ever known getting smaller in the distance as his tear-stained face gazed over my shoulder.

At the hotel, my mother was joined by my sister, who had just arrived too. Vic and Kyle and I, in our own room next door, were now a family of three for the first time. Kyle had tried to hold Vic at the orphanage, but Vic had just wailed and protested. Our stop at the clinic for a chickenpox vaccine—mandatory to help prevent Vic from becoming part of the local outbreak in progress, which could have delayed his entry into the States for weeks—probably hadn't improved Vic's mood, nor had the long, hot drive from the orphanage to the hotel.

Then, at bath time, Kyle and Vic finally connected. From the next room, I could hear them splashing and giggling as Kyle poured cups of water over Vic's back and chest. Stepping into the doorway, I watched Kyle soap our son with bubble bath, wash his hair gently with a facecloth, and snuggle him in a towel. Vic was smiling for the first time since we'd met him. Soon he was fast asleep, sprawled across the starched white sheets of the hotel crib.

For all our preparations, we marveled at how unprepared we felt. The contrast between what we'd expected and what we encountered was as striking as the contrasts in India's landscapes. We had brought bottles and baby-food pouches to feed Vic, but he was already drinking out of regular cups and eating spicy Indian curries. We had brought a whole suitcase of clothes because we didn't know what would fit him, then we discovered that he didn't own any shoes. We had never changed a diaper, and we suddenly found ourselves learning on a twenty-pound toddler who kept trying to stand up and run away.

When the time came to go home, after two weeks of more paperwork and legal proceedings and the inevitable waiting all that entailed, we traveled backward across ten and a half time zones, arriving in the States the day before we'd departed India. When Kyle finally carried Vic into our house and set him down on the entryway floor to meet our tiny white-haired poodle, who'd spent the last few weeks with our neighbors, Vic's eyes grew wide.

"Bah! Bah! BAAAAAH!" he yelled. He scowled and pointed at Charlie, who sniffed his foot enthusiastically. We didn't know what he meant, but in India, stray dogs roam the streets everywhere, and I think Vic was astounded to see one allowed inside. Or maybe he thought Charlie was a sheep. Within two weeks, his first word in English was *doggy*.

We were continually surprised by what surprised Vic: Seeing himself in a mirror and startling, then trying to play hide-and-seek with this fun new playmate. Reaching for our hands to walk us outside, then wrestling against the injustice of being strapped into his car seat. Tasting peppermint ice cream, his dimpled, expressive face registering confusion and delight in equal measure.

Launching into parenthood abruptly, without the gradual progression of pregnancy to newborn days to infancy to toddlerhood, was sometimes just as baffling to us. We felt like we were constantly learning what Vic was capable of. When we put him on the shortest slide at the playground, he'd fall off at the bottom. When we tried to help him slip his arm into a jacket, he'd topple over, since he'd never learned this maneuver in the heat of Mumbai. When we guessed at his abilities, we were wrong as often as not. It didn't help that we were all exhausted from grappling with his inverted India Standard Time sleep schedule. We half-heartedly joked that he'd have to adjust soon, since there was no such thing as night preschool.

Still, after a few months together, we were getting used to the rhythms of family life. We spent the summer before I started residency indulging in family adventures—visiting playgrounds and libraries, strolling along a paved trail behind our house, renting a cabin in the mountains of New Mexico with friends—and taking care of slightly less fun tasks, including catching up on immunizations and treating Vic's plethora of intestinal parasites. We loved bringing Vic to new restaurants because, being used to the intense flavors of traditional Indian fare, he seemed much more open to trying new foods than the average kid his age.

As he explored his new community, Vic rarely encountered people who looked like him. And, although we shared our Indian heritage, Vic's skin was much darker than mine. This wasn't particularly surprising to me. In keeping with its vast cultural diversity, India's people have a wide range of appearances. Patterns of exploration and invasion dating back five thousand years explain, at least in part, why northerners tend to be tall and fair skinned, southerners of medium height with darker complexions, and tribal groups with distinct physical differences scattered east to west throughout the middle of the country. None of this is simply a neutral result of history. In India, those with darker complexions are often made to feel inferior, judged less desirable for marriage and employment, and pressured by their families to change their appearance with chemical treatments. With its rampant prejudice toward fairer skin, colorism maintains deep roots and problematic consequences to this day.

But in the United States, no one commented on the difference between my skin color and my son's. People seemed genuinely shocked when I told them Vic was adopted, then equally interested in our story. In our majority-white community, casual observers didn't seem to give weight to gradations in darker-toned skin. And no one ever questioned my very pale husband when he and Vic were together. I guess they just figured Vic had his mother's coloring.

Before our adoption, I'd heard about all sorts of staggeringly insensitive questions fielded by other adoptive families: *Didn't you want to have your own children? Why couldn't his real family keep him? How much did he cost?* My friends who had mixed-race children or whose families were created via transracial adoptions seemed to face the most awkward moments. One close friend of mine—a Black woman with a fair-skinned biracial son—told me that she's asked almost weekly if she's her son's nanny. She's still taken aback every time. We both wish people would just say "What a beautiful child!" and leave it at that.

From the beginning, I was absolutely not opposed to talking frankly about adoption. I wanted Vic to know his story and to embrace it. In our pre-adoption parenting classes, several instructors had stressed that adoption should be a proud part of a family's history. Kids shouldn't remember the day they were told they were adopted, like some shameful secret revealed. They should have a natural understanding from a young age about how their family came together.

Every year on Vic's birthday, we talked about how grateful we were to his birth mother for helping him come into our lives. We watched to see what he understood, tried to gauge what he was ready to hear. We hoped she was at peace with her decision as we imagined who she might have been. Every year, we bought her a flower, which sat in a vase on the table as Vic drew her a picture or, once he was able, wrote her a note in a card that couldn't be mailed.

As Vic got older, knowing so little about his birth family and his background seemed more relevant—and more distressing. My understanding of adoption kept evolving too. I had always been keenly aware of the grief and loss that must be part of his birth mother's story, and of Vic's, but I was beginning to see how fraught adoption could be in more subtle ways too. I was intensely grateful for our son, even while I resented the implication that Vic himself should feel lucky to have been removed from the life he would have had in India. I was concerned that our actions as adoptive parents supported a market that sometimes profited unscrupulous investors, but I firmly believed that international adoption was not charity. I wished that societies had the resources to keep biological families together, yet I knew that we wouldn't have Vic if they did. I'd read accounts written by adult adoptees that described the pain of not knowing more about their backgrounds.

When Vic was eight, we reached out to the social worker we'd worked with in India. Her hasty reply confirmed, in no uncertain terms, that there was no trail leading back to Vic's family of origin. His birth mother had made a deliberate choice from the limited options available to her and had elected that this part of her life remain undocumented, inaccessible, unknown. She was protecting herself. I respected the privacy she chose, but I wished we could learn more. I felt such a loss for my son.

So we've built our own history together. If we couldn't know Vic's past, we could at least preserve memories of his childhood going forward. From the day we'd received that single photograph of him at nine months old, we'd been collecting articles about life in Mumbai and clippings from newspapers published around the world on the day he was born. When we'd brought him home from India, we'd started a scrapbook, adding pictures of our time there together. The adoption agency required regular updates—first every three months, then every six, then every twelve—so we produced beautiful newsletters full of glossy prints and detailed text to capture his days. We made extra copies for ourselves and kept creating them far beyond the agency's last requested submission when Vic was seven years old.

Vic keeps this compilation, this life book, beside his bed. Now in middle school, he doesn't ask many questions about his origins, though sometimes I notice him, bedside light on late into the night, flipping through the pages we've crafted. We try to hold on to pieces of our shared culture by watching Bollywood movies, reading Indian comics, and lighting lanterns for Diwali. He likes to summarize the story of his adoption by telling people that, although we're pretty nice as parents go, the first thing we did after meeting him was take him to a doctor's office and make him get a shot, which he didn't enjoy. He's turned what he knows into a funny punch line, reinventing it as his own. He's starting to claim the parts of our story that are his, which helps me begin to see them as distinct from the parts that are mine, even as the years fly by like months. I blinked, and he grew up.

Vic knows a little about my medical history, and he's noticed my scars. But things that happened before he was born register only as remote and unfathomable to him. The first twenty-five years of my life, before illness invaded our family, seem easy in retrospect, and sometimes I still feel bitter about the loss of my father, my health, my fertility, my innocence. I'm grateful for all that I have, but there's a sadness that doesn't go away. I think that's just part of the human condition. We get through things even if we don't get over them. We do what we can with what we're given. We endure hard times and happy times, then we try to make sense of it all and move forward. Our children might become our lives, but they should never be our only purpose.

Though I love my career, I'm planning to retire much earlier than I might have had I not been sick or watched my father die too young. I still want to see more of the world. In the pathology lab, when I place a drop of contrast stain on a surgical slide and lower my eye to the microscope lens, I watch color drift through the magnified cells, outlining boundaries between them like countries, like topographic lines on a map sketching mountains and rivers and valleys. I think about the huge range of experiences—both perfectly unified and starkly contrasting—that have come together to create my life as it is now. I think of our family's ties to India, in all its jumble of complexity and diversity, of old and new, of rich and poor, of tradition and innovation. I think of inhabiting both sides of medicine, as a patient longing to be healthy and as a doctor taking care of the sick. I think of all the terrains I've traversed to get here.

We haven't been back to India since the adoption, but I'm eager to travel there with Vic someday. When we visit the Taj Mahal, see the Golden Temple, and ride the Maharajas' Express, I will know that the story he writes with his memories may look very different from the story I would have written for him. When I bring him to my father's hometown of Pune and to the orphanage outside Mumbai where we first met, I will wonder if what he chooses to take from his experience will be the same as what I've imagined. Traveling together, we will be tourists and we will be natives. We will be citizens of the space between. We will be a family, both like and unlike any other, unifying our contrasts, seeking our homes, traversing this vast and amazing landscape where my son and I both began.

III:

SERVING

CHAPTER 5

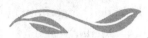

After three pregnancy losses in a row, I was disoriented by the intensity of my feelings. I vacillated between a looming cloud of despair and a defiant sense of optimism, sometimes almost hourly. Even while I prepared our home with vibrant paint and picture books and tiny shoes, I recognized that more than a year had passed since we had started trying to have a baby.

I had to admit the possibility that I might never have a successful pregnancy. Statistics predicted that my chances of giving birth to a living biological child now hovered in the thirty percent range, but even this felt impossible to calculate, since there were no studies of women who'd had a first-trimester miscarriage followed by two rounds of failed methotrexate treatment and a surgically excised ruptured ectopic then a molar pregnancy and who were now down to one tube and one ovary. The uncertainty of our situation loomed large.

Still, whatever else might happen, I desperately wanted something positive and purposeful to come out of my experiences. I felt compelled to honor the attentive, lifesaving care that Devorah had given me by using what I'd learned to help other women—and to serve as the informed and compassionate clinician I had wished for when other doctors were belittling my concerns.

Throughout the spring, I'd been talking with my department's director about the possibility of joining the family medicine residency. He'd supported and encouraged my interest, but the program was full. On a Wednesday afternoon in mid-June, he called to confirm that they wouldn't be able to offer me training this academic year. He hoped I would apply to start the next summer instead.

This news was both a disappointment and a relief. Having decided to undertake additional clinical training, I was ready to move ahead with my plan. But I was also okay with having more time before committing. One week earlier, after six months of post-molar-pregnancy monitoring, I'd been medically cleared to try to get pregnant again. Maybe this timing would work out perfectly for having a baby, wrapping up my current research projects, and starting the new program right after maternity leave.

Then, on Friday morning, less than forty-eight hours later, my phone rang again. The program director told me that one of the incoming residents had just submitted her resignation—ten days before orientation was set to begin—and he wondered if I might like to fill her spot.

I was surprised, excited, eager, and grateful. I was also terrified.

In some rotations, the doctors and staff whose misjudgments had put me in danger during the ectopic pregnancy would be my direct supervisors and assistants. As much as Shreya's story had inspired me to be more open with friends and family, I felt uncomfortable that those who would be evaluating me knew so much about my history—especially since they had been partly responsible for my less-than-ideal outcome.

Accepting the position would also mean starting over at the bottom of medicine's professional hierarchy. I thought back on a time during the first year of my first residency when I'd gone to pick up my mother for a visit and had realized, in circling the airport to await her flight, that the short-term parking spots garnered substantially higher hourly wages than I did. Pursuing other options to build our family, including assisted reproductive technologies or adoption, would be difficult on a resident's salary and with a resident's extremely limited free time.

But most daunting was the fact that I would be spending much of my time conducting prenatal visits and assisting in deliveries. Maternity care training was a strength of this program and precisely the reason I'd sought the position. But the leap of faith was unimaginable. How would I be able to cope with showing up for my patients each day if I kept getting pregnant and having complications, or if I never got pregnant again?

Nine months had elapsed between the beginning of my first pregnancy and the end of my third, which seemed both a poetically fitting and a terribly cruel amount of time to frame our experiences. Nine months: The essential measure of a healthy, ordinary pregnancy. The conjurer of images as embryo becomes fetus becomes newborn. A mirage of normal that had retreated further into the distance for me with each passing day. It wasn't so much the loss of the pregnancies themselves that weighed on me. I knew that none of them had been viable conceptions that would have led to a child. It was the loss of the idea, the dream, the potential.

But the awareness that had crowded out that innocence had one incredible benefit: for the first time, I truly understood what it meant to be a patient. And it was only in becoming somebody's patient, in being cared for while being cared about, that I had begun to comprehend the enormous privilege of being somebody's doctor. I couldn't control whether I'd ever have a successful pregnancy. But I could control whether I embraced this opportunity or let my fear limit me. I decided that finding a way for my experience to benefit others—finding meaning beyond how these losses impacted me as an individual, no matter how my story continued to unfold—would help me build myself back up against feeling broken.

With newfound resolve, I accepted the position.

I found out I was pregnant for the fourth time a few days after starting the family medicine residency. But after three ways of pregnancy gone dramatically and dangerously wrong, the notion of correlating that little pink line to expecting to have a child struck me as both charmingly quaint and exceedingly arrogant.

After the first miscarriage, and even after the ectopic, I had found some comfort in knowing that at least I could get pregnant. I would have been offended if someone else had said this to me, but I had clung to it myself as evidence that if I persisted, we would probably have a baby eventually. Now, as I stood at my bathroom counter in the low morning light, the positive result felt like little more than an abstraction. An empty idea that didn't guarantee any specific outcome. A nudge toward parenthood that made our odds of having a baby slightly better than, say, a negative pregnancy test. A suggestion much more than a promise.

I moved through the early days of pregnancy along with the early days of residency. We scheduled our prenatal appointments with the hospital midwives, disappointed that my schedule wouldn't allow me to travel off campus for appointments with Devorah at the community clinic she'd joined after graduation, but optimistic that this pregnancy might be uncomplicated enough to avoid involving obstetricians. As I met my new classmates, I was happy to learn that most of them had followed nontraditional paths to medicine and several had young children. Orientations, conferences, and welcome barbecues blurred into blood work, morning sickness, and—miraculously—a six-week ultrasound that revealed our tiny embryo's beating heart exactly where it should be. With more than a little trepidation, we decided to tell our friends and family, joking that the pregnancy was planned but the residency had been a surprise.

By twelve weeks, I was amazed that I had made it through the first trimester and the first three months of training, balancing half-time work finishing projects from my research job with half-time work in the hospital. Even while enduring relentless all-day nausea, I thought that maybe the pregnancy would seem more real once I could feel the baby move.

By seventeen weeks, I was sensing flutters while I spent my days counseling women in a family planning clinic. I decided that I would believe things might be okay once Ian could feel the baby kick from the outside.

By nineteen weeks, Ian could sense faint movement along my abdomen when he held his hand in just the right spot, and I'd begun a challenging pediatrics rotation. As I took care of my tiny patients, with their histories so much more complicated than their short lives would predict, I wondered if any milestone existed that would truly allow me to feel more secure. The edge of viability at twenty-three weeks? The beginning of the third trimester at twenty-eight weeks? The gestational point at which Nick and Emily's son, Leo, had been born at thirty-two weeks? Being officially at term at thirty-seven weeks?

In a moment of dark-humored optimism, I suggested that we call our baby Lefty, in honor of their indisputable origin from my lone remaining ovary, and tried to believe that maybe we were going to have a child after all.

Our anatomy scan in the middle of the second trimester was routine. We watched with rapt attention as the black-and-white monitor revealed ten fingers, ten toes, two kidneys, two lungs, and a perfectly formed spine attached to a perfectly sized brain. Everything looked normal except for a bright spot on the baby's heart.

After I was dressed, the radiologist came back into the room to synthesize our clinical information. Overall, this bright spot—this echogenic intracardiac focus, as it was referred to in the medical literature—did double our odds of having a baby with a chromosomal anomaly. But that brought the estimate only from around a one percent chance to around a two percent chance. In the context of my reassuring recent blood tests and an otherwise normal ultrasound, the EIF was most likely a harmless variation. She handed us a packet with information about invasive procedures such as amniocentesis, which would be the next step if we chose to seek a formal diagnosis beyond these initial screening tests that offered only probabilities. I filed the papers into my bag and wondered how worried we should be.

At home later that night, I tried to convince myself that a spot on the heart really could mean nothing. As I reviewed research studies, Lefty hiccuped along enthusiastically. My reading proved unhelpful, linking this marker to genetic disorders then noting that it also occurred in a small percentage of fetuses with typical chromosomes. I pored over journal after journal, as if I might stumble upon some hidden data point that would give us definitive information about our own particular baby rather than just extrapolations, statistics, and conflicting results.

Offered the chance at the anatomy scan, we had opted not to learn the baby's sex before birth. I wanted to meet this tiny new person without imagining that I knew more about them than I really did. I didn't believe that biological sex was the greatest determinant of identity anyway. And I relished the idea of preserving a little mystery in a realm that I'd become accustomed to scheduling, planning, and exhaustively researching. So many times before my own pregnancies I'd heard well-meaning parents-to-be express that they didn't have a preference for a boy or a girl. *As long as they're healthy!* was the usual cheerful sentiment that accompanied this declaration.

But what if they're not? What then?

The ultrasound finding had called this possibility starkly into question for us. We wanted a healthy baby, but we also wanted *this* baby. We knew we would continue the pregnancy regardless. We'd endured enough to understand that this might be our only chance at parenthood, and we were prepared to make room in our lives for whoever this child might be. Although the risk of miscarriage with invasive diagnostics was small, it wasn't zero. I knew I'd never forgive myself if I caused the loss of what could have been a fully viable pregnancy just because I was impatient.

In these first few months of family medicine residency, I'd watched other young parents grapple with so many of the same kinds of concerns, decisions, and uncertainties we'd faced. And I'd watched them loving their children and each other, no matter how complex their medical histories became. I'd begun to realize that my experience of pregnancy wasn't just shaped by my own losses. Taking care of women like Erin and Rachel, before they became mothers and then through their pregnancies and beyond, served as the most powerful reminder that everything about this process was inherently full of doubt, with no guarantees and few measurable endpoints.

Ian and I declined further testing as we sat with the unknown, cautiously counting the days, tentatively marking the milestones, guardedly waiting to meet our baby.

Erin ~ Blood and Promises

When her son was born on her brother's birthday, my mother knew that the tests had been wrong. Because her brother had severe hemophilia, my mother had chosen to undergo genetic analysis before getting pregnant to find out if her own future children would be at risk of the disorder. She had breathed a sigh of relief when the results were clear: she was not a carrier. But now, looking down at her baby, she knew that her son and her brother shared more than a birthday. She watched as a nurse pricked her tiny newborn's heel for routine testing and the blood just flowed and flowed. She understood what it meant all too well.

When my mother's brother, Joseph, was diagnosed with hemophilia as a child in the 1940s, his family learned that the disorder is linked to the X chromosome, which means that almost all affected children are male. They learned that Joseph's blood didn't clot normally, so when his blood vessels were damaged by ordinary bumps and scratches, they couldn't seal themselves and he could develop life-threatening bleeds into muscles and joints with very little warning. They learned to navigate the world of doctors' offices and emergency transfusions, accepting blood from unknown donors as the only available treatment.

Each time he bled, a transfusion would grant Joseph small relief for a short time, as the internal bleeding slowed just enough for his body to begin to resorb it. Joseph would walk out of the hospital, where he felt like the doctors couldn't do anything more for him, and go home, where he felt like his family couldn't do anything more for him. Day after day, he curled up in a chair in the living room, shivering under a pile of blankets and ice packs, waiting for the deep-tissue pain to abate. As they grew up, my mother watched Joseph suffer, each feeling their own helplessness. Treatment options remained limited, and they lost dozens of friends to infectious diseases from contaminated transfusions.

My brother, Gavin, was born when I was almost five years old and Joseph was thirty-six. It was the 1980s, the height of the AIDS crisis, the beginning of a hidden hepatitis epidemic, just a few years after a young Midwestern teen's tragic story of contracting HIV from a transfusion made hemophilia nearly a household word. It was an era of poorly screened blood supplies from questionable sources.

From the moment Gavin was born, my mother fought tooth and nail to protect him. She wanted him to receive transfusions only from my father, who had the same blood type. The clinics tried to convince her that the pooled supply was safe and refused to give Gavin special treatment. But she didn't trust the system that had failed to diagnose her as a carrier of the disorder Gavin now lived with—and she didn't want special treatment for her son. She wanted safer treatment for all children with hemophilia. So she and my father fought to change the protocols, working with other families and medical teams across the country to expand the reach of their programs. They felt grateful to be part of the movement that helped spare a whole generation of boys from transfusion-related diseases.

Unfortunately, Joseph didn't benefit from my mother's efforts. He died in his forties from complications of AIDS. Our parents must have kept Gavin and me pretty sheltered from what was happening with our uncle at the end because I don't remember much. At twelve years old, I was so self-absorbed that I might not have noticed anyway, and Gavin wouldn't have understood much of it at seven. I do clearly remember standing up at Joseph's wake to read a poem about love and loss and spirit and connection, feeling calm and collected before starting to sob. When I looked over at my mother and watched her watching me struggle, with tears in her own eyes, I suddenly glimpsed the real impact this might all have. My grandmother was never quite the same after her child died too soon.

When we talked about AIDS in my middle school health class that same week, our teacher's explanations were laden with stigma, implying that people who suffered from this disease brought it upon themselves. I felt vulnerable and confused, indignant on behalf of my uncle, his wife, his daughter, my mother, and everyone else affected by this poorly understood immune deficiency. I didn't see why the way someone acquired a disease should matter—or change how much compassion a person was allowed.

Around that same time, Gavin and I went to a summer camp for kids with hemophilia and their siblings. The girls in my cabin had traveled from all over the country, and we had different accents and favorite foods and hairstyles, but every other detail paled in comparison to this crucial thing that we shared. We almost never talked about our families while we made friendship bracelets and played field games and waited for our turn on the waterslide. Just being together was such a comfort.

I knew some of the girls' siblings weren't doing well, but I didn't ask a lot of questions. Gavin was in such perfect health that, to my almost-teenaged mind, hemophilia didn't seem like a big deal. Gavin's life looked like any other kid's. The blood supply was much safer now than it had been for Joseph. Recombinant clotting factor VIII, a manufactured form of the protein that stops bleeding, was becoming widely available, and with it came an emerging promise to eliminate the risk of exposure to diseases spread by sharing human blood. My uncle's experience of hemophilia seemed worlds apart from my brother's.

That must have been the summer I got tested too, because I remember my parents sitting me down a few months after camp to tell me, with solemn faces, that I was a carrier. I remember it didn't seem like any sort of tragedy, or even particularly relevant to my life. Gavin returned to camp for a week every summer, but I didn't give my results much thought as I grew up, maintaining a steady conviction that everything would work out as it should.

When I met Michael more than ten years later, I immediately felt this same sense of trust and security. We were travelers together by chance, strangers seated in the same row on a small commuter flight. When he retrieved a bookmark I'd dropped on the airplane floor, a casual conversation led to the two-hour flight passing in minutes.

Our relationship got serious just as quickly, and I told Michael early on about our family's medical history. The only person he'd ever met with hemophilia was my brother—and Gavin was an incredible rock-climbing, motorcycle-riding, adventure-seeking, all-nighter-pulling college student. So Michael wasn't too concerned about hemophilia having big implications for our relationship. My carrier status just seemed like a sidenote about me, like my lifelong fondness for historical romance novels or my inexplicable aversion to mayonnaise, not something that needed to shape our decisions.

A few years after we got married, we began to imagine we might want to be parents. We planned a road trip for our next vacation and headed to Yellowstone National Park, knowing that the vistas of wilderness and less-traveled byways would help us gain perspective.

Across hours framed by snowcapped mountain ranges, winding roadside rivers, and bubbling pools of rainbow hot springs, we pondered what building a family might look like for us, what being a carrier meant to me, and whether we should consider options other than getting pregnant the old-fashioned way. The conversation swirled around in vitro fertilization, preimplantation genetic diagnosis, adoption, taking chances, and choosing to live without children.

As we talked through our worries, we realized that if my parents had been in our position and had used technology to select out embryos considered defective, Gavin and I would have both qualified as undesirable. We wouldn't exist. Suddenly, Michael and I both knew we had answered our own question. We just needed to have a little bit of faith that if we did bring a child with hemophilia into this world, he would thrive. He would have my mom, who lived nearby and was a fount of knowledge. He would have my brother, who was an amazing role model. Our family held so much history, and we understood—as much as anyone can before actually living an experience—how we would deal with it. We knew we had a one in four chance of having a child with hemophilia, but we also knew we had all the resources he would need.

Once we decided we wanted to be parents, I was intent on controlling what I could. I learned how to chart my cycles, watch for fertile days, and maximize the chances of conception each month. I read about factors that affected sperm health and considered theories on how to influence the sex of the baby conceived. I told Michael we should try for a girl, thinking gender swaying might be a simple solution to our worries. But when we'd been trying for six months without a pregnancy and I developed erratic menstrual cycles, I started to get concerned. After a series of blood tests over three more months, I was devastated to learn that I had an ovarian hormone imbalance that could severely impact my fertility.

But just one cycle later, I sensed I was pregnant even before I missed my period. I was so sick so soon that I knew in my bones what was happening—which was, I came to realize, a testament to the incredibly strong life force of our child.

My pregnancy was immediately deemed high-risk because of my carrier status. And being saddled with this label overshadowed how great I felt physically and undermined the trust I had in my own body, as if one careless move could send the whole thing tumbling down. Our doctors, our families, Michael, and I were all holding our collective breath. Throughout the pregnancy echoed the question *Is something wrong, is something wrong, is something wrong?* instead of starting from the assumption that development was progressing normally until proven otherwise.

I was amazed by how much a label could change the way I was treated. Yes, I was a carrier of a genetic disorder that I might have passed down to my child. But fetuses aren't affected by hemophilia because maternal factor VIII, the normal clotting protein, keeps them healthy before birth. The extra attention and extra ultrasounds that our doctor encouraged weren't helping Michael or me, since we were both already the worrying type. I was cautiously happy but kept wishing I could just relax and enjoy what felt like a perfectly ordinary pregnancy.

By the second trimester, we were looking forward to our upcoming anatomy scan. Although we were eager to learn the sex of the baby, we knew we wouldn't consider terminating a male fetus, as some other families in our hemophilia support networks had chosen. If we were having a boy, we didn't even want to try to find out ahead of time if he had hemophilia. We just knew reaching this milestone and getting more information would help us feel less scared of the other unknowns.

I remember being giddy with excitement and laughing about the fact that the ultrasound had been scheduled for my brother's and my uncle's birthday, somehow oblivious to what the universe was trying to tell me. In an even stranger twist, when the ultrasound technician welcomed us into the dark exam room and read on my chart that I was a carrier of hemophilia, she remarked that she used to know a little boy with hemophilia. As she scanned and we talked, we realized that the little boy had been my brother. The tech was the daughter of my parents' friends, and we had all played together as kids. When she told us we were having a boy, we received her congratulations with mixed emotions. We could no longer pretend that everything was going to be smooth and simple.

With the sex of the baby confirmed, our obstetrician again brought up the option of diagnostic testing at our next visit. Although amniocentesis is considered very safe, we didn't want to accept even the slightest extra risk of losing our son. After he was born, we decided, we'd have them sample the blood from the umbilical cord, then we'd have the results within a day. But the question of what should happen in the space between this moment of ambiguity and that definitive newborn testing was more complicated.

Our doctor told us that when hemophilia is confirmed prenatally, a cesarean delivery is typically scheduled to minimize potential trauma to the baby—because a difficult vaginal delivery can lead to using a vacuum or forceps on the baby's head, and the hardest bleed to treat is a brain bleed. But he also said that if we wanted to try for a vaginal birth, he could set up for delivery in the operating room, being ready to convert the plan quickly if my labor didn't progress. He acknowledged that research studies had yet to settle the question of which mode of delivery was truly safer for babies with hemophilia and mothers who were carriers of the gene. Not even knowing if our son actually had the disorder, we went back and forth about what we should do from the moment we knew he was a boy.

When I took a childbirth class, the instructors asked each of us to write a birth plan. Although a part of me wanted to give us a chance to have a vaginal birth, if only to recapture some sense of the ordinary we'd lost, I expected to end up delivering by cesarean—and I was okay with that. Many others in the class seemed set on an unmedicated delivery and leery of surgical interventions, but I didn't hold any preconceived notions that birth had to happen a certain way. I remember the uncomfortable silence when I said that I didn't have a plan. That I knew what I envisioned for my baby's birth but didn't know what would happen. That I'd been coming to realize I couldn't control everything. I didn't want to write something down on paper like a contract, only to have my hopes dashed when birth didn't unfold as I'd expected. I had witnessed too many friends be crushed with disappointment, devastated when reality deviated from their well-intentioned plan, feeling like failures even while holding a beautiful, perfect newborn.

When I reached forty-two weeks, everyone agreed it was time for an induction. At the hospital, the nurse connected me to the monitors and surprised us both by picking up strong contractions immediately. I was thrilled. If labor was already underway with no pain, maybe this would be easier than I'd anticipated. The on-call doctor gave me some misoprostol to help soften my cervix and to encourage labor to progress. As the medication bolstered my contractions, I started to sense them more, but my dilation hovered at barely two centimeters for several hours. The doctor offered to break my bag of waters, but I decided to walk around the ward instead.

By the time I'd made it to the end of the hallway, I had transitioned into full-blown labor. I was suddenly drenched in sweat, and the nurse and Michael had to carry me back to the room. I felt like I would split in half. The pain was so severe that my nurse was worried something was wrong. She called the anesthesiologist as soon as I requested an epidural, and he was there by the time I had repositioned myself in bed. The relief I felt once it was placed was indescribable.

The doctor came by to check me again, and the reason for my level of distress became clear: my cervix had dilated to ten centimeters in less than thirty minutes. He hurried out to call my obstetrician, to tell him he needed to come in. *Now.* Meanwhile, in the sweet calm of the epidural, I lay down on my side and took a moment to rest.

The next thing I knew, there were eight nurses in my room. They were pulling cords and cables out of the wall. They were tightening monitor straps across my pelvis. They were shouting at me to get on my hands and knees and unlocking the wheels on the bed as I scrambled to try. Michael watched with frantic eyes, asking what was happening. I was kneeling face down, asking what was happening. My mother arrived and started asking what was happening. Nobody explained anything as they raced my gurney down the hall. When we got to the doors of the operating room, they told Michael he couldn't come with me. I saw the panic rise up within him.

As we'd gotten ready for this day, as we'd talked over endless variations of how birth might go and what decisions we should make, the one plan we'd agreed on was that we would not get separated. *Don't go into an elevator and get stuck in it,* I had made him promise, laughing. *Just stay with me the whole time. The whole time. No matter what happens.* The last thing I did before they wheeled me away was look at him steadily and say, "Michael, it's okay. I'm going to be okay." He was distraught because he was being forced to let me down. I had to be the strong one and show him I had released him from his promise already.

As the operating room doors swung shut, the nurses guided me onto my back and placed my legs into the stirrups, and my obstetrician quickly scrubbed in and joined us. He told me the baby's heart rate was dropping dangerously low with each contraction. But the baby was stuck. Stuck in the birth canal, somewhere between where they could go in and pull him out with a cesarean from above and where he could be eased out with hands from below. "What I need you to do," my doctor said, "what *he* needs you to do, is to push him out."

I couldn't feel anything below my waist. But I focused on my doctor, on my baby, on my body. I tried to visualize my muscles deep within, tried to summon memories of doing a squat, tried to bear down on my baby with the bright lights bearing down on me.

A nurse brought Michael, now in scrubs, back to my side. He grasped my left hand as the nurse held my right. My doctor told me that I needed to keep pushing and that he was going to have to use forceps. He locked eyes with me and said, "I think we can do this." So I agreed. And while he pulled, I pushed three times. Our son came out screaming, and Michael and I both burst into tears of relief.

The whole process, from the time I had gotten out of bed to walk the hallways until the time he was born, had taken less than an hour—less time than it had taken me to drive to each of our prenatal appointments. Every other woman in my family had had long, drawn-out labors, and I really had been expecting to end up with a cesarean. I was still reeling as I watched the nurse carry our baby over to the warming station.

I turned to Michael, who stood dazed beside me. "Go," I implored. "You need to go! I can't go to him—and I'm fine!"

Michael was so conflicted, so unsure where to place his attention. I felt nothing but the awe of new love as I watched my husband, suddenly a father, walk over to stand beside our squirming, screaming, breathing son for the very first time.

As we waited for the cord blood tests to be run and took in the enormity of what had just happened, we decided to name our son Cooper, a strong and masculine name that Michael and I had both come across and liked independently. Cooper was perfect, with no evidence of head trauma from the forceps and not even a single visible bruise on his body. We passed the time staring at our son, giving him his first bath, visiting with extended family members who sat around my room awkwardly as this child and I made our first clumsy efforts at breastfeeding. I don't think I slept that night, but at one point Michael and Cooper were both snoring and I had to laugh to myself, sandwiched between them, at my new lot in life. I remember holding tiny blond Cooper in the crook of my arm and not wanting to put him back in the bassinet.

Every time the nurses came in to check on us, we asked them again if the hemophilia test had come back. With eyes averted, they kept saying we had to wait for the doctor, making it clear to me that they knew the answer but couldn't reveal it. Michael was desperately trying to hang on to his last shred of hope.

"But Michael," I said, "don't you see? If they're waiting for the doctor, the answer to the question is yes. And we already knew it was yes. He has hemophilia. You have to know, in your heart, that that's what they're going to tell us." I just wanted Michael to be prepared.

Finally, a doctor we'd never met came in and stood solemnly at our bedside. She delivered the results of Cooper's blood test like he had inoperable cancer, like some sort of tragedy, like hemophilia was something we hadn't been expecting all along. Like this was the first time she had ever shared difficult news with a family.

"I know this isn't what you wanted to hear," she continued, with a pained look on her face, seeming at once both overly concerned and terribly misinformed. She offered her sympathy, and I politely refused it.

"We're fine," I said firmly.

She looked down at the floor and shook her head slowly. "I'm so sorry," she said again.

I stared at her, somewhere between startled and offended, until finally I said, "Do you even know anyone with hemophilia? We don't need your misguided pity here. It would have been great if he'd been born unaffected, but we knew what we were getting into."

Her words and her tone were deeply upsetting, especially for Michael, who already loved this child so much and was utterly terrified. He had been traumatized by everything that had happened over the last twenty-four hours and felt a renewed helplessness with this confirmed diagnosis. He hadn't quite moved out of the stage of denial that had allowed a glimmer of hope that Cooper would be born perfectly healthy. I had landed solidly on an optimistic version of denial where what I'd expected had come to pass, and now I'd rallied to believe there was nothing we couldn't handle. But to hear the test result in this unsupportive way from someone who had so little understanding of hemophilia made it that much harder to take in the joy that surrounded Cooper's arrival. And now I, the exhausted puddle of blood and sweat who had just given birth, was managing everyone else's feelings and reactions too.

After the doctor left, Michael turned to me. His eyes were filled with a mixture of fear and acceptance, of doubt and confidence. And I looked down with amazement at this new creature who was at once complicated and simple, who embodied the traditions of our families as well as the promise of a future that would make his life with hemophilia so much better than it would have been years ago, and I let it all wash over me.

To this day, more than six years after Cooper's birth, other people's lack of understanding remains one of the toughest things about dealing with hemophilia. Affecting about one in five thousand newborn boys, it's rare enough that even most medical professionals don't know much about it. Many doctors and nurses meet only one or two people with hemophilia over the course of a career, and many meet none. Any time we see a clinician other than Cooper's hematologist, we feel like we're back in that place of good intentions and poor communication. Every time we're in the emergency department—and this is not a rare event for our family—I find myself trying to explain what's going on and what treatments are needed. I often feel like they're just nodding and writing down whatever I say because they've never taken care of a child with hemophilia before. I'm constantly dispelling misconceptions. "He's bleeding really fast!" a nurse might say. "Hurry! We've got to get him his medication now!" But people with hemophilia don't have accelerated blood. They're not going to bleed out from an ordinary cut. They just don't clot well to stop the vessels from bleeding once they start.

There's so much guessing and anticipating and anxious waiting for the parents of a child with hemophilia. I have to let Cooper be a child, but I feel such an urge to protect him too. I don't know if it's more than what any mother feels, but the stakes seem higher. When Cooper stumbles over a toy and falls on the carpet, when he hits his shin on the playground slide, I hold my breath. Even a simple headache—which would be written off as hunger or fatigue in most kids and treated with a graham cracker and a nap—consigns us to a brain scan to make sure Cooper doesn't have an intracranial hemorrhage. We need to be willing to err on the side of caution, to insist on imaging for the vague discomfort that is probably just indigestion but could also be a life-threatening intra-abdominal bleed. Nothing can be taken for granted. My son relies on me to know his body almost as well as I know my own, to understand all its signs and strengths and limitations. I am constantly trying to imagine what he is going through.

To understand Cooper's experience better, I talk to Gavin about what it feels like when he has a bleed. He explains to me that muscle bleeds hurt more than joint bleeds but joint bleeds are scarier. Blood in a joint can erode the bones and connective tissue required for flexibility and movement. A damaged joint can start rebleeding even as it's healing and become a target joint—one that develops bleed after bleed, each one harder to control, leading to stiffness, chronic pain, and loss of function. Gavin warns me that life will only get harder for us when Cooper is a teenager, when he doesn't want to use his medication, when he rejects anything that makes him feel different from everybody else— when he is in that invincible phase I was in when I first learned I was a carrier, thinking that this part of my story wouldn't change the way I led my life.

When I talk to my mom about what it was like to raise Gavin, she reminds me about the early years of fighting for safe transfusions and making prophylactic treatment more common, of learning to prevent bleeds rather than just respond to them. She gives me lots of practical tips: When Cooper falls, *factor first*. Mix the freeze-dried clotting factor powder with the sterile water in the vial and load it into the syringe immediately. Get it into him before calling the doctor, before calling Michael, before anything else. She reminds me to question assumptions and to be my son's advocate. The heaviness in her voice reminds me of all that she went through, of the fact that many mothers of sons with hemophilia in the past didn't get to see them grow up—and that this in itself is a privilege. I thank her again for everything she did. Intellectually, I've always known what she did. I'd heard the stories from my family for as long as I could remember. They were part of our lore, the legends of our history. But now that I'm a mother, I really feel the impact of her actions. I'm in awe of how much she had to fight for.

My lens on the world has changed completely since I became Cooper's mother. I've come to realize that everyone is dealing with something that's hard for them, even when I can't see it. I listen to one friend's complaints about her husband's long work hours while our boys play together in a corner of her kitchen, and I hear another's laments about her aching back in her second perfectly healthy pregnancy. Their words fall flat, and I feel angry, isolated, lonely in my experience of having a child with a complex chronic disorder. My first thought is that these women just don't have perspective on what matters. But I've known both of them long enough to remember that they've had other struggles. And I know we'll all face new challenges as life progresses. I hope that the next time they need a friend I'll be able to tell them that, although I haven't been through the same things, I can help. I can try to understand. I can listen.

I used to think that life followed a path, sometimes smooth and sometimes bumpy, but that everyone traveled together. When my life started to get harder, I believed that each complicated event would eventually be explained away as a temporary anomaly. But those days of sitting in sterile exam rooms and listening to discouraging test results about my ovaries blurred into days of sitting in sterile exam rooms and waiting for another ultrasound to monitor my pregnancy, which, in turn, have blurred into days of sitting in sterile exam rooms and holding my son close while he gets his next IV treatment.

Now I feel like I've stepped off the path altogether. The path is no longer even in sight. I have to figure out how to navigate these unmarked edges, with no road maps and no directions and with very few other parents I can relate to. It's both liberating and terrifying to stop comparing myself to others. It allows me, like in the days leading up to Cooper's birth, to reject the idea of a plan and relinquish the conviction that life has to unfold a certain way. But it also means I'm left with the admission that I have no idea what's going to happen.

Michael and I have experienced parenthood very differently too. In our partnership, I continue to be the one driven by cautious optimism, while Michael absorbs more of the worry. When we first face something difficult, I push headlong into the challenge. I am a whirlwind of activation, energized by strife, reading and researching everything I can dredge up. Michael's first impulse is to withdraw, feeling defeated, while he takes time to gather his strength. But once the crisis is over, I fall apart—usually at just about the point that Michael has had the time he needs to process our experience and collect his thoughts. He's ready to step up when I'm suddenly lost in despair. I used to think that I'd always want us to be in the same emotional space at the same time, that to be synchronized in our experience was the only way to be truly unified. I used to get frustrated by our different styles of coping. But now I see that when we each work through things at our own pace, we can better support each other in our times of greatest need. There's power and compassion in letting ourselves grow separately before we come back together.

I'm still struggling to find ways to describe our experiences that don't make Cooper sound broken. But every time I tell our story, I feel the love a little more and the losses a little less. I do believe that everything in our lives has happened the way it needed to happen. Now that I can see all the events in a line leading to where we are today, I feel hopeful.

A friend once pointed out to me that Cooper's name, with its reference to the barrel crafters of years gone by, marks him as a repairer of containers and vessels. It's incredible to me how perfect this meaning is for him—an allusion to the blood vessels that he cannot heal normally but that we support him in protecting every day—and even more incredible to me that I hadn't realized this meaning when we chose his name. It's a nod to the strength of the vessel that is our family, our history, our future moving forward boldly even in uncertainty.

Cooper, Michael, and I are in this together, even when we're each facing our own challenges. Our vessel is whole, even though it's damaged. Blood keeps flowing. Family endures. We've had to learn new definitions of unity, of being there for each other as a family of two and now a family of three. Our bonds of love are more resilient than ever. We've forgiven ourselves for some inevitably broken promises. We've realized that those promises were never really ours to make.

Rachel ~ Enough for Today

On the day of the procedure, my toenails shimmered with iridescent magenta polish. I'd treated myself to a pedicure earlier that week, reveling in the indulgence, thinking I had something to celebrate. Now, my feet stuck out awkwardly from beneath my hospital gown. Their cheerful shine only reinforced the darkness and imperfection I felt inside.

As I rolled into the operating room, several nurses commented on how pretty my nails looked. I wished I could be more grateful for their attention. They were trying to notice what was different and special about me, to remind me of beauty when I couldn't see it. I held on to their small kindnesses as I faded into the haze of anesthesia.

Nearly a year earlier, Joel had come home from sharing a beer with a friend and had woken me up in the middle of the night. He couldn't wait to tell me, after spending the evening looking at pictures of his friend's adorable newborn daughter and hearing him marvel over becoming a father, that he thought he might be ready for a family too.

I'd wanted to be a mother my whole life. But my partnership with Joel hadn't come easily, even after we'd known each other for nearly thirty years. Joel and I had attended the same schools and church services since we were four. Photo albums in both our childhood homes included pictures of us with arms around each other's shoulders, grinning over drippy orange slushies at the county fair and giving goofy thumbs-ups on the sidelines of high school football games. Joel was my best friend, even after we'd moved away to go to college in different states. As we got older, I realized that I was only half kidding when I said that I didn't want to date Joel—I just wanted to marry him. Outspoken life of the party that I was in many ways, I was never brave enough to push beyond my standing joke to see if it might hold some truth.

I was devastated when Joel married someone else. But their marriage ended quickly in divorce, and Joel and I found ourselves face-to-face with a second chance. Joel decided that he'd gotten married too young and for all the wrong reasons. I admitted to myself that I still loved him—I just wasn't sure what that meant after so many years. I tested the waters, teasing him gently about his starter marriage, saying that practice makes perfect. Gradually, we began to explore whether our friendship might be the foundation for a life together. We struggled with whether we were ready to commit to each other. We finally found that we were.

At our wedding, the minister shared a reading from the Old Testament's Book of Habakkuk: *But these things I plan won't happen right away. Slowly, steadily, surely, the time approaches when the vision will be fulfilled. If it seems slow, wait patiently, for it will surely take place.* Everything good in my life had taken longer than I'd expected, and the promise in this verse resonated perfectly. My faith was deep.

I was pregnant nine months after we got married, on the third cycle we started trying, and I felt giddy with excitement. Many people in our circles of family and friends had struggled for years to have a baby. We told everyone close to us as soon as the home test showed a faint positive. I counted down the days until our first prenatal appointment.

At that long-awaited visit four weeks later, Joel and I beamed at each other as the doctor pointed out a pulsating white line on the bedside ultrasound screen. She listed the baby's measurements as she marked them, commenting that the embryo seemed smaller than my calculations would predict. But no worries, she assured us. Just come back in two weeks for a recheck.

I passed my time at the local flower shop where I worked, crafting elaborate displays to celebrate engagements and new babies and Mother's Day. I loved watching the arrangements come together, then presenting our customers with bursts of color balanced in the perfect vase to accent their natural beauty. I loved holding this amazing secret as I went about my ordinary days, dreaming of tiny socks and onesies.

At our next appointment, our doctor said that the heartbeat looked slower than it should. She confided that this had happened with her first baby too and he was a healthy toddler now. As she reminisced about those early days, so fraught with uncertainty, we drank in her confidence. I didn't hesitate when, at the front desk, her receptionist offered me my next follow-up at a different clinic with unfamiliar staff on a day that Joel had to work. I was so eager to see the baby again that I didn't mind being on my own for this routine check.

But when that day arrived and the monitor flickered on, a faint gray shadow lay motionless across the screen. The nurse announced that there was no heartbeat. Her voice was so flat, so casual, as if this was what we had both been expecting to find.

I gathered up my things and stumbled out of the room. It didn't make sense. I was still queasy and tired, and my breasts were still tender. I still felt so pregnant. Now feeling foolish to have accepted my doctor's reassurance, like I'd been tricked into an unfounded optimism, I barely got myself to the car before I fell apart into uncontrollable sobs.

When I called Joel, I couldn't get the words out. He kept telling me to take my time, saying that everything was going to be okay. He left work to meet me at home, where I collapsed into his arms and cried as we leaned together. I suddenly realized how many people we'd already told about this pregnancy. I didn't know how I'd find the strength to tell every one of them what had happened.

As instructed, we returned to my regular obstetrician the next day to discuss our options. When we checked in, the receptionist grinned at us and teased, "Well, you sure are here a lot lately!" Sitting in that waiting room, in that sea of swollen bellies, felt awful, interminable, wrong.

Finally, the nurse called my name. I followed her to the scale and stepped up, cringing at the numbers that I knew had started quite high before pregnancy but now should have been rising if this pregnancy were healthy.

"Hmm. You've lost weight," she observed, admonishing me loudly in the echoing hallway of exam rooms. "That shouldn't be happening when you're pregnant." I was mortified. Another patient passed by us, averting her eyes.

I was both too much and not enough.

I'd struggled with being heavier than I wanted to be my whole adult life, and I felt extremely self-conscious that she was drawing attention to my weight loss now, without even consulting my chart to realize that my baby had died.

The discussion with the doctor was a blur of technicalities. She wasn't unkind, but she focused on the risks and benefits of letting things resolve on their own versus using medications or a dilation and curettage to speed up the process. I followed her lead in concentrating on practical matters. I chose the D&C procedure and scheduled it for two days later. Then I went home to wait.

A couple of hours after I got home, I started to bleed. It was sudden and heavy and painful and scary—and all the more so because I had no idea what to expect. Having decided to have the D&C, I hadn't prepared myself emotionally to handle my body beginning the process on its own.

When I called the clinic for advice, they scheduled me to come in the next day. I spent most of that night in the bathroom with Joel by my side. Every few hours, I would retreat to the living room, only to be driven back by the nauseating sensation of an impending gush, a golf ball–sized clot the visceral reminder of what was not to be.

Somehow we made it to the clinic the next day. A different nurse led us to the exam room and congratulated us brightly on our pregnancy. "How far along do you think you are?" Too shocked to contradict her, I heard her start reviewing an unfamiliar medical history. When she asked how my last delivery had gone, I found the words to interrupt. I told her I had lost my baby at home yesterday. Why was I the one apologizing as her eyes darted away from mine to inspect the chart? Only then did she confirm my last name and realize that she had the wrong Rachel. She shuttled me back to the waiting room sheepishly and disappeared.

When it was finally my turn—while some other Rachel in a room nearby was surely smiling over the image of her perfectly formed baby—Joel and I watched the silent screen at our bedside confirm an empty uterus.

"The good news," said the doctor quietly, "is that you should be done bleeding. And no need for the procedure." We were fortunate to have gotten pregnant so quickly, she said. This happens all the time. We could try again soon. The platitudes spilled forth, warm but somehow hollow.

At home, the bleeding continued. Then, four days later, the doctor's office called to inform me that they had overlooked a recent test result—my Rh-negative blood type—and that I should get a shot to prevent my body from making antibodies that could jeopardize the health of the baby in any future pregnancy. I dragged myself to the clinic for a shot and a blood draw later that afternoon, where the phlebotomist beamed and added her congratulations. I stared straight ahead, too numb to correct her.

The doctor's earlier assurances of this ordeal being over also proved false. I bled and bled for weeks. I thought the bleeding would never end, that it would drain me until I disappeared. Feeling so mistreated by people I had trusted magnified my suffering. I wasn't mourning the loss of the pregnancy so much as feeling the frustration of all the misunderstandings and mistakes. I tried to remind myself that

I'd gotten pregnant easily. I told myself it would happen again, and I pushed my grief away.

I knew I needed to find a new clinic—but I also needed a break to recover from my emotional and physical exhaustion. When Joel and I were ready to try again a few months later, I met with the obstetrician my mother and grandmother had been seeing for years. At my first appointment, her nurse listened without turning away while I told my story through tears. She even cried a little with me, reflecting on her own struggles. The doctor herself had an offbeat sense of humor but seemed eager to help. "I'm trying to get your daughter knocked up!" she said to my mother during one of her own gynecology appointments, cackling conspiratorially. I had told her that my mother knew why I was coming to see her. I loved that she was caring for three generations of my family, and now she would be a link between us all as I tried to build a fourth.

After several cycles passed with no sign of pregnancy, she offered me fertility drugs in hopes of strengthening my ovulation. I was pregnant again almost immediately. But at eight weeks, there was no heartbeat. There wasn't even a faint white line of possibility. Coldly clinical terms floated by me in my shock: *Missed abortion. Blighted ovum. Anembryonic pregnancy.* I had a form of pregnancy in which a fertilized egg attaches to the wall of the uterus, generating a small sac of amniotic fluid and the beginnings of a placenta, but doesn't develop into an embryo. I had never heard of such a thing. I couldn't believe that a pregnancy without a baby could feel so real.

This second miscarriage was much more devastating than the first, which I had been able to dismiss as bad luck. Now I had so many questions I was terrified to ask: *Did I do something wrong? Am I too fat to stay pregnant? Is this all my fault?* I was silent as my doctor closed my chart and offered quiet condolences. At the front desk, I scheduled a D&C for the next morning. I couldn't imagine letting the bleeding stretch out again as it had the first time. The loss alone was more than enough to bear.

So that was how I found myself rolling through a long hospital corridor, magenta toenails recalling the happier times of just a few days earlier. Empty as I felt when the nurses complimented my style, that shimmering polish did remind me that I could find beauty even in the most difficult situations. It helped me hold on to the essence of who I was. I wasn't just a patient undergoing a procedure. I was a good friend, always known as both a sensitive listener and the vibrant woman full of flair at every party. I was a hard worker, widely respected as an extroverted business ambassador eager to connect with new clients. I was a devoted partner, and I knew that I was blessed to be married to my best friend.

The D&C and recovery proved mercifully uneventful. At least having anesthesia, with its minimal physical pain and complete lack of memory, felt like some small victory over our last loss that had dragged out into weeks and weeks of cramping and bleeding. I was ready to move on. From the first moments of the first miscarriage, I'd found it easier to look forward than to look back. Behind us was a trail of disappointment and loss. The landscape ahead glowed with possibility.

But these things I plan won't happen right away. Slowly, steadily, surely, the time approaches when the vision will be fulfilled. If it seems slow, wait patiently, for it will surely take place.

I trusted that we were going to have a baby someday, somehow. I never worried that I wouldn't become a mother. I reminded myself that everything in my life seemed to take longer than it should but that it always worked out for the best eventually. I didn't know if I would give birth to my baby physically or if someone else would have to hand a baby to me, but I knew we were meant to be parents.

Considering adoption came naturally to us. Joel had always felt that there are so many children in this world needing a family that we should be open to that option. I had grown up as the middle child between one older brother, adopted, and one younger brother, biological. My parents had decided to pursue adoption after being told, in the wake of their own two miscarriages, that my mother would never get pregnant again. After fourteen months, they were matched with an expectant mother and her unborn baby boy. For weeks, they kept thinking that the phone call to announce his arrival should come any day, but it never did. Finally, my dad reached out to the agency. The caseworker told him that, after a series of labor complications, the baby's biological mother would never be able to have another pregnancy, so she'd decided to take him home after all.

That was when my grandmother swept in, having watched her daughter's anguish for as long as she could bear. "Put on your best suit," my parents remember her saying. "We're going to get you a baby." I'm sure none of this was as simple as family legend would suggest, but my parents did adopt my brother shortly after that. Eighteen months later, I came along as the first surprise, and, five years later, my little brother as the second. If the three of us had lined up, you would have guessed that my older brother and I were twins. Although our family always discussed his adoption openly, we were such a natural pairing that it wasn't until I was in college that it occurred to me that I was the first baby born to my mother.

I thought of my parents' patience as Joel and I endured our own hopeful wait. My obstetrician offered to start me on a medication called metformin. She said that it could help improve egg quality and strengthen ovulation in heavier women. I agreed without hesitation even though I didn't know how metformin worked. Secretly worried that my weight was the cause of our problems, I was not eager to ask questions that might lead to more shame and guilt about the possibility that the miscarriages were my fault. I was willing to try whatever she suggested—especially if it took attention off the weight itself.

Pregnant for the third time a few months later, I was sure it must be our turn: *Slowly, steadily, surely.* But the eight-week ultrasound again revealed an empty sac with no embryo. I sighed, too numb to cry this time. Though nothing seemed to be coming easily for us, I held steadfastly to my faith that when the time was right all would fall into place. Even at my lowest moments, I recognized that there was always someone whose pain was greater than mine: Joel's friend, who had hit her abdomen when stumbling on a curb and lost her unborn daughter just two weeks before her due date. Joel's mother, who had suffered multiple pregnancy losses before delivering her second son, who died at three days old of extensive birth defects while she drifted into and out of consciousness, recovering from a severe postpartum hemorrhage. My friend from church, who went into premature labor at the end of her second trimester and lost both her twins. My parents, who spent three years with a nursery in their home, sitting with open hearts but no baby.

Listening to the stories of the strong women around me helped me mourn while keeping my own struggles in perspective. My eyes teared up when I realized that we hadn't even gotten far enough into any of our pregnancies to have a printout of an ultrasound. But the abstractness also helped me cope—or at least rationalize enough to keep seeing my cup as half full. I had never felt the flutter of first kicks from someone I'd never get to meet. I had never endured labor to deliver a baby who wouldn't grow up. I had never named a child, only to engrave that name on a stone. Still, I knew that minimizing my feelings because I believed that others had it worse made no sense in the context of loss. *Worse* implies a hierarchy, a ranking, an ability to measure. Grief is not a contest.

I felt despondent when faced with the decisions I needed to make yet again. I didn't want to go through another loss at home, but the substantial expense of a D&C made managing with medication my only reasonable choice. I knew I'd rather put that money toward seeing a specialist to figure out why this kept happening than spend it on a procedure that wouldn't improve our chances of taking home a baby. I left my appointment feeling empty already but determined to move ahead.

That very afternoon, as I waited for the medications to kick in, I called the fertility clinic and scheduled an appointment for the following month. As I bled at home over the next few days, I felt sad but hopeful, anticipating that the help I needed to maintain a pregnancy—and an explanation for why I hadn't been able to in the past—might finally be close.

One month later, the reproductive endocrinologist greeted us with kind eyes, then walked through our story methodically. When I told him about the metformin, he asked if I'd ever been tested for insulin resistance. I didn't really know what that meant. When he explained that it's essentially on the continuum of diabetes and is a marker for being at elevated risk of developing the disease, I mentioned that my father and his sister both had diabetes and that I thought both of their parents probably had as well but had never received a diagnosis.

He paused for a moment, taken aback. He told us that this was very concerning, but he encouraged us to stay optimistic. We were already ahead of many of the families he worked with because I was getting pregnant. Now we had to figure out why the pregnancies kept ending almost as soon as they had started.

When the doctor called me at work the next morning with the results of my blood tests, he told me right away that I wasn't simply insulin resistant—I had severe diabetes with a blood sugar level more than four times the normal range. I realized as we talked that since my obstetrician had put me on metformin, she must have suspected that insulin resistance, at the very least, could be playing a role in our losses. I felt so misled. Why had I been prescribed medication without being tested for the condition it was supposed to be treating? Why hadn't I asked questions before accepting a proposed solution? At my weight and with my family history, why had I needed to suffer three losses and get sent to a specialist before anyone suggested basic blood work to look for common metabolic disorders? I had written off being tired and thirsty and running to the bathroom all the time as markers of pregnancy. Now I realized that those symptoms had been the result of my dangerously elevated blood sugar. In a moment, the doctor's words, compassionate but insistent, pulled me back to the present. I needed to see my primary care doctor immediately, he warned me, to get control of my own health before we could even think about pregnancy again.

Just one problem: I didn't have a primary care doctor. I had been so focused on pregnancy, and on supporting the health of an imagined future child, that I hadn't been thinking of my own health outside that context. In the past three years, I had consulted with only those two obstetricians, and—naively, I now saw—I'd trusted their guidance implicitly. Suddenly, I didn't know what to believe.

I thought back to a friend I had confided in, discouraged in the midst of our losses. While listening to my litany of worries about running out of various forms of resources, from financial means to mental determination to physical energy, she had interrupted me gently. "Rachel," she had asked, "do you have enough for today?" With that revelation, *enough* shifted from signifying a burden, a pressing to the limit of what I could tolerate, to affirming instead my own resilience. Her words reminded me that I was capable of getting through this challenge. I remembered a family medicine clinic in my neighborhood that I'd driven past countless times. I called them and scheduled to go in the next day.

I arrived in the late afternoon, just in time for my doctor's last appointment. Incredibly, though, she never made me feel rushed. She understood immediately that my ultimate goal was to have a healthy baby, and I sensed that she was deeply invested in my story. Our time together seemed to last for hours while I cried and she listened. When I left her office, the reception desk was dark and the clinic was closed but my heart was full.

The next morning my phone rang with follow-up calls from her office. Two days later I was back in the clinic discussing a plan for medications, hearing the reasons behind what she recommended, and feeling for the first time like a partner in my own health. When I told her I hadn't been able to schedule with the dietitian she'd recommended because she was about to go out on leave, the doctor excused herself. She returned to the room a few minutes later to let me know that she had spoken with the dietician, who had agreed to meet with me as soon as we were done with this appointment.

I'd never been treated this way before. These people cared, and their care inspired me to take better care of myself. Within a few months, I had my average blood sugar down to within a few points of the normal range. In the past, I had been reluctant to ask too many questions or to read too much on my own, fearing I'd make things worse by creating new worries. But now I began to realize that it was up to me to dig deeper. I deserved to make informed choices about things that affected my body. Being proactive was incredibly empowering after years of feeling like I was going through the motions without any real understanding.

Soon Joel and I felt emotionally ready to try again, and my doctor agreed that we were medically ready too. At the beginning of my next cycle, we scheduled another appointment with the reproductive endocrinologist. Though an ultrasound at his office had shown a few promising follicles, the pee sticks I'd tested with at home suggested that I had stopped ovulating, likely from the long-standing lack of balance my body had been enduring. He gave me a hormone injection to trigger ovulation, and we followed through on our homework to have sex twice in the next twenty-four hours. We could hardly believe it when our fourth pregnancy was confirmed at the five-week mark.

Now every stage felt like an even greater hurdle—something to be thankful for moving past successfully, but also with so much more to lose. I cried more through that pregnancy, blessed and burdened by my ever-growing hope, than I had cried for the ending of any of my first three pregnancies. At the first ultrasound, I chanted under my breath, "His will, His way," over and over. *I trust You*, I thought. *You're going to make this happen*. It was the first time I had prayed for a baby. The embryo came into focus with a strong, clear heartbeat.

With guarded optimism, we moved from the reproductive endocrinologist to the high-risk obstetrician. I counted the days and watched the hours, monitoring my blood sugar closely, giving my-self three insulin injections per day, and wondering if failure might lurk just around the corner. I found myself visiting my primary care doctor between prenatal appointments, seeking the reassurance of her encouraging words and one more chance to listen to the baby's heartbeat. Crying with anxiety while I waited for her to bring in the bedside Doppler and crying with relief after she found the spot that revealed the quick, steady rhythm, like magic on my belly, I wasn't sure if I was setting goals for myself or making bargains with God: *Just get through the first trimester*, my thoughts would whisper, *and everything will be fine.*

Joel and I attended every appointment together, cautiously ap-proaching the second trimester and meeting with a genetic counselor. As we learned about technologies that could help us predict the health of this tiny person, we realized that discovering a problem wouldn't change our plan. We were already working with high-risk doctors at a hospital facility equipped to care for a baby with special needs right from birth. "My wife is going to bed at eight o'clock every night just to make it through another day," Joel told the counselor as we declined extra testing, "so I think we'll take a pass on something else to worry about." We were committed to this baby, no matter what obstacles we might encounter. We didn't need to know more than this essential truth.

Getting halfway to our due date, marked by the twenty-week anatomy scan, felt huge. Joel had been hoping for a girl, so we were over the moon with excitement when the ultrasound technician con-firmed that it was a girl indeed and that her measurements and or-gan development all looked normal. But our unblemished relief was short-lived. She had only two blood vessels in her umbilical cord, rather than the typical three, and the radiologist who reviewed the report with us said this could indicate complications. Though I tried not to read much about pregnancy other than following the growth and development charts that told us when our baby would reach the size of a large avocado, Joel wanted us to be prepared and understand all possibilities. He sent me an article that described heart defects and genetic anomalies associated with this finding. The bottom line, as we understood it, was that either the problem would be really bad or everything would be fine. There wasn't much middle ground.

Our excitement remained tempered with uncertainty as we waited two weeks for a more detailed ultrasound—an echocardiogram—of the baby's heart. Even when she passed with flying colors, I couldn't relax. I had thought I would tap into a deep well of gratitude if we could just get past this exam. But I still found myself reluctant to believe that everything would work out. Then I remembered that someone had told me that more than half of babies born after twenty-four weeks survive, so this became my new goal. When twenty-four weeks came and went, my flutters of doubt continued, even more persistent than the intermittent kicks and rolls of the growing baby girl inside.

Our friends and family were undaunted by my worries, bargaining, and rationalizations. Their excitement for us could hardly be contained. With our due date fast approaching, they celebrated us with three baby showers. We came home each night to a house full of flowers and gifts and home-cooked meals, and I'd been writing thank-you notes for days. The rest of our village had been hoping and praying for this baby as much as Joel and I had. Everyone knew our story and wanted to be part of it.

Early on in our pregnancies, I had wondered whether we should tell people right away or wait until things felt somehow safer, further along. In the midst of our losses, I had sometimes judged friends for sharing their own news too quickly. I had misunderstood their motivations. Now, surrounded by so much love, I saw how personal and individual a decision this is for every family, with each new pregnancy. And—whatever the outcome—I realized how much I needed this community of friends and family around me, lifting each other up in times of joy and holding each other together in times of loss.

Finally, after months of worrying and waiting and hoping and doubting, it was time to meet our daughter. Because of the diabetes, ten days before my due date marked our deadline for an induction. I had envisioned that once I made it to the hospital, everything would go smoothly. I'd pop in, and she'd pop out.

Instead, after forty-one hours of halting progress, we started to talk about a cesarean delivery. My family was worried about me and couldn't believe how well I was adapting to this change of plan—that now involved major surgery. But I was ready. My high-risk obstetrician cleared his clinic schedule to come deliver her, saying that, with everything we'd been through, I was a special patient and this was a special baby. He wanted to be there for her birth.

Elsie Marie arrived an hour later and weighed just seven pounds. She is named for my grandmother, my mother's mother, who dragged my mother to that adoption agency almost forty years ago, determined to help build her family's family. For my grandmother who, still alive at ninety-seven, took in the news of this honor with a crinkled nose, then said, "Are you sure? Because I never really liked my name."

My grandmother is strong and stubborn and creative and kind. She is one of the most persistent people I know. She now brags to anyone who'll listen about this amazing little girl—out of thirty-six grandchildren and thirty-four great-grandchildren, the only one who bears her name.

I hope Elsie lives to be ninety-seven too and has a life as full and as wonderful as my grandmother's. But Elsie also saved *my* life. If it weren't for wanting Elsie, I have no idea how long it would have taken me to realize I was sick or to discover the motivation to take control of my own health.

These days, I feel empowered to ask hard questions. I've learned that I can—that I must—be an advocate for myself and my family. My diabetes is under excellent control and my body is in such better balance that I ovulated on my own and got pregnant again just six months after Elsie's birth. It took half a dozen home pregnancy tests—and Joel's refusal to buy me any more—to convince me of this incredible news. Staring down at all those pink lines, even in the shining light of the joy of Elsie, I felt memories of loss creeping in to fill me with doubt. If I could have sped ahead to a safe delivery at that moment, I would have.

Two months ago, we celebrated Elsie's first birthday surrounded by the remarkable friends and family who have seen us through everything. And today, thirty-six weeks pregnant with our second daughter, I still fight the fear of losing this baby. Even though I might not cry at every doctor's appointment, I won't believe she's okay until I can hold her in my arms. The one baby item I bought when we didn't know how we'd ever become parents—a tiny pair of cheetah-print sneakers—still sits, unworn, on the girls' dresser. Our lives keep coming together, slowly, steadily, surely.

Before Elsie, I was always holding on so tight, like I was afraid of losing something I didn't even have. When she was finally placed upon my chest, with her quick, birdlike heartbeat nestled beside my own constant rhythm, all my worry dissolved. She was perfect, the answer to my prayers. And everything I'd had to wait for was a hundred times better than what I had thought I wanted.

My life is filled with small, beautiful things. This is enough. I am enough.

CHAPTER 6

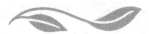

From the moment the second line on the pregnancy test had revealed the faintest trace of pink, I'd felt like I was holding my breath, willing myself to expect things to go well while allowing myself to remain detached. Something in me doubted the likelihood of taking home a baby even as I worried about hazardous viral exposures in the hospital, long hours on my feet that could induce premature labor, and possible effects on the placenta from an occasional cup of coffee during a thirty-plus-hour shift. I paced the wards on morning rounds and again each evening, wishing for a chair—or, in a fit of exhausted post-call whimsy, wheels like the ones that transported our mobile computer stations. Sometimes I lingered in the bathroom just to catch an extra moment's rest.

Well into my third trimester, I was still wary of calling attention to what was happening. I feared that some force in the universe might presume I was taking too much for granted and revoke it without warning. Through a remarkably smooth pregnancy, I often saw people look confused when I mentioned that I was expecting a baby, watched them wonder how they hadn't noticed earlier. The heavy coats and cozy sweaters of winter in Oregon explained their oversight easily enough. But I also liked traveling under the radar. I liked pretending that nothing unusual was going on so I could hope that nothing even more unusual would interfere to stop the good unusual of this pregnancy actually—maybe—succeeding.

My mid-March due date arrived without fanfare. I'd briefed the colleagues who'd be caring for my patients while I was on maternity leave. I'd written up the results from a yearlong research project that shared its due date with the baby so I'd be ready to focus on residency full-time once I came back. Ian and I kept going on longer and slower walks through the damp green woods as winter stretched toward spring. The night after my due date, we were about to get ready for bed when I realized I might be going into labor.

At first I just felt a little queasy. Then the sensation faded and returned at least three distinct times over the course of an hour. When I noted the time, the next three cycles were fifteen minutes apart. By two o'clock in the morning, the contractions were overwhelming. I had been in labor for nearly six hours, moving from couch to tub to hallway to bedroom, swaying and walking and leaning on Ian, determined to stay at home for as long as possible to avoid extra interventions or the recommendation to go home and come back later that might be offered if I arrived at the hospital too soon.

In the full moon's light, we made our way to the car. I curled on the seat while Ian tried to steer delicately over our neighborhood's potholes and navigate the same school-zone speed bumps that had caused me so much pain during the ectopic. At least once along a winding, shadowy side street, I asked him to pull over while I rode out an intense wave of contractions.

When we arrived at the hospital, I insisted on walking from the parking lot to the labor and delivery unit. But I couldn't move very far very fast. Many times I had to stop in the empty fluorescent corridors along the way, squeezing Ian's hand, pressing my side to the wall, lowering myself to the floor with no idea how I'd get up afterward but with no power to prevent myself from sitting down.

Somehow we signed in at the nursing station. Somehow I got into a bed. Somehow I held still enough to be connected to a monitor. The baby's heartbeat was strong and steady, and my contractions were coming every five minutes. When the midwife checked me, I was seven centimeters dilated. I was relieved that my labor was moving so fast, and even more relieved to hear her say that I should be ready to push very soon.

Morning light came. The nurses changed shifts. I continued to move restlessly around the room, seeking comfort in the tub, on the bed, in the bathroom, on the chair, all the while knowing that I had to go into the pain to get past it. The midwife checked me again, and her news was discouraging: four hours had passed, and I was still at seven centimeters. Now she suspected that the baby's head was tilted, not putting enough direct pressure on my cervix to dilate it further. But with the heart rate galloping along at a solid one hundred fifty beats per minute, everything seemed reassuring, so we were in no rush.

By midday, when I'd still made no progress, the midwife broke my water. Nothing changed—except a sudden and enormous increase in the pain. At four thirty, I closed my eyes and wondered if the epidural and oxytocin I'd reluctantly accepted after more than twenty hours of unmedicated labor might encourage my body to open up while I slept.

Instead, I awoke to a nurse hastily adjusting monitor straps across my abdomen. Ian stirred in the blue plastic recliner beside me, where he had dozed off too. The next thing we knew, the nurse was leaning into the hallway, shouting, and several more people were rushing into the room. One of them grabbed my arm and maneuvered me onto my hands and knees. Another held an oxygen mask to my nose and mouth and urged me to breathe deeply. Still another repositioned the monitor again to confirm that the heart rate it was registering wasn't my own and was truly the baby's—at fifty beats per minute, only one-third of what it was supposed to be.

Face down on a gurney with my gown hanging open and my

bottom in the air, I heard myself agree to a cesarean as we rolled toward the operating room. I kept asking if the baby was okay and was told—I have no idea who was speaking—that the heart rate had come back up and I should try not to move.

Less than five minutes later, I lay flat on the operating table as a crying and flailing and very alive baby was lifted from my abdomen. Ian, now standing beside me in scrubs, peered over the surgical drape to exclaim that we had a boy. I was overwhelmed with relief and shaking with cold as Ian followed him to the warmer where a team of pediatricians huddled around him.

"Does he look like a Zach?" I called over to Ian. Although we'd never settled on a name for a girl, we'd decided on a boy's name shortly after the anatomy scan. *Zachary Liam* means *God has remembered* and *strong-willed warrior*, and we appreciated the connotations of memory and persistence and hopes ultimately fulfilled that came with these names, tracing their origins far back through the Middle Ages and to my family's Irish heritage—but mostly we just liked the nickname Zach. Agreeing on the name had been easy. Allowing ourselves to believe that we'd actually have a baby to give the name to had been much harder.

Information reached me in snippets as the obstetricians delivered the placenta and sewed me up. The baby seemed normal. He'd had the umbilical cord wrapped tightly around his neck—twice—but now he was alert and crying. Ian confirmed that yes, he definitely looked like a Zach. But he was working harder and harder to breathe. His oxygen saturation levels had dropped from nearly one hundred percent into the mid-sixties, and no one knew why. Within a minute, he was wearing a scaled-down version of the oxygen mask I'd had on just before his birth.

The neonatologists took Zach into a nearby room to evaluate him more closely. When X-rays revealed bilateral pneumothoraces—air trapped inside the chest cavity that had led both of his lungs to collapse—the doctors inserted needles along our baby's rib cage to release the displaced air and allow the lobes to reinflate, drew blood for lab testing, and pushed a round of broad-spectrum antibiotics. Ian told me later about watching with equal parts gratitude and horror, marveling at the deft movements that allowed these skilled clinicians to insert an IV into such a tiny hand, as Zach clamped his other tiny hand around Ian's outstretched finger. We rolled past each other in the hallway as I was moved to the recovery room and Zach was transferred to the neonatal intensive care unit, pausing just long enough for me to touch his wisps of reddish-blond hair. I shivered uncontrollably beneath three layers of heated blankets, reeling from the sudden hormonal shifts and stress of delivery. I still hadn't held our baby.

Soon it was nighttime, exactly twenty-four hours from when I'd gone into labor at home. A nurse delivered me to the postpartum wing of the hospital as I drifted into and out of sleep. We called our families to announce our news and were surprised by how worried they'd been. The eight-plus hours since we'd last spoken to them had, to us, passed in such a chaotic blur that we hadn't noticed a logical pause for an update—much like two years earlier, when we'd also felt so much uncertainty but had a very different outcome.

Through the night, Ian went back and forth between the NICU and my bedside, trying to relay details that he only half understood. Zach was under close observation but seemed stable. He was breathing normally on his own. His heart rate was steady. He hadn't developed any signs of infection. When a lactation consultant brought in the breast pump—a rounded yellow box perched atop a lanky five-wheeled post—I managed to extract two drops of colostrum into a tube around midnight.

By daybreak, the good news arrived that we could bring Zach to our room. As Ian rolled us away from the NICU in my wheelchair, I snuggled our baby close against my green fleece bathrobe, grateful and incredulous and bewildered—and still more than a little surprised—to finally be holding a living, breathing infant in my arms.

But my relief was soon replaced by new worries. Just after Zach and I had settled in for a nap, a phlebotomist woke us to collect another vial of blood from his miniscule veins. When we tried to breastfeed, a medical assistant arrived to run a bedside electrocardiogram to evaluate his heart rate and rhythm. As Ian stepped out of the bathroom in only a towel, fresh from his first attempt to shower in three days, we were all startled by the cardiology fellow rolling a portable echocardiogram machine into our room to check Zach's heart for structural defects. We kept asking why he needed all these tests, but no one seemed to know. All we could glean was the noncommittal answer that they were just making sure everything was okay.

Finally, when the on-call pediatrician came by the next day to tell us that all the results had come back normal, we pieced together what had happened. Three factors had coalesced into a perfect storm of unnecessary testing: the incidental cardiac marker on Zach's second-trimester ultrasound, other clinicians' desire to give me the best possible care because of my role as a fellow physician, and the sympathy of all those involved for how much Ian and I had been through to have this baby. The elaborate workup was a side effect of well-intentioned but overblown efforts to put my mind at ease about unlikely possibilities I hadn't even thought to consider.

I tried to be gracious as I explained to the pediatrician that all the extra attention was actually making us more anxious. What I didn't say to her was this: *There are no tests that can answer unanswerable questions anyway.* My doubts hadn't faded as much after birth as I had expected them to. Even taking in her reassurances, I was only slightly less daunted by the unknowable future.

What I did know was that Zach was here, sleeping in my arms. He wore adorable tan pajamas stitched with baby lions and an orange cap that our neighbor had knit for him—the same neighbor who had driven us home from this very hospital after my ambulance ride for the ectopic pregnancy and who was now pregnant again herself after her own complicated losses. I knew that our worries paled in comparison to those of many other families in the NICU—like the families of patients I would soon take care of, including Anna and Maya. I knew that many of these families would be keeping vigil over their babies for weeks and months and that some wouldn't get to take their babies home at all.

Our son seemed fine, for now. *For now* was all we had anyway—and is, I was coming to realize, all any of us ever really have. Just like every other parent who's longed to protect a child, I would need to learn to accept that the best we could do was live our lives and see what came next.

Anna ~ Fairy Tales

Under the warm spray of the shower, I whispered to my baby that he was going to be my hero. I soaped my growing belly as I spun tales about monsters that only this child could save me from: A tyrannical boss at my dismal job. Childhood memories layered with disappointment and dysfunction. A nagging inner voice insisting that security and stability were out of reach, that happy endings were only for fairy tales. I was convinced that motherhood would empower me to change the narrative that had been unfolding beyond my control for so many years. I was determined to write my own story.

Peter and I were cobbling together our lives as a hopeful young couple one makeshift chapter at a time, and our baby's conception was one of the first things that had come easily for us. After sacrificing all nonessentials for nearly three years, we'd just managed to buy a quaint ranch-style house. The first few months of my pregnancy passed effortlessly as we unpacked boxes, talked about a home birth, prepared healthy meals together, and envisioned welcoming our baby into the world in the most peaceful way possible. I felt like we were finally building something for ourselves that was all our own, a continent's breadth away from my past.

At my routine twenty-week scan, the ultrasound tech squinted at the screen and scowled. She rolled the probe across my gel-smeared abdomen to repeat all the measurements. Again she confirmed the date of my last period and asked when I thought we'd conceived. By dinnertime, Peter and I were sitting at our favorite neighborhood restaurant and staring wide-eyed, first at each other, then at the center of the table, where an unassuming envelope lay ready to reveal its secret. Flushed with excitement after having waited all day to learn the sex of our baby together, I tore it open.

The blocky lettering proclaimed its message across the grainy ultrasound printout: *IT'S A GIRL!*

Suddenly all my convictions fell out from under me. I was instantly burdened with the gravity of raising a daughter. As I held the thin sheet of paper, my mind flooded with thoughts of my own shortcomings and failures, and the myriad lessons I would need to teach her for her to avoid the mistakes I'd made. A few days before the ultrasound, when my mother-in-law had told me about a dream she'd had of walking along the beach with her granddaughter, I had shrugged off the image. Since the moment I knew I was pregnant, I had pictured my baby only as a little boy. How could my intuition have been so wrong?

My phone rang at work the next morning. My family medicine doctor, who had known me for years and wasn't easily ruffled, had received the radiologist's report and wanted to schedule me for an urgent visit. Now I understood why the tech had kept repeating the measurements and asking to confirm my dates. The baby was measuring two full weeks behind.

When we met in her office that afternoon, I could tell that my doctor wanted to be optimistic. But a cloud hung over us. We smiled hesitantly at each other while the steady beat of my baby's heart echoed through the exam room like footsteps racing away from my hopes for a healthy pregnancy and an uncomplicated birth. Then, as my doctor sat down with me to go over the ultrasound findings in detail and explain her concerns about my daughter's development, my attitude shifted. I remember thinking that my baby was just small. That her growth would catch up. That Peter and I aren't very tall and that we both come from long lines of not-very-tall people. Feeling skeptical as she spoke, I couldn't accept the fact that my doctor's experience was telling her something was wrong. I didn't want to believe that I could possibly not know what was going on in my own body, with my own child. I walked out of the room a little shaken but mostly convinced that my daughter was going to be fine.

We waited two weeks, then went to our next ultrasound to repeat the measurements. She was still tiny. Doubts crept into my mind. If my mother-in-law had been right about our baby's sex when I wasn't, was the doctor right in her concerns too? If I couldn't trust myself to know such an essential thing, how could I be sure that I knew anything about being a good mother? Was I already hurting my baby somehow?

My questioning stirred up memories of past hardships. I certainly hadn't had an idyllic childhood. My parents' divorce had upended my world when I was eight, as had the accidental revelation, when I was ten, that my dad was gay. The oldest of my four sisters, thirteen years my senior, had been adopted at age six out of a home full of trauma and had been unable to escape the cycle of abusive relationships ever since. Our family was plagued by mental illness as we each struggled to repair the damage in our own way. Growing up in the fishbowl of working-class small-town Maine, I'd spent years feeling trapped and hopeless, while all my challenges had seemed magnified. There had been no break in the grief.

But even if my insecurities were fueled by my past, the concerns raised by the ultrasounds were real and present. Suddenly, twenty-two weeks into my pregnancy, the tenuousness of our situation was palpable. When we met with our new team of high-risk maternal-fetal obstetrical specialists, I took diligent notes with the hope of uncovering that one elusive detail that would solve the puzzle we had become. As we talked about chromosomal disorders, placental problems, and medical conditions that might be causing the baby's growth restriction, along with the tests that might reveal them, I reeled. I couldn't imagine what kind of information—what kind of terrible forewarning—could possibly prepare us to survive if our daughter didn't.

We chose the name Miranda, and naming her gave us hope. Twelve long days later, when Miranda was just under twenty-four weeks' gestation, the results of an amniocentesis came back normal, and we were overwhelmed with gratitude and relief.

Only two days passed before I lost sight of the reassurance the test had offered—because that was when the pain started. But the concept of *pain* is far too simplistic to capture the massive physical anguish that assaulted me without warning. After dinner one night, a squeezing ache rose up in the middle of my chest and escalated to excruciating within minutes, stabbing me repeatedly in the heart. On it went, every night, relentless for ten, twelve, sixteen hours, then vanishing suddenly each morning. I dreaded each evening, fearing that the agony would return. I would describe the pain as *unbearable*, but that wouldn't be true because I did bear it. I worried that Miranda might be suffering like I was. I remember thinking, *What could be so wrong that I could feel this bad?*

The only thing worse than the pain was its complete lack of explanation. My doctors were at a loss to find a cause, and I tried everything I could think of to get rid of it. I practiced controlled breathing, meditation, and relaxation techniques from our childbirth class. I sat straight upright for hours after meals. I stood. I stretched. I bounced. I hummed. At one point, I found the slightest improvement by lying upside down with my legs dangling over the armrest of the couch. I imagined Miranda desperately grasping for purchase as she slid up into my rib cage, tumbling through a landslide in my uterus.

Even as I visited the maternal-fetal specialists twice a week, following their close monitoring schedule and hearing constant admonitions to call them immediately if anything changed, I had a hard time accepting that my pregnancy was precarious. If all these brilliant people with all these advanced degrees couldn't figure out what was going on, then it couldn't be that big of a deal. I focused on my deepening connection to my daughter and my growing excitement to meet her. Far off though it still seemed, Miranda's birth held so much promise. Like the triumph of an unlikely hero over the forces of evil, it offered the reprieve I'd been waiting for, complete with a vision of birds singing out in joyous melody and the sun shining brighter throughout the land. Miranda's arrival would be my rescue.

Then, suddenly, at twenty-six weeks and two days' gestation, direct from our routine Saturday-morning monitoring session, I found myself admitted to the hospital with my entire team of doctors on high alert. The hours dragged on and turned into days. Each time the thing Peter and I thought we were supposed to be worrying about stabilized, the doctors became convinced that something entirely new posed the gravest danger instead. Blood pressure, liver tests, fetal heart rate, cell counts—I didn't understand how it all fit together. Every time we ran a test to assess one concern, the result would come back reassuring but with a hugely out-of-range value popping up for something else that happened to be included on the panel, like a high-stakes version of some twisted carnival game. At all hours, dozens of staff members with furrowed brows scurried into and out of our room, adding to the sense of mounting but unfocused urgency. I was at once baffled, frustrated, disoriented, and terrified.

Late Monday afternoon, we received a diagnosis: severe atypical preeclampsia with HELLP syndrome. My doctors explained that HELLP—hemolysis, elevated liver enzymes, and low platelets—was destroying the blood cells I needed for oxygen transport and blood clotting. Preeclampsia was causing blood vessel constriction throughout my body, leading to high blood pressure and compromised blood flow to my vital organs—including the placenta.

We needed to deliver Miranda. But if the delivery went badly, I would begin to hemorrhage and the doctors wouldn't be able to stop it. All my systems were failing, but my liver was failing the fastest, and the distress calls it sent in its collapse radiated into my chest to manifest as the crushing ache just below my heart. The fear behind my pain was finally quantifiable. My body had been trying to tell me for weeks that Miranda and I were in serious peril.

As we prepared for an emergency cesarean, I felt responsible for how complicated everything had become yet powerless to change the course of events. My daughter was about to be born a full trimester early because my body wasn't a safe place for her. I wanted so badly to believe that my doctor would soon walk in and declare this whole thing a big misunderstanding. That I could somehow keep Miranda inside until her due date. That I could protect her.

Instead, the nurses transferred my fluids and medications to a rolling pole and whisked me to the operating room. Under glaring overhead lamps, they gave me a spinal anesthetic, inserted a catheter into my bladder, shaved the upper edge of my pubic hair to prepare for the incision, and splayed out my arms on planks perpendicular to the surgical table. I felt like I was being crucified. The on-call obstetrician arrived and, after introducing herself quickly, stepped behind the blue drape. A moment later, I sensed an intense tugging, as if someone were rummaging around for keys and my uterus had become a purse. I was chilled to my core. Gripping Peter's hand, I began to make low, guttural noises, trying to vocalize the disturbingly visceral sensations, drawing on the strategies we had learned together for coping with labor.

The surgeon paused and asked if I was feeling any pain. She sounded very worried.

"No," I groaned. "This is just really awful."

The anesthesiologist had advised me that I would still be able to feel movement in my abdomen, but I was shocked by the crudeness of the whole process. I heard the surgeon and the anesthesiologist in anxious discussion as I continued to moan, as I tried to step outside this moment and remind myself that it would end soon—and that when it did I would have my baby. Misinterpreting my agitation, the anesthesiologist dosed me with more powerful pain medication. All I felt as I slipped into unconsciousness were my own warm tears and an overwhelming sadness.

When I woke up three hours later, I was in the recovery room. Swirling concentric circles blurred my vision, like a movie fantasy sequence in reverse, spinning me back into reality. Concerned faces peered down at me. "She's awake," someone whispered. My focus sharpened, and I saw Peter huddled in the corner with his mother and sister, all of them looking exhausted and shell-shocked.

"Miranda's okay," Peter said quietly, stepping toward me to kiss my forehead. "She's tiny, but she's okay." Tears welled up in his eyes as he leaned close. "I thought I was going to lose you both."

A dim orange-yellow light illuminated the cramped space, casting an unwelcoming, antiseptic glow. The air was heavy with defeat. Everyone kept patting my legs and telling me how relieved they were that I was okay too. It was true that Miranda and I had both survived. But I wasn't sure I knew what being okay meant anymore.

After three more hours, our nurse finally told us we could go see Miranda. My whole body moved into the wheelchair in slow motion, hot and itchy, weighted by a lethargy that made my chest heavy and my breathing shallow. Intravenous magnesium—running to prevent my severely elevated blood pressure from causing a seizure—left me queasy and uncomfortable in my skin, like I was coming down with the flu. I ran my tongue across my sticky teeth and winced at the metallic taste in my mouth. I tried not to be self-conscious about wearing nothing but a pair of white mesh underwear lined with a bulky pad and a flimsy cotton hospital gown that I'd already sweated through twice over. I had the distinct impression that if I stood up I would pass out immediately.

The first thing we noticed as the doors to the neonatal intensive care unit closed behind us was the quiet. Rolling down the hallway, I imagined a ghost town with tumbleweeds blowing along the floor.

There were no smiles from proud grandparents cradling swaddled babies. There was no laughter coming from groups of delighted friends bringing gifts. There was just the vigilant attention, wordless and solemn, of each family standing guard. Peeking through a cracked door, I heard the muffled sobs of another new mother, her back turned toward me. Each self-contained habitat held someone else's experience, distinct and isolated, decidedly uncelebratory and vaguely untouchable.

Outside Miranda's room, one daunting sign above a gleaming white sink implored visitors to stay away if they were feeling the least bit sick, while another instructed us to take off rings and wash for three full minutes. As I scrubbed meticulously between every finger, under every nail, and up to my elbows, my heart ached at having to wait even a few more moments to meet her. But if I got any of this wrong, I could actually kill my baby. I knew that preemies are much more susceptible to infection than babies born at term. Their immune systems haven't fully developed, which means they have smaller reserves of the cells that defend against bacteria and viruses. Even the babies in the NICU who aren't preemies are dealing with a host of medical problems and complications. Combine the invasiveness of the procedures that many of these babies undergo with the immune-lowering steroid medications often given just prior to birth to boost lung maturity, then add a layer of inflammation from stressful delivery conditions and aggressive respiratory interventions, and the NICU becomes a terribly vulnerable little microcosm.

When we finally crossed the threshold into Miranda's room, we were immediately panicked by the flurry of activity surrounding the clear plastic box that dominated the scene. Bodies in scrubs and their jumble of hands converged on it—on her—as monitors flashed and beeped over low lights and hushed voices. With no language to describe anything I was seeing, I felt helpless to interpret what was happening.

One person broke away from the group and stepped toward us. She told us that Miranda had narrowly avoided intubation and that she had received a blood transfusion just a few minutes ago. She gently but firmly suggested that it would be best if we came back later.

Feeling devastated to be turned away, Peter and I retreated to my room. On our way to the NICU, I had steeled myself for the complete unknown of what I might see and feel. Now I was stuck, unable to move into the crucial moment that we had prepared for. Miranda was six hours old, and I still hadn't met her. Although I desperately needed to rest, I fumbled with the breast pump the nurse had left at my bedside and somehow collected a few drops of milk—the only thing I could think of to do to help my baby.

An hour later, Miranda was stable enough to visit. We went back to the NICU and scrubbed again. This time, when Peter wheeled me to the doorway of Miranda's room, it seemed strangely empty and inordinately huge. Monitors still beeped, throwing soft echoes, as a single nurse sat working on her computer. At the center of this vast expanse was the incubator. Peter maneuvered my wheelchair as close as he could to Miranda's little plastic crib. I tenderly lifted the handmade pink patchwork quilt that had been draped across it to keep out the light and peeked inside.

Nothing could have prepared me for how small my daughter was. My eyes searched for her in the nest of lambswool blankets that the nurses had constructed around her to simulate the womb. Born at twenty-six weeks and four days' gestation, Miranda weighed five hundred grams—just over a pound—and measured ten inches long. The foreignness of the whole experience made it difficult for me to connect it to anything else I'd been through, which sparked the strangest comparisons in my mind: She was about the weight of a pack of butter. She was barely the size of a squirrel. Because her growth had been severely restricted by preeclampsia and HELLP syndrome, she weighed only half as much as a typical micropreemie born at her gestation, teetering on the edge of viability. I knew immediately that this was not the size a human should be. It boggled my mind that she could be a complete person.

Wires seemed to spring out of her everywhere. A breathing mask dwarfed her face, and her head hardly stretched the knit cap that helped hold the apparatus in place, rigged up as it was with safety pins and rubber bands. Surgical tape led from cheek to nose, positioning a nasogastric tube that delivered drops of my breastmilk directly into her stomach and released excess air. Half a golden heart sticker covered her smooth torso, which hadn't yet developed visible nipples. A tangle of black and white wires radiated from beneath it, tracking her vital signs and relaying the results to the monitor overhead. A central intravenous line pierced her mosquito-bite-sized navel to deliver fluids and medications directly to her heart. A pulse oximeter illuminated her foot in an eerie glowing red. A foam identification bracelet had been wrapped twice around her ankle but was still too big. As Peter and I stared, frozen, Miranda's nurse reminded us to speak quietly and approach her cautiously, advising that stimulation could upset rather than comfort a baby this delicate.

I was afraid to touch my own child—and it was the worst feeling I had ever experienced. Slowly, I reached my arm into a porthole in the incubator and spoke to her softly. I told her that I was her mother. I told her that I was so happy to meet her. I told her that she had been born a fighter, that she was brave and strong and powerful, that I was so proud of her already for all she had overcome. When I offered her my thumb, she amazed me by clasping on with her whole hand. Her fingers didn't quite reach around it.

Later that evening, resting in my own hospital room while Miranda rested in hers, I started to process all that had happened. Peter had stepped out to get something to eat, and I was alone for the first time since we'd left home for our prenatal monitoring appointment just two days earlier. I realized that I felt kind of numb—relieved, certainly, but also hollow and disappointed. I didn't feel any of the storybook euphoria that I'd been taught to expect after childbirth. Birth hadn't offered me a glimpse of the majesty of the universe, with all the beauty and hope and wonder of life made manifest in the purity of a new being. I didn't get to look down at my baby or weep tears of joy as my doctor placed her, wet and squirming and completely mine, upon my chest. In fact, I didn't feel like I'd given birth at all. There'd been a birth, and my baby was now outside my body, and I certainly felt like crying. But I didn't feel directly responsible or even very involved. All the promise inherent in birth had been replaced by self-doubt and inadequacy.

One of the hardest things about having Miranda so early was that no one was jubilant—not even me. Any kind of celebration seemed foolhardy and farcical, an insensitive affront to the precarious balance that was suddenly our daughter's life. *Congratulations* was a word people carefully avoided, perhaps reluctant to seem naive to the realities of the struggle ahead, perhaps worried that declaring her arrival a victory could tip us all into disaster. We didn't share photographs. Any welcome presents that might have been planned were abandoned. Nobody came bounding into my room with chocolates or surprised us with oversized balloons in the shape of baby bottles, and flowers weren't allowed in the NICU for fear of introducing contaminants into its fragile ecosystem. I wouldn't have felt comfortable accepting gifts at that moment anyway, my own happiness far too tentative to hold up against gestures of unreserved joy.

When Miranda was three days old, I was finally allowed to hold her for the first time. I positioned myself in the rocker as the nurse methodically disconnected her nonessential monitors to move her out of the incubator. I lifted one of the flaps of my blue hospital gown, and the nurse set her gently on my bare chest. As soon as this tiny, incredible person nuzzled against my heart, I knew she was mine. After all the chaos and trauma of her birth, after all the grief of our abbreviated pregnancy, after all the anxiety and all the pain, I finally believed that she was meant to be my daughter, that I was meant to be her mother. I practically held my breath for the entire twenty-five minutes she spent nestled against my skin.

From her first moments of life, Miranda's routine was intensely regimented, repeating in four-hour cycles through the day and night. I was discharged five days after she was born, grateful that delivery had almost instantly shifted my physical condition from being near death to having just a healing scar on a tender body. Each morning, Peter and I returned in time for her eight o'clock care routine. With fingers like clumsy giants', we changed her miniscule diaper and took her temperature in the birdlike pocket of her armpit. After spending a few minutes together, Peter kissed us both goodbye and left reluctantly to bike to his office downtown.

I spent all day, every day, at the hospital. I pumped milk as the nurses collected blood samples, tracked vital signs, and recorded chart notes. I consulted with Miranda's doctors to get updates from their rounds. I paced the corridors to clear my head and forced myself to eat something before each cycle began anew. Once a day, I gingerly snuggled her on my bare chest for just a few minutes, then placed her back into the incubator before she could become overtired or overstimulated.

When I was at Miranda's bedside, I sang and talked incessantly as if she could understand me. Leaning close to her clear box of a crib, I marveled as her heart rate slowed and her breathing stabilized at the sound of my voice. I spent hours reading her tales of magical far-off lands of enchantment and wonder, about unlikely heroes overcoming great hardship. I recounted the story of how Peter and I had met, about how I had known I was going to marry him long before we were engaged, about how I'd undertaken the quest to win his heart after it had been badly broken by someone else. I reminded her that she came from a long line of strong and determined women. I told her about all the adventures she and I would have together once she was big enough to come home.

Hidden in my promises was the worry that, in failing to carry Miranda to term, I had brought this fate upon myself and my baby. Each moment I spent in the NICU reinforced my awareness that what she was doing—eating and growing and sleeping most of the day—was what other babies were still doing inside their mothers. I had failed the first test of motherhood by letting her come into the world before she was ready. In fact, I had specifically asked her to come as soon as she could. Early in my pregnancy, when I'd first started talking to my belly, hadn't I told Miranda that her arrival would mean my salvation?

After Miranda's birth, the doctors had explained to me that preeclampsia, with its foundations in shaky implantation of the placenta along the uterine wall, begins just after conception, even though its effects typically appear later in the pregnancy. And the disorder is related as much to the father's genetics as the mother's. If a man's own mother had preeclampsia while pregnant with him, any pregnancy he's responsible for is more likely to be complicated by it as well. Still, I was just as vulnerable to crafting faulty narratives for myself as for Miranda, and my self-blaming logic kept me awake at night in fear. I couldn't imagine the grief I would feel if I lost her.

But Miranda surprised us all by thriving. Peter and I, reunited every night to be with her, learned to rely on numbers to measure her progress, even when those numbers felt disheartening—or outright terrifying. We knew that her Apgar score at birth had been a grim three on the ten-point scale. We counted and recorded her episodes of apneas—cessations of breathing—and bradys—or bradycardias, abnormally slow heartbeats. As she slept in her darkened incubator, nurses and respiratory therapists perpetually adjusted her machines when her oxygen level was too low or her respiratory rate too high. When her white blood cell count dipped, I worried more about infections. When her hematocrit dropped, she received a transfusion—four times in the first few weeks alone. I knew the temperature of her incubator, the weight of her last wet diaper, the depth of her stomach tube, and the caloric value of the supplements the staff used to fortify my pumped milk. Every measurement, every expectation, was recalculated with each gram of weight she gained. I knew her day of life and adjusted age to the hour.

As Peter and I grew accustomed to the rhythms of the NICU, we learned to interpret this astounding array of data and to watch our daughter and her monitors without panicking if something shifted slightly. Gradually, the number of wires attached to Miranda decreased. But each time I got lulled into a sense of safety, our course would change just enough to be unsettling. I would arrive ready to hold her, then learn that she couldn't leave the incubator because she had just received a transfusion or had stopped breathing several times that morning. I would be asked to set her down after only two minutes of snuggling because a specialist was coming by to do an eye exam, assessing for the retinopathy of prematurity that could blind her. I would be waiting to connect with her medical team after morning rounds to hear their report, then they would postpone their evaluations because she was receiving an ultrasound to check for intraventricular hemorrhages, distressingly common bleeds caused by the rupture of delicate veins in preemies' brains. I tried to squelch the sense that we were all just waiting for a catastrophe.

By the time Miranda was a month old, we had accepted this roller coaster as normal. We had even begun to allow ourselves to enjoy the blissful monotony when things were going smoothly, all the while acknowledging that despair could be just around the corner. We spent a lot of time being hopeful, and almost as much time guarding against hope. We were reassured that, tiny as Miranda was—the smallest baby that many of her doctors and nurses had ever met, even in their long careers of caring for thousands of preemies—she seemed to have no other significant medical problems. Every night before we left the hospital, Peter and I held hands over her incubator and sang lullabies, the same lullabies my father had sung to me when I was little. When I said good night, I really did feel at peace with leaving her at the hospital. I recognized that I was doing all I could for her as her mother, that she was in the capable hands of an amazing team of doctors and nurses, and that there was nothing more we could do for her at home.

In fact, our home held almost no evidence that we had a newborn. All our friends who were expecting a baby had prepared a nursery ahead of time, but we just had a bland guest room still waiting to be painted. Deep in my closet were the only two items that hinted at the moments we had thought we were planning for. At the beginning of my second trimester, I had sewn a maternity dress to help get myself excited about the looming prospect of feeling huge. The piece was simple and cozy, with an empire waist, elbow-length sleeves, and a twist at the bust. Now, when I ran my hands along its soft heather-gray fabric, it struck me as a sad reminder of an imagined self I wouldn't become. I had gained less than ten pounds through my whole pregnancy, barely enough to stretch its gathered waistline. The one piece of clothing I had begun fashioning for Miranda, a red sack sleeper sewn from Peter's favorite old hoodie, sat poignantly nearby on a shelf, marked and pinned and turned inside out. Five Mirandas would have fit inside—if I had even had a chance to finish sewing it.

My days, too, felt patched together, the fabric of four-hour NICU cycles overlaid with rare fragments of time spent anywhere else. Even as Miranda became stronger and more stable, thinking about any life outside the hospital seemed a disservice to the enormity of what was going on within it. While I was at her bedside, my focus was clear. As soon as I stepped away, I didn't feel like a parent. Everyone had told me that becoming a mother would change me immediately and color how I saw everything in the world thereafter. Now that assertion felt like a myth. Wandering around in a grocery store, I would suddenly remember that I had a baby, as if I had been living in a parallel fantasy world. I couldn't quite grasp how the smiling cashier, the woman in line behind me, and the man restocking the produce couldn't instantly understand my life when they looked at me. I was so raw, so defenseless. I felt like I should be see-through.

By two months, we had become keenly aware that Miranda's course in the NICU would be considered routine. Easy, even. She was doing far better than her doctors had predicted and showed no indications of significant disability or delay. Twice the doctors talked about how close she was to being ready to leave, but then she would have a bad night, with enough apneas and bradycardias to make us all hesitant to broach the topic again for several days.

Slowly, Peter and I started to share pictures of her with friends and family and to allow a few other NICU parents to meet Miranda. I welcomed visits from our family doctor and our maternal-fetal medicine specialist. Relieved as I was to be able to take these steps, anticipating others' reactions was sometimes even harder than managing our own. I bristled whenever I heard anyone call her a miracle. The term made me feel vaguely incensed—a little bit indignant and a little bit afraid. Wasn't every child a miracle? Why should the world call out my child's life more than any other's, more than the fact that any person ever exists and grows and thrives?

The truth is that Miranda *was* a miracle. She absolutely was in so many ways. Yet she couldn't be. Because to admit that Miranda was a miracle would be to admit how close we'd come to losing her—and how close we might still be some days. Even as we sensed ourselves inching closer toward bringing our baby home, we knew that nothing about her outcome was guaranteed, or even foreseeable. We imagined daily that we were barely avoiding alternate futures full of devastations, unknown and unthinkable, that cast only the briefest shadow as they passed by.

When we named her, some part of me must have understood all this. *Miranda* translates from the Latin as *worthy of admiration*, with origins in the word *mirandus*, meaning *miraculous, that which is to be wondered or marveled at*. Perhaps I felt that it was my right alone to acknowledge the improbability of her survival, linked as it was to my own. But if the world marveled at her, why should I take offense?

Finally, after eighty days in the NICU, eighty days of reading stories and singing lullabies and watching her grow, two weeks before her due date, we were told that Miranda was ready for discharge.

We put her in a car seat and drove away from the hospital, thrilled and terrified to be leaving together as a family. Alone with our tiny daughter, untethered from the safety net of the NICU, we found it hard to believe that she was okay. I couldn't help but keep telling myself the story of my inadequacy, and with each retelling it became harder to push away. I bounced back and forth between my narrative of guilt and fear and my narrative of hope and triumph. I worried about missing something crucial in Miranda's development, all the while realizing how fortunate we already were in how well she was doing.

During Miranda's first six months at home, doctors' visits punctuated our schedule like little platforms of safety to be leapt to one by one. Between appointments, we stood near the edge and peered into the abyss of uncertainty below. Traditional measurements and milestones seemed unreachable, like illusive quests in a far-off land. She couldn't pass as normal yet—because she wasn't normal. She was the exception. The survivor. The unlikely hero who had triumphed. As a micropreemie with growth restriction caused by severe HELLP syndrome and preeclampsia, Miranda didn't even track on the preemie growth charts.

Every day that Miranda had spent in the NICU, I had longed for her to be done. To be safe. To be ready to move on from that world of two steps forward and one step back. But once she was home, I couldn't recover from the not knowing, from being told that my child had been struggling with complications I was completely unaware of. My mind spun, desperate to decipher what immense misfortune she would someday face as payment for beating the odds. I kept thinking that if I could move ahead to a moment when our fate would become obvious, then I could accept the inevitable retributions. As often as I'd recounted hero tales to Miranda, I wasn't sure I always believed in them—or maybe I was just skeptical of endings that seemed too good to be true.

During my pregnancy with Miranda, what I had felt in my heart physically was pain, sharp and gnawing and constant, with no explanation and no relief. But what I felt in my heart metaphorically was trust that we would be okay. My intuition kept telling me there was nothing wrong with Miranda. Maybe, in spite of the doubts I was feeling as she grew, that first instinct had been right all along.

Because Miranda *is* fine. At two years old now, she is thriving. Though the future is unknowable, in this moment she is utterly perfect. The smug, obstinate part of me wants to keep believing that she was just small, she was bound to be small, and there wasn't anything anyone could have done to change that. She survived. We survived. Together, we endured it all.

But I do recognize that I was also wrong. The reality is that my pregnancy wasn't healthy. Miranda couldn't have stayed inside me safely for forty weeks, no matter how strong my desire to protect her. If she had been born even a few days earlier, she almost certainly would have died. If we had waited any longer to deliver her, I might have. We wouldn't be here without the urgent collaboration of a team of experts and a whirlwind of interventions I'd never even known existed. We both needed every bit of help we received. But we also turned out to be more resilient than I could have imagined.

Miranda still loves fairy tales. She asks me to tell her stories of daring rescues and of brave heroes defeating monsters. When I curl up beside her, I think back on the stories I told her before she was born, and I think of all that we've been through. Her struggles seem so unfair when measured against her cheerful grin, her seventeen-pound frame, her squeaky toddler voice singing a tune about the starry sky as I hand her a cracker and buckle her into her high chair. She doesn't seem to remember any of her past. Now, when my heart aches, it's because I see the magic of the strong and delicate and capable and vulnerable and wondrous creature that she is today. I see a glimpse of the happy ending that just might be our beginning.

Maya ~ So Far

Pregnancy was a magical time for me. Growing another being made me feel like a queen, with the power and dignity to take on anything in this world. No other woman had ever been me, pregnant with this very baby, and no words seemed adequate to convey our time together. As I watched my belly grow week by week, I felt the peace of being in this moment, with every experience unique and new and yet somehow deepening our connection to all the families who had traveled this road before us.

We had a smooth, fun pregnancy, my son and I. Enthralled by every little kick and wiggle, I daydreamed about a dark-haired boy running around the backyard, playing baseball with my husband, Daniel. I pictured all of us cuddling up together to read bedtime stories. Most of all, I imagined having a tiny little baby, just born and still almost a part of my own body, snuggling and nursing at all hours of the day and night. Even nearing my due date and feeling large and awkward, I loved every minute of it. I never tired of reading books and hearing stories about other women's experiences with labor, breastfeeding, bonding, and parenting. I was fascinated with this new world that was about to become my life.

Five days before my due date, just after dinner, I began to sense a low cramping in my pelvis as I was heading out to my prenatal exercise class. I thought back to every time I'd heard that first babies are usually late and that false labor happens all the time. I weighed my options, considered the frequent but mild sensations, and decided I had plenty of time to fit in the hour-long session.

By the time class was over, I could hardly stand. My instincts insisted that I drive myself home, and the contractions ramped up faster than I had imagined possible through the fifteen-minute trip along the neighborhood streets of our Phoenix suburb. I clutched the steering wheel and breathed through each stoplight. A streak of July sunset lingered above the mountains at the edge of town as the red glowing clock on my car's dashboard lit up the night, telling me that my contractions were now coming every three minutes.

When I got home, I careened straight through the front door and past the living room couch where Daniel sat. In the bathroom, I was strangely grateful to have only the diarrhea that I had heard could herald early labor, without the vomiting. Just as Daniel came in to check on me, I leaned around the corner, head spinning, and told him he should probably call the hospital and tell them to expect us tonight.

Back in the car, Daniel guided us with a steady hand as I gripped the door handle and whimpered with each contraction. The slightest bumps on the road sent waves of pain through my body as the bucket seat restricted my movements in a way I'd never noticed before. When we arrived at the hospital, I scribbled my signature on some paperwork that I had no patience to read, then threw up immediately upon walking into my labor room—and almost laughed when it occurred to me that my experience now precisely matched what I had read about. The doctor checked my cervix as the nurse started filling the tub. When I stepped into the water, its warmth and buoyancy relaxed every muscle in my body.

Then, almost immediately, the urge to push overtook me, distorting the passage of time. I imagined it must be getting close to morning as I bore down over and over. Daniel whispered that I was doing great and that I'd been pushing for half an hour. A few minutes later, I heard the nurse tell him that it had been more than two hours now, and she was concerned my progress was slowing. She asked me to climb up onto the bed. I emerged from the water reluctantly and tried every position we could think of. I was all over that room, crouching on hands and knees, squatting on a towel, sitting on the toilet, rocking in a chair, everywhere at once. After another two hours—or so I was told later—grasping at a sheet wrapped around a bar at the foot of the bed for counterbalance, I summoned one final push before dawn.

Ethan slipped out, silent, soft, and completely blue. He wasn't moving as they placed him on me, the rise and fall of my chest a stark contrast to his stillness. Daniel reached up to cut the cord with shaking hands, then the doctor whisked Ethan across the room to a counter I couldn't quite see. A dozen other people poured in and crowded around him, struggling to get him to breathe. My doctor returned to my bedside, coaching me to push out the placenta as I strained to listen for Ethan's cries.

At last, one of the unknown faces smiled as she handed me my son wrapped in a striped baby blanket and a stretchy white hat, looking warm and pink and staring straight at me. I was overwhelmed by his beauty. He was rooting, so I put him to my breast. He seemed just as exhausted as I was, but he began to nurse ever so gently, exactly as I had envisioned him for so many months in my dreams. He was here, and he was perfect. After the panic surrounding his birth turned into elation and relief, Daniel stepped out of the room to update our anxiously waiting families in the visitors' area. Finally, we were alone as mother and son.

For ten minutes, Ethan and I and this single room were the whole world. Tears of joy rolled down my cheeks as he looked at me with curious gray eyes. I kissed his forehead, his nose, his whisper of dark hair. I tried to memorize his every feature, his every sigh.

After such a difficult start, Ethan was being watched carefully by the hospital staff too. The pediatrician had mentioned a concern about his muscle tone, then a couple of hours after he was born, our nurse noticed a subtle twitch in his left arm. It lasted less than a minute, and we all hoped maybe she had been imagining it. But an EEG—an electroencephalogram, or brain wave tracing—showed a slightly abnormal pattern, indicating that the twitch had indeed represented a seizure.

The parade of unfamiliar faces began again. Ethan was poked and prodded for blood tests, urine tests, spinal taps, and an ultrasound of his brain. My placenta was sent off to the pathology lab for examination. We waited with hope and helplessness. Finally, about four hours after his birth, the pediatrician came to our bedside to give us the good news that, so far, all the test results looked encouraging. No explanation for the seizures had been found, he said, which was generally a good thing. Sometimes this just happens in normal, healthy babies. Sometimes it's about getting off to a rough start. Sometimes there's something else going on that doesn't reveal itself until later. For now, Daniel and I were content to enjoy our baby, ready to dismiss this as an isolated incident. But as the nurse readjusted Ethan's diaper and set him back into my arms, his left arm began to move again. We silently watched the slow, rhythmic jerking silhouetted against my belly. As the twitches settled down, the pediatrician slowly met our gaze, his eyes now registering deep concern. Perhaps more treatment would be needed after all.

Two doctors from the neonatal intensive care unit came to our bedside and proposed hooking Ethan up to a continuous brain wave monitor while giving him medication to decrease the risk of further seizures. We were confused and exhausted, but of course we accepted their advice—of course we wanted to do whatever would give him the best possible chance of avoiding problems and healing from any complications we couldn't see yet. They set up his intravenous lines and started an anti-seizure medication called phenobarbital.

Soon, he was resting in the NICU on his tiny bed, nothing more than an elevated white square among a pod of other babies, with tubes coming out of his hands and feet and belly button and a video monitor perched nearby to record any abnormal movements. He had a bright red light taped to his finger to measure blood oxygen levels and a display of wiggling green lines that traced his heart rate and breathing patterns along the screen over his bed. They warned us that he'd probably need to stay there for a few days and that he couldn't be held much, since that would interfere with the monitors and, even more importantly, with his brain's need to use all its energy to recover.

Through more than seventy hours attached to these machines, Ethan was allowed to leave the confines of his bed for only a few minutes at a time, which also meant he couldn't nurse. I pumped milk every two to three hours around the clock so we could feed it back to him later through a tiny tube. I longed to comfort him, but the anxious glares of the nurses reminded us that the brief moments we spent holding him in our arms meant a risk of overstimulation and a sacrifice of accuracy in monitoring, a dilemma impossible to reconcile.

One nurse watched Daniel placing Ethan delicately back into his NICU bed and suggested we take some pictures. "I know this is a really difficult time for you," she said, "but you're going to want to remember it later." The thought of having photographs of Ethan in this setting was unnerving—and I didn't think it was possible that these images could ever fade from my mind. We snapped a few pictures, struggling to find a good angle to capture his peaceful face among all the tubes and wires. These, we thought, would be the hardest days of our lives, barely being able to touch our son. And they certainly were, so far.

Ethan lay exposed, vulnerable, and pumped full of fluids while Daniel and I spent our hours driving back and forth from home to hospital, wishing for guarantees that we knew were impossible to have. This was the best thing for him, everyone promised, and we believed them with all our hearts. As the days crawled by, the doctors grew more optimistic about his prognosis. His brain imaging showed no sign of bleeding or tumors. His EEG hadn't recorded any residual seizure activity at times when he wasn't having a visible seizure, which we were told was a strong predictor of doing well in the long run. One by one, the tubes and monitors came off, and he began to look more like a normal five-day-old baby—a baby we could imagine bringing home.

Welcoming him into my arms after the last tube was out felt like a second birth. As his next dose of phenobarbital was prepared, Daniel and I were thrilled that this might be one of the last treatments he'd need. I tried to feed him again, but he was having trouble latching. He just couldn't seem to get comfortable. He alternated between being really fussy and falling asleep instantly when he stopped moving.

I was disappointed, since having a few good feeding sessions was one of the milestones he had to meet before leaving the hospital. The nurse told us that many babies had trouble coordinating their suck and swallow after the kinds of things he'd been through. With her reassurance, we felt better again. She had seen this before. Our baby was going to be fine. We stepped out of the NICU to use the bathroom and collect ourselves for a moment.

But as soon as we walked back in, less than five minutes later, I knew something was very wrong. Ethan's color was terribly strange. He looked pale and blotchy and slightly yellow. I asked what was the matter with him. The nurse glanced at us and smiled as she finished entering his most recent set of measurements into her computer. Then she walked casually over to his bed.

As she placed her tiny silver stethoscope on his chest, I saw her face turn ashen. She sprinted to the hallway and shouted for the doctor. A flood of people arrived and someone started giving Ethan chest compressions. Daniel and I stood in a corner, hugging each other, desperately wanting to understand what was happening but afraid of what the answers might be if we asked. We could no longer see Ethan within the growing crowd of medical personnel that moved with frantic energy as time all at once sped up, slowed down, and stood still. The NICU doctor rushed in. I heard his shouting voice demand more epinephrine just before a woman's softer voice inquired if we'd like a visit from the chaplain.

The chaplain? Why would we need a chaplain? Just a split second ago, it seemed, we had been talking about stopping Ethan's anti-seizure medicine and joking with the nurse about introducing him to our cat. Now we were being told that the team had been doing CPR on him for thirty-four minutes. Someone in scrubs finally stepped out of the crowd to explain that something had gone wrong with his phenobarbital dosing and that he'd received more of the medication than indicated for his weight, which had caused his heart to stop suddenly. These kinds of medicines could suppress a baby's urge to breathe, she said, suggesting that this had been a risk of treatment we should have understood. We were speechless in our disbelief.

As the layers of doctors and nurses peeled away, we could finally see our son again. He was still alive, looking smaller than ever on the white bed that was now splattered with his blood and littered with used green surgical gloves. His chest was rising and falling with the whir of the ventilator. He was under a tangle of wires again. Daniel held his hand while I silently wondered if it was even possible to recover from what had just happened—for any of us.

They found us a call room and urged us to get some rest. So Daniel and I huddled on the narrow single bed and cried together through a sleepless night. As we stood awkwardly beside Ethan the next morning, again not allowed to hold him, his nurse asked casually if I'd seen him wiggle his legs recently. Well, no. I actually hadn't.

"What does that mean?" I worried aloud.

"I'm not sure," she said slowly, opening a new chasm of uncertainty.

That was the moment I realized that he hadn't been moving much since last night—and that we'd been so relieved he'd survived that we'd forgotten to notice how his behavior had changed. A neurologist came by to examine him and ordered another EEG. After tapping and prodding and repositioning his limbs, he told us that Ethan had essentially had a heart attack and that it had lasted so long that he had ended up with a stroke in the part of his brain that controls leg movement. He would be paralyzed from the waist down.

We were devastated and furious. We already loved Ethan so much, and we knew nothing could change that. We would strive to give him a life of happiness and fulfillment with or without the use of his legs. But the weight of what the future might hold for our family began to sink in as we grappled with the impact of their medical error. Daniel and I stayed by Ethan's crib, talking to him, trying hard not to admit that he had stopped looking back at us. His deep gray eyes held a distant gaze, like he had moved on to somewhere else.

The doctor approached Ethan's bed and said he wanted to talk to us in the family conference room. A feeling of doom settled heavily down on me. I knew that good news would have been delivered at the bedside. My mind was full of ominous, useless clouds as I walked numbly along the fluorescent corridor with Daniel at my side. We sat down on padded chairs in the spartan room with a doctor and a neonatal nurse practitioner.

"As you know, Ethan's been through a lot these past few days. And we've been running a lot of tests," said the doctor. "By far the most concerning results," he continued slowly, "are from the EEG."

I broke down in tears before he had finished the sentence. For a long time, no one spoke. I was irritated by their silence. The doctor shouldn't stop explaining what was happening just because I was crying. *Just tell us!* I wanted to shout as I tried to stifle my sobs. Finally, the doctor went on.

"Ethan is showing virtually no brain activity."

I asked if he was ever going to get it back, if he would walk or talk. The nurse said most likely not. And if we kept him on the breathing tube for a few more days, his lungs would probably become strong enough to breathe on their own, but he wouldn't ever be likely to do much more. She paused to let us take this in. Then the doctor spoke again.

"It might be too soon to say this," he ventured kindly, quietly, "but at this point some families would consider removing the breathing tube and letting nature take its course, whatever that may be."

A moment later, they stepped out of the room and left Daniel and me to cry some more. We talked about what Ethan would want and how much harder the decision would be to make later if he started to breathe on his own. We called our parents to tell them, but I couldn't get myself to say that Ethan was going to die, only that he wasn't going to live. Word spread among our families as they reached out to one another to spare us from repeating the news.

We told the doctors our decision. We were numb as we watched the machines get switched off and removed, one by one, again. The NICU nurses moved delicately around us, as if their attentive efficiency would call less attention to how suddenly the goals of their work had shifted. No one ever said they were sorry for what had happened. There was no apology, and no lament.

Our parents and Daniel's sister arrived and tried to join us. At first, I asked the nurses not to let them in. I wanted this to be a private moment. I thought back to gazing down at Ethan after delivery, when everyone else had stepped out of the room. Could I have captured his essence any more deeply then, if I had known it would be the only time I would ever have him all to myself?

My mom was very upset, demanding to see me and to meet her grandchild, and finally I agreed. We didn't pass Ethan around to let everyone hold him—the minutes were just too precious for Daniel or me to be willing to share any of them, except with each other—but they did all give him a kiss.

As his breathing became more labored, we asked for some time alone, and our families respectfully left. We held our son, close and warm in our arms, and told him we loved him, over and over, until he took his last breath, more than two hours after the ventilator was turned off. We set him on the cold white sheet one last time and filled out some paperwork I can barely remember. *Yes*, we said in monotone, to handprints and footprints. *Yes* to autopsy. *Yes* to cremation. I don't think Daniel and I talked much to fill the darkness on the drive home. The clock still glowed red on the dashboard, as the numbers rolled past midnight and into a new day.

The next morning I awoke dazed and uncomfortable as I realized I was in my own bed. It took me a moment to find the source of a deep new pain that had sprung up among my many forms of suffering. My breasts were rock-hard and my clothes were covered in milk. No one had warned me about this, and I hadn't thought to ask. I called the clinic and was put on hold. I didn't know exactly what my question was or how to preface it.

When the advice nurse finally got on the line, all I could manage was "How do I stop breastfeeding?" She hesitated, then said I could wrap everything up with an elastic bandage and not feed the baby or pump, because stimulation would make more milk come in.

Then she asked, "Is this something you just decided not to do anymore?" She sounded so young and naive to me.

"No," I managed in a quivering voice. "My son passed away yesterday." Then I started crying again. I could hear in her silence that she was stunned by my answer and couldn't think of anything else to say. So I hung up the phone, wrapped my chest tight, and tried to contain my body's instincts to feed a baby who would never come home.

Almost immediately, I found myself yearning desperately to be pregnant—and feeling desperately guilty about this. I didn't want another child. I wanted my son. I longed to turn back time, to return to that place where he'd moved around inside me with all the promise of childhood. More than anything I'd ever wished for, I wished to be pregnant again with Ethan so I could find a magical way to prevent his death. My heart was in such agony that I thought it might collapse with just one more thought of him.

A few days later, we were called to the hospital to pick up his remains. When we arrived, the clerk behind the reception desk asked us, with a look of pity, to have a seat. After what seemed like too long, a solemn-looking man stepped out from a doorway and handed us two boxes. The first, a disarmingly utilitarian white foam block, contained Ethan's ashes inside a clear plastic bag. The other was filled with things Ethan had used at the hospital. Small and wooden, this second box was intricately hand-painted, a soothing turquoise along the sides with delicate orange flowers on the lid. The grace of its embellishments and the gesture itself, in fact, were so striking that I was immediately angry. What right did the place that had caused Ethan's death have to turn his belongings into a neatly packaged thing of beauty and present them to us in this way? We went back to our car and sat staring down at both boxes through tears, with wounds that had just begun to heal torn open again.

At first, it was too painful even to think of looking inside that painted box. After about a week, while Daniel was sleeping one night, I decided to go open it alone. Inside I found Ethan's white hat, a green pacifier, a tan umbilical cord clip, and a tiny doll made out of a handkerchief with ghostlike tails hanging down from its little round head. The doll was the one I had slept with to transfer my scent, then had given to Ethan to snuggle with until he could be at my side again. Holding these objects, my son's only possessions, wrecked me. He had seen them. He had worn them. He had felt them. I could still smell his sweet baby smells on them. I pressed the doll against my chest and cried for a long, long time. This was the lowest low I had ever felt.

Sitting alone with that box on the floor of his empty room, in front of his empty crib, allowed me to let everything out without judgment or witness. It was the one thing I did by myself, with myself, for myself. I don't know if Daniel ever looked in the box. I don't know if he knows that I looked. Yet that moment, in its devastation, became a turning point for me. I had fallen into such a whirlwind of emotion that the surrender was a relief in some ways, giving me permission to begin to heal. Because I was so broken as my tears fell upon all that was left of Ethan, nothing since has ever seemed quite as bad in comparison. The pain was still very real, but the days started to become slightly more tolerable. I didn't feel better yet, but somehow I started to feel not as bad. The road before me was long and uncertain. But I had come so far.

For a long time, I wanted to stay deep within my own grief, where the pain was overpowering but somehow comfortable in its familiarity. Reading the stories of others who were sad let me wallow in sadness, absorb memories of loss, and fulfill my unspoken promise not to move on too quickly. I feared that letting pleasure back into my life would be some sort of betrayal. Dancing, one of my passions since childhood, had always made me feel vibrant and alive. So when my dance instructor encouraged me to come to the studio to dance with her, confiding that losing herself in movement had really helped her to heal emotionally after her miscarriage, I declined. The physical memories of dancing rose up: How radiant it had made me feel. How fluid my body had been. How I had felt Ethan's kicks and rolls as I gracefully stepped across the polished floor in those joyful days of pregnancy. I wasn't ready to go there. I didn't want to feel that good.

The night Ethan had died—after less than a week outside the safety of my body—and every day after that, Daniel and I had cried. Well-meaning friends had warned us that the death of a child could tear a couple apart, but Ethan, in life or in death, only deepened our partnership. Daniel and I worked through devastation, rage, and disbelief, and we did it all together as our world kept crashing down. We had the same conversations over and over, utterly unproductive yet somehow exactly what we both needed. We held each other as our hearts broke anew each morning, when we woke up from another night of restless sleep and remembered that our son was gone.

Finally, after about two months, Daniel declared that if we didn't start getting out of the house we were just going to get worse. I was still mentally and physically exhausted, weakened further by a month of heavy bleeding after Ethan's birth. But I knew he was right. If we didn't get outside, we would continue to spiral downward into a dark, empty space that felt like it would obliterate us. We started going on hikes in the wilderness to get away from our daily reality and figure out how we were going to live our lives from now on.

We found that keeping our bodies in motion kept our minds moving forward somehow too, and Daniel threw himself into the distractions of remodeling projects around the house. One day he single-handedly demolished the moldy cracked-tile bathroom we'd been talking about redoing for years. Friends showed up bearing the gifts of their time and skill to help rebuild it. As Daniel toiled side by side with one friend who was a plumber, then one who was an electrician, then one who knew tile work, they talked about tools and fixtures, not loss and suffering. But I knew that cooperating with others on something so straightforward and tangible was helping him to heal.

While I mostly alternated long hikes with long naps as Daniel worked on the bathroom, one trip to the hardware store together to select a toilet stands out in my memory. We were talking with the salesman, asking questions about different models, comparing features and prices to decide what would suit us best.

"Do you have kids?" he asked us.

We both froze. I didn't know how to answer as a million thoughts flooded my mind. With no word in my language for a mother who is left behind after her only child has died, every possible response felt untrue. I didn't want to say no, because Ethan was my child and he did exist. I couldn't say yes, because then a question would follow about how old he was, and I couldn't go down that road either. Then Daniel just said no, and I'm not sure the salesman even noticed the pause. But I was totally unnerved by his innocent question. I had never imagined that Ethan could come up in a toilet conversation, that I wouldn't be safe from the torrent of memories on such a practical, ordinary errand.

The first day that I didn't cry, I felt incredibly guilty. I thought that

I was somehow betraying my child's memory, that he would think I didn't miss him, that somehow I had stopped caring. Then a friend told me about her favorite aunt, a strong and stoic woman in her eighties, who had lost her first child too. Her son had been sick, and they had taken him away right after birth. He had died a few hours later in an incubator, before she even got to hold him. She had always wanted six children, and had become pregnant again right away and gone on to have the large family of her dreams. Still, as she had told my friend this story, she had sobbed, remembering who he was and who he might have become, transforming in an instant back into that young mother who had lost her baby nearly sixty years earlier. Her story helped me to realize that thinking about Ethan is always going to hurt. I'm never going to get over it. And I don't have to feel like I should.

Six months after we lost Ethan, I became pregnant again. It was not an accident, but it still felt like a surprise. We knew we would never get back that blissful innocence of the days when senselessly tragic stories were just abstract ideas that happened to people we didn't know. We were so grateful to have a second chance at creating a life together. The baby items in our house, which I had refused to clear out despite the gentle but persistent encouragement of family members, again became something I looked forward to using. Hearing the word *baby* triggered feelings of hope and optimism instead of pain and emptiness. My bitterness began to fade, and my desire to understand and to reach out to others deepened. When strangers asked me if this was going to be my first child, I would pause, unsure again of what to say. How many times had I asked people that I met in passing if they had any other kids? How many truths did I never witness, hidden beneath casual answers?

Now, on Ethan's birthday each year, we stay close to home and I write in my journal, reflecting on what we do have. We walk along winding trails and remember those long hikes that helped us heal, back when our despair was so raw. When we travel, we bring a small tin with some of Ethan's ashes and scatter them in a beautiful place so he can be part of the world with us. Holding his younger sister and brother in our arms, we watch pieces of him drift away. At home, we keep the rest of his ashes in an elegant yellow glass bottle and store the box of his belongings on his sister's bookcase.

We cherish the time that our family had with Ethan, and the presence that he still has in our lives. We miss him on ordinary days and feel his absence on special occasions. We think about him as we share his story with his siblings, passing on the legacy of all that he taught us about love. This is how we honor his memory, so far.

CHAPTER 7

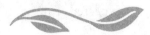

Zach had arrived nine months to the day after I'd been offered the residency position. He had been born in the hospital where I'd spent his entire gestation tending to children and families and bearing witness to the stories of other women. He was alive. He was beautiful. I knew exactly how fortunate we were, and I was beyond relieved to be on the other side of childbirth.

But even after we were safely home, with Zach's cardiac evaluation remarkably unremarkable and NICU stay blessedly uneventful, I couldn't shake the feeling that I'd failed. I'd failed my son, and I'd failed myself. Needing a cesarean to bring him into the world—and in distress, at that—I felt defeated.

Before Zach was born, I'd almost convinced myself that my body was strong enough, capable enough, to get through one pregnancy and birth without elaborate interventions. I had wanted to do it all under my own power. Now I felt a complicated and self-conscious gratitude for the lifesaving care we had both received. Without modern medicine, my son and I might not have survived this pregnancy either.

The protective layers I'd wrapped around my own story were much more fragile than I'd realized, the wounds from my losses fresher. Yet I would never have judged other women as harshly as I judged myself.

When my friends had babies, I admired their strength and determination. I was happy for them no matter how they'd given birth. Unwaveringly supportive of my patients, I empathized with the complex decisions they faced when delivery wasn't going as expected. I never felt critical when they asked for help.

The contrast confused me. If I had committed to becoming a family medicine doctor to help others, why should I feel inadequate when I was the one in need? Why did I see myself as weak when I was vulnerable? Why couldn't I grant myself the same compassion, the same respect, that I tried to offer everybody else?

By the time I returned to work, ten and a half weeks after Zach's birth, I hadn't resolved any of these questions. Juggling a difficult start to breastfeeding, an exhausting recovery from labor and delivery, several bouts of plugged ducts and mastitis, and the frequent wakings of a hungry newborn left little time for reflection. To add to the challenge, I would be starting back with three of the hardest rotations in residency, spending a month each on the adult medicine hospital wards, in the intensive care unit, and on the obstetrics and gynecology service.

I wasn't ready. But I packed up my pumping supplies and my snacks and some baby pictures, and I put on my scrubs.

During my first weekend call shift back on the medicine wards, I met Kelly in the emergency department. As our team's supervising physician briefed me on what he knew of her history, many details resonated with me immediately: She was a young mother with a worried partner. She had recently developed a series of poorly understood medical problems. Many of the doctors who'd evaluated her before that night had dismissed her concerns.

Now Kelly and I sat together as the bustle of illness and injury carried on outside our narrow doorway. Atop the angled gurney in this brightly lit space, she labored to breathe as she repositioned her too-thin blanket. She had spent the past twelve hours here, just down the hall from where I'd waited all day for a methotrexate injection two years earlier and a lifetime ago. I brought my black rolling stool closer to her and adjusted my clipboard.

And I listened. I listened to her fears about what had happened and what might happen. I took in her worries for her partner and her children. I felt her desperation for answers to questions she didn't know how to ask, and I hoped that I could help her find those answers.

As Kelly told me her story—and as we spent hours together over the weeks and months and years that followed—I understood that this person, these questions, and these hopes represented exactly why I had chosen to do this second residency. I felt the same way when I met Victoria, on the day that her daughter was born, and Marissa, as she first considered starting a family. These three women were just a few of so many I would care for in training and beyond—so many amazing, struggling, resilient women—who showed me that pregnancy and delivery, monumental as they may be, are just the smallest of moments in a lifetime of motherhood.

Kelly ~ Breathe

When we first set out to have children nearly twenty years ago, I had unwavering confidence in my body. I got pregnant on our first try and had a healthy, uncomplicated pregnancy. The birth of our son, Avery, reflected the person he would become, starting with a peaceful but powerful labor that rose up over the summer heat. Scribbled notes were posted on the walls around me: *Use your voice. Trust yourself. It will never be too much. Breathe.*

But I have very few visual memories of that evening. I was deep within myself with eyes closed, my connection to others maintained only through the sounds of their voices. Words of encouragement drifted through my home from the beloved women who surrounded me to witness this event: my mother, my aunt, my midwife, and my partner, Dolores. Water splashed the sides of the birthing tub as I shifted the weight that would soon emerge as our child. My aunt inhaled and exhaled calmly in a corner of the room, her breathing purposeful and rhythmic for me to follow.

We had not named him, had not even discovered if he would be a boy or a girl before his birth. I took in how lovely it all was, holding this unknown creature in his first hours, sitting with Dolores in the stillness of the night, staring in awe at this new being who hadn't been here before.

Life with a child suited me immediately, and our family felt complete as we fell into the joyful chaos of those early years of parenthood. But when Avery turned three, I realized he wasn't a baby anymore—and I began to want another. Dolores and I had never talked about a second child. I truly didn't know what she'd think. Then one day, when we were sitting in a restaurant, Avery asked us, "If my sister was here, where would she sit?" Taken aback, I replied, "Where do you think she'd want to sit?" Every so often, he would look at something and say, "I think my sister would like this." Then he would smile as if he knew something we didn't. Little by little, a conversation about growing our family began.

With our daughter, Evan, everything about pregnancy and birth was different. We went through eight inseminations over a year and a half. I threw up every day until she was born while I tried to muster enough energy to chase four-year-old Avery. Each time we went for an ultrasound, she was spinning so much that no one could capture a clear image of her, and each night my restless sleep was filled with dreams of a baby who seemed just as elusive to me.

On the eve of my due date, Dolores and Avery and I were relaxing over a cozy winter dinner at a friend's house when my water suddenly broke, spilling across the kitchen floor. We piled into the car, and I sat on a stack of towels and newspapers as the contractions mounted with an intensity I couldn't believe. I remember thinking how funny it was that we were driving past two hospitals in rush hour traffic in pursuit of a home birth. But with every contraction, I thought of home and yelled, "Tub!"

Our midwives met us at the house, urgently setting up the birthing area. This time, there was no gradual labor, no time for me to go deep within myself to a tranquil, assured place. Two hours and thirty-three minutes after I'd taken my last bite of dinner, and with the tub barely a third full, our daughter came screaming into the world. Her intense, rapid delivery left me tremoring in such shock that hours passed before I was able to really look at her.

But soon our expanded family fell into easy new rhythms—until Dolores was diagnosed with breast cancer when Evan was four months old. I remember trying to digest the news while going to the store to buy a knobby red pacifier and a snuggly duckie blanket, very intentionally grasping at material objects that I hoped would help us get through this time. With Avery, I had been so opposed to these props, too quick in my judgment, I now realized, before I had understood why a child—or a parent—might need them. But I knew I would not always be available to offer my own breast when Evan wanted soothing. I remember the grieving thought, *This child is going to need a comfort, and it is not always going to be me and my body because I'm going to be taking care of Dolores.*

As we moved into the mysterious and frightening world of cancer treatment, we noticed that forty-one-year-old Dolores was often the youngest patient in the chemotherapy infusion room, and usually in the oncology waiting room as well. There would be a nod, a sigh, a quiet acknowledgment of this when we entered. During her first infusion, I thought I was imagining it. But at the second visit, I felt it again, then overheard someone whisper, "She's so young." I wondered just how old you have to be before a cancer diagnosis is not difficult, unexpected, traumatic.

But something else happened—with the staff as well as Dolores's fellow patients—on the days we brought Evan with us. I couldn't quite put my finger on the swirl of emotions that surfaced when we walked in as a family. Maybe it was the unbridled joy of a smiling, drooling baby in stark contrast to the plight of her young mother. Or maybe it was the symbol of the silky purple batik scarf over Dolores's bald head, telling part of her story in a single glance. Or maybe it was simply the presence of this young child, this embodiment of growth and renewal, that lent the fight a new dimension for everyone. Somewhere in the transformation, I felt a huge Hail Mary of hope being lobbed our way, and I wanted to share it with every single person in that room.

While we held our breath, the world moved forward, and our children grew. We chased Avery through the house in his superhero pajamas. Evan giggled and rolled on the floor, blowing big wet raspberries until her shirt was soaked. The intensity of childhood kept us grounded, even as all our ordinary milestones became somehow tied to threats to our family, a balance of celebration and trepidation. Dolores had taken herself in for that fateful mammogram on Avery's fifth birthday, just six months earlier, right after noticing the lump. Then, as Evan wobbled her first steps, Dolores finished chemo. Evan turned one, but the cupcakes also celebrated that Dolores had completed her radiation treatments the day before. *If we weren't all so tired*, I thought, *we'd really live it up!* But, for the moment, we were just thrilled to have some cake, wear silly hats, and bask in the relief of having made it this far.

Cancer consumed our days in a big way. But it also reflected back how rich and wonderful our life together was. Evan's sweet smile became a little more fabulous. Avery's quirky observations seemed slightly more brilliant. The never-ending kindness of our friends and family filled me with even more gratitude. And the exquisite boredom that prompted Dolores's wonderings about how string cheese is made and her ideas for potential projects with dryer lint made me happy in a way I didn't think possible. I loved letting these everyday pleasures hold my attention.

Our lives went on like this, in waves of commotion and constancy, for another two years. In some ways, parenthood had uniquely prepared us for the unpredictability of illness. We were in a fog of exhaustion, much like early days with an infant, getting through the moments but barely able to focus enough to see them as any coherent picture. Just when I got used to some sort of order, our family's needs would shift and we'd have to figure things out all over again. Still, as intravenous chemotherapy and daily radiation transitioned into simplified oral medication regimens and then the brief, infrequent checkups of remission, I never suspected that all the hours I spent beside Dolores would be just the beginning of our hospital days.

The following April, our family got a mild cold. Usually I was the first one in the house to recover from any illness, but this one lingered in me for weeks, along with a nagging fatigue. As Evan and I worked in the yard to build a garden bed one morning, springtime flowers pushing up all around us, I kept dropping things as I transported stones from the wheelbarrow or picked up a trowel to turn the soil. My hands had suddenly lost the strength I'd relied on for years as a trained massage therapist. Persistent coughing fits triggered a migraine-like headache and left me struggling to breathe.

My doctor, who had seen me through two pregnancies and all manner of ordinary illnesses, thought the recent virus and spring pollens had reactivated my latent asthma. She reassured me, encouraged me to take more time for myself, and prescribed an inhaler. Her advice resonated. For a long time now, I had been working very hard to put myself on the list—to carve out time to attend to my own needs while emerging from the haze of supporting my partner through a life-threatening illness and managing the ever-changing demands of two young children. But the exhaustion was making it difficult to take care of anyone, emotionally or physically.

One afternoon, I drove Evan to a nearby park. As soon as I unbuckled her car seat, she scurried away, and my panic swelled as I lost view of my toddler over a small hill. My pounding heart amplified the rustle of bark chips beneath my feet. My breathing got heavier as I tried to keep up. I couldn't. By the time I'd covered the fifty or so steps to the playground, Evan was happily going down the twirly slide. I felt an overwhelming urge to lie down right there, driven by a weariness heavier than any I'd ever imagined possible. The only thing that kept me upright was the fear that I wouldn't be able to get back up.

A sudden storm hit during the first week of June, and the kids huddled on the porch with our neighbor, eating pizza and watching the great oaks sway. While they distracted themselves with rain boots and puddles on that cool, windy night, Dolores and I sat in the emergency room as I struggled to move air at all. I felt like something was taking over my body. My lungs ached and my heart raced from misguided efforts to use my inhaler again and again as my breathing grew increasingly strained. But after a handful of blood tests and nasal swabs that ruled out infection, hours of reassuring oxygen levels, and a bafflingly normal chest X-ray, the attending physician told us that I was probably having panic attacks. That I should make another appointment with my doctor. That I should cut back on stress and make time for myself. Now that I was two months into this illness, his advice just rang hollow.

The rest of June was a blur of end-of-school festivities and planning for Avery's eighth birthday. I had a constant headache from the relentless coughing. I could sleep only sitting up. My follow-up tests had all been inconclusive. When friends came by to visit, I would send the kids out with them, shut the blinds, and try desperately to get a little rest. Realizing that solving the mystery I had become was going to require additional expertise, my doctor called in a consult to our local teaching hospital.

The specialist I saw there sent me for a series of breathing tests and informed me that my pulmonary function was down to forty-seven percent of normal. *Forty-seven percent.* When I heard that number, I had the strangest reaction. Happiness, almost. I was so relieved that something had finally confirmed what I had been feeling for so long that, at first, it didn't occur to me to be afraid. The pulmonary clinic scheduled me for their next available new-patient intake appointment—in three months.

A few days later, at Avery's birthday party, I managed to rally for a little while, hiding behind those garden beds that Evan and I had built in our backyard, laughing as I took aim with my orange-and-yellow plastic squirter and drenched Avery and his friends. Then, soaked by their jubilant retaliation, I retreated into the dark house, leaned back, and slumped down against the wall, too exhausted even to stand. How was I going to survive until September with no further evaluation or treatment of whatever was happening?

The next week, after walking two blocks to watch Fourth of July fireworks at a friend's place, I couldn't sleep and I couldn't breathe. I started to feel feverish. It was ten o'clock at night. I needed to go to the ER, but I was afraid they'd just send me home like the month before. Still, desperate for answers and for any reprieve, I gathered up my binder of every test I'd undergone and every note I'd taken since this had started. Dolores arranged for my dad to come to the house to be with the kids and field their questions if they woke up before we were back in the morning.

When we walked into the waiting room, I must have looked as sick as I felt because they whisked me to the back immediately. My blood oxygen levels, which should have measured close to one hundred percent, were drifting down into the high seventies when I was seated. Each time I moved, even with an oxygen mask on, they dropped lower still. The doctor ordered a high-resolution scan, which finally revealed what X-rays alone had missed. When I saw my lungs on the screen, two-thirds whited out by some unknown shadowy substance, I had the same reaction I'd had to hearing my abysmal pulmonary function test results: Validation. Relief. Hope. Now that we could see the problem, we could begin to figure it out. We waited in the ER for fifteen hours for an inpatient bed to become available.

Once I was settled into my cramped shared room on the wards, a parade of specialist teams consulted on my case one by one. Nobody seemed to have any idea what was wrong with me. I underwent still more blood tests and more lung-function measurements and more imaging studies. The doctors were reluctant to try a course of steroids to decrease the inflammation my scan had revealed, rightly fearing that if the cause were infectious, steroids would allow it to flourish. They were hesitant to offer antibiotics, which might cause unnecessary side effects and promote resistant bugs, since no clear infection had been identified and one of my blood tests had hinted at a possible immune system disorder. There was talk of a lung biopsy because, being unable to agree on appropriate treatment, the doctors were giving me nothing but oxygen and my lungs were getting worse and worse. One team of specialists felt they needed the information to move forward in helping me. Another team was convinced I wouldn't survive the procedure, or at the very least would end up in intensive care on a ventilator for weeks afterward, vulnerable to all sorts of other complications.

Dolores and I diligently wrote down everything that happened, keeping my medical binder close at hand. I asked her to bring in pictures of the kids and of all of us together, and I slid them into the clear sleeve on its front cover. Looking at snapshots of my children's mischievous smiles and bright eyes drove my determination. When the doctors hovered over my bed during rounds, I would intentionally leave the binder with its photo side facing up, prominent on the rolling tray beside me. I wanted the people taking care of me to understand that I was a mother with a family I needed to get back to.

As the days wore on, I struggled to breathe sitting still. I struggled to walk along the flat hospital corridors, even with a tube pumping pure oxygen up my nose. I struggled to integrate this sudden shift in my physical capabilities into my identity as a can-do person whose primary coping strategy tended toward barreling through obstacles while calling out silver linings. I wasn't ready to let myself think about how this illness was going to affect my experience of motherhood, my work as a massage therapist, or my ability to be as active as I liked to be.

My blood had been sent to research and academic labs all over the country to be tested for obscure diseases and complex syndromes. As I lay tangled in the stiff white sheets, waiting for results and listening to monitors beeping through the night, I longed for home in a deep and visceral way, with a need as raw as the one I'd felt for the comfort of those familiar surroundings as Evan's birth had approached. In labor, though, I'd willingly sped by hospitals to get home. Now I would have to learn to reconcile my wariness of modern medicine with my surrender to a system that was my only hope for answers and for healing.

After twelve days, we finally had a name to give this intrusion: anti-synthetase syndrome, a rare autoimmune disorder that had tricked my body's defense system into attacking its own tissues, with a particular affinity for the oxygen-transferring membranes in my lungs and the small muscles of my hands and feet. When my hospital team called the busy pulmonary clinic to schedule a follow-up, they were advised to keep my September appointment. By now, my laments about whether I could make it two more months until that appointment were not a matter of simple exasperation. Some of my doctors didn't think I'd be alive in the fall. As they stood outside my door on morning rounds, I heard them whisper about lung transplants and desperate measures. They discharged me from the hospital on the paradoxical cocktail of medications that had caused such ardent dissent among them when I was first admitted—high-dose steroids to suppress my immune system, antibiotics to fight off opportunistic infections that could easily kill me because of my suppressed immune system, and a jumble of other less memorable pills to counter the side effects of each—along with a seventeen-pound oxygen tank that drained rapidly on our way home. While we had finally settled on a way to treat my symptoms, I wasn't convinced we were addressing the underlying disease.

When we drove into our neighborhood and pulled up along the curb, Evan came running out of the house to greet us dressed only in sandals and sparkly blue underpants. She offered her tiny hand to help me out of the car. Dolores and my mother supported my slow walk up the five porch steps, then switched my tubing over from the portable oxygen cylinder to the newly delivered oxygen concentrator churning loudly in our living room. Even with constant supplementary oxygen, my lungs felt pushed to their very limits. Within minutes of my arrival, Avery had managed to fall out of our claw-foot bathtub, smacking his knee and elbow loudly on the hard tile floor, while Evan had wailed herself into a tantrum about Dolores making the trip to the pharmacy to pick up and review the complicated instructions for my half dozen new prescriptions without her. There is nothing like the immediacy of children to remind you that you're finally home.

Within a few doses, the side effects of the steroids stripped away any ability to filter or regulate my emotions, and riding these extremes made me all the more determined to participate in our family's beautiful ordinary moments. One evening, I became suddenly compelled to inspect my garden. My mother obligingly relocated my oxygen concentrator to the back porch, then guided me outside while she rerouted fifty feet of tubing. She watered all my plants while I inquired about their blossoms, fruit growth, and needs for pinching back or trimming. Dolores found my clippers. Avery lugged my chair toward the plant I wanted to prune. When I spotted some perfect green beans, heavy on their climbing vines, Evan charged inside to grab a basket. Since my hands had the strength to reach up for only a few minutes at a time, my mom pulled the stalks closer while she continued to water beside me. An hour later, as Dolores washed the beans and put them away, I was feeling flattened by the effort, but productive—thanks to my extensive crew of helpers to achieve what I used to consider the simplest task. Adjusting my expectations was going to be a long and arduous process. Dolores wasn't sure if my goals were reassuringly optimistic or discouragingly unrealistic.

If my family didn't know what to make of me, my doctors seemed equally perplexed. My lung function dipped to thirty-three percent of normal. The pulmonary clinic managed to bump up my appointment to August, but they were just watching and waiting, bewildered, and made no adjustments to my medications. I felt like my disease was being undermanaged. The specialists' fascination with a condition they'd never seen didn't translate into much action.

In truth, I have always credited my primary care doctors for my real care, and even my survival. As the months miraculously crept by and my health somehow stabilized, they helped me fine-tune medication and exercise regimens that kept my lung function reasonably steady and my energy level better than anyone would have predicted when I'd been first diagnosed. They connected me to the right people at the right time and advocated for the evaluations and consults I needed. They appreciated that I was a mother long before I was a patient—and appreciated why that distinction mattered. They knew that the side effects of whatever plan they proposed had to be more tolerable than the disease itself. They understood that their treatment needed to leave me functional enough to be a parent.

As much as my doctors did for me, I understood from the beginning that my outcomes would be very much tied to my own efforts as well. I spent hours wading through dense medical journals, hours attending clinic appointments and pulmonary rehabilitation programs, and hours trying to figure out how I was going to get to all these appointments and get my kids back and forth to school. I couldn't drive. I certainly couldn't walk. Dolores was working on construction sites as an industrial electrician with zero job flexibility, zero vacation days, and zero sick time. If she didn't work, she didn't get paid. Her job provided our sole income and the health benefits for our whole family. I needed to ask for help, and lots of it.

I had long been an active cultivator of friendships, but my physical limitations—and my fear that I might not be around as my children grew up—now made me acutely conscious of the need to invite other people in. I grappled with the paradox of wanting to live a full life with my family in the present and plan for our future together while simultaneously weaving a net to catch them in case I couldn't be there. Reaching out to trusted friends, I asked them to take on specific roles during milestones my kids might experience without me: first crushes, school performances, driver's licenses, graduations. I reframed my beliefs, adopting the mantra that strong people ask for help and that that's how we stay strong.

Many of my relationships grew deeper as I initiated these frank conversations. But my illness didn't magically make every friendship better or more honest. As the months of the initial crisis were replaced by years of redefining priorities, some people quietly fell away when I stopped actively seeking out opportunities to connect. Some were scared of what they didn't understand. Some were wary of letting their children get close to my children because of their feelings about illness and ability, and some worried about burdening us with their own problems.

I did not want this disease to be the center of our universe. I frequently found myself reminding friends that it was more than okay to tell us what was going on in their lives. I wanted to explain that, while we were immensely grateful for their unconditional support, we felt left out when they withheld the very real details of their own struggles. I wanted to reassure them that what made our friendships so vital, vibrant, and comforting was the way we carried each other's pains and celebrated each other's joys. I wanted to beg them to share, because their sharing made us feel more normal.

Adapting to my limitations changed our family dynamics even more than it changed my friendships. Before I got sick, I was the one who arranged our days. I was the stay-at-home parent while Dolores worked long hours in a male-dominated profession that expected its employees to be available at all times while their spouses took care of their children. When I suddenly transitioned from being captain of our ship to being grateful to still be one of the passengers, Dolores was forced to manage the details in ways she had never wanted to and in ways I wouldn't have been willing to concede to her in the past.

At first it was painful for me not to be in charge of everything. Dolores was overwhelmed. The kids became unhinged when she tried to step in as I sat right there beside them, looking fully available to their young eyes but being physically unable to tend to their needs. Every once in a while, Dolores would say she wished things would go back to the way they used to be. But I didn't. Of course I wanted to be well. But I was beginning to appreciate sharing the journey in a way we never had before in our twenty-plus years together, for the balance it created in big and little decisions alike. I felt so fortunate that all the challenges we were facing had only brought us closer together.

One night, as Avery and I talked about some of the ways my illness had changed our lives, he confessed that he had thought I was going to die when I was in the hospital. I reassured him that I hadn't thought that. I'd been sure I would come home to my family. "But if you thought you *were* going to die," he asked slowly, "would you tell me?" I promised my pensive third grader that indeed I would, so we could talk about it. So we could say things to each other. Because he had a right to know. And I told him we don't always have that chance, but if we do, it's a gift.

Parenthood has taught me a lot about how little in this life I control. But that's the one thing my children crave—some control. They want to believe that everything is going to be okay. So how do we tell our children that everything might not be okay? Is it enough to teach them that bad things will happen and that they are resilient? To tell them that they are strong enough to experience great sadness and still feel great joy? To hope that they will learn to manage their fears—or at least that their fears will not paralyze them entirely?

Both Avery and Evan are old enough now to worry that I'm not always telling them everything. They know my health is still very precarious. With Dolores, they were younger and the treatment felt clear: *They're going to cut out that lump, Mama's going to get better, and life will go back to normal.* My illness has never held that certainty. Occasionally, when I've been feeling brave, I've reflected on the differences between my experiences and Dolores's. Because cancer evokes so many associations and images, people understood the gravity of her diagnosis implicitly. Everyone accepts that when a person is told she has cancer, her world stops. Everyone tries to be patient with her and her family as they absorb a terrible new reality.

Almost no one has any context for an atypical presentation of a rare autoimmune disease. They don't realize that I will forever need debilitating chemotherapy to keep my overreactive immune system from killing me or that the immune suppression that was an un-wanted side effect for Dolores is a benefit for me. They don't know the quiet despair I feel as I watch the clear toxic potion drip into my veins like a ghost, like tainted magic, its creeping fatigue a trade for more life. They don't understand how much I worry that people think I'm just lazy or withdrawn or exaggerating my symptoms when I can't commit to plans until I wake up and see how well I'm functioning each day. They haven't felt the anguish I felt when I first read the only comprehensive article I could find about my disease and discovered that it has a sixty percent mortality rate within ten years—or how that grim statistic was overshadowed by the relief of finally, mercifully, having a name to put to my symptoms.

This summer, unbelievably, marks my tenth anniversary of living with this illness. Although I've learned to breathe on the equivalent of half of one lung, losing strength and dexterity in my hands still feels cruel. When my niece had her first baby, I couldn't hold him safely for more than a few minutes. I am no longer the massage therapist offering a healing touch, the skilled soccer goalie defending the net with arms outstretched, the person in our house who can open any jar. That's the version of myself that I miss the most and that I wish my children knew.

I never want to tell my children that my hands are too tired to make their breakfast, to tie their shoes, or to hug them close when they're crying. I never want them to hear me say I can't—because I don't want to believe it myself. But also because I don't want them to give up on me. So when I'm utterly exhausted, when I know the task ahead is not something this body is going to do easily, I work hard to keep those words out of my language. Instead, I'll enlist their help: "If we want to do this," I'll say, "we're going to have to work as a team. Let's figure it out." *I can't* is heartbreaking for all of us. There's a panic of fear and deprivation that comes with realizing your mother can't take care of you.

If I have any grief about my illness, it's for the loss of security and innocence for my family. I remember one day early in my recovery, when I decided to wash my hair but didn't have the strength to reach up to my head. Dolores was at work and my mom was busy helping Evan. That left then-eight-year-old Avery the most qualified person available for the job. We talked through a plan. He held the curtain in place so we wouldn't spray the wall, then he helped me soap up my hair. When the water ran down my face and into my oxygen tubing, he grabbed a dry towel and sweetly blotted my cheek. I was grateful that he couldn't distinguish my tears from the wash water—or that if he could, he didn't let on. Gentle and patient caregiver that he was, never did I expect to switch roles with my son at such a young age. I hope that, as they grow, each and every way that my children have been forced to be self-sufficient and compassionate beyond their years will turn into a gift rather than a wound.

Motherhood does feel like my life's best work, and the motivation to be present for my family, to witness their lives, has kept me alive many times over. But in many tangible ways, I'm not the mother I planned to be, in this tender space where we are living. I thought I'd be kayaking, hiking, and adventuring with my children rather than inviting someone else to lead them on expeditions I devised. But being on the sidelines has forced me to shift my focus from a place of doing to a place of being. And to inhabit a place of being is a privilege in itself. To parent in this way is to watch my children unfold, to shelter their voices, to release my expectations as they become who they are, beyond who I wish they would be.

Serendipity has always been one of my favorite words, conjuring a little bit of planning and a whole lot of fate. I hope I've put the right pieces into place, and then however things come together, I've got to let them be. I strive to make myself obsolete while fighting as hard as I can to be here. Uncomfortably aware of my mortality, I wrestle with a self-imposed pressure to get it right—for how I parent and for how Dolores does too—so that if I'm not here, they'll all be okay. That's a heavier weight to carry than the oxygen tank that sustains my breath.

I've spent so many hours over the years just waiting. Waiting to be better. Waiting to grow stronger. Waiting to heal, and falter, and heal again. I've spent so many hours in the recliner in the living room of the same house where my powerful body twice birthed my children into quaking water, and I've watched my family go about their lives all around me. The fatigue has long arms.

Some days, it would be really easy to make a list of all the ways that life has not gone along with everything I expected of it—and even easier to make a list of all the things that don't work or that hurt in this version of my body. Instead, I try to remain in a place where I can remember how capable I was, and how capable I still can be. I lie in bed, breathing deeply to stretch my scarred lungs, sending grace to my sore muscles, acknowledging how much my body has endured, and marveling at its strength to see me through.

My children always seem to ask the big questions while we're driving: *What's the difference between Democrats and Republicans? Where do babies come from? Is Heaven real?* Dolores half jokes that this is why she avoids running errands with them. Once, a few years ago, Evan and I were coming home from a soccer game when her voice broke a dreamy silence from the back seat.

"Mommy, what will happen to me if you die?"

I reflexively took a sharp breath and thought, *I'm not going to lie to my daughter. I'm not going to tell her that everything will be okay.* The duckie blanket I'd given her as an infant when Dolores was sick, when she needed a comfort in my absence, flashed through my mind.

As I stared straight ahead at the road through silent tears, I steadied my voice and answered calmly, "Well, it will be hard. And you will be sad. Things won't feel right for a long time." I told her she would be surrounded by people who would also be feeling these things and who all love each other very much. "You and Mama and Avery will figure it out," I promised. "You will miss me, but you will have each other."

Then I remembered the advice I'd given myself in labor: *Use your voice. Trust yourself. It will never be too much. Breathe.* I said, "It will get better. You know, it will be different, but after a while you won't be as sad." I told her that when I've lost people I love, I always miss them, but the way I keep them alive and keep feeling their spirit is by telling their stories. So I said to her: "I hope that you know enough of my story and that you keep telling the stories of our times together. I hope that whenever you tell our stories, it gives you more joy than sadness."

Then she asked me if she could have a Popsicle when we got home. And I just smiled. And breathed.

Victoria ~ Body Of

As I stand on the edge of the river and look down, I can almost feel the water hitting my flesh before I jump. I imagine its chill invading my every crevice, mapping out the ravines of my thighs, tracing the topography of my breasts, darting into my navel to seize my core. I gauge how deep it is, how cold it is, how long it would take me to swim from center to shore. I consider what I would do if I were swept away, battered by errant boulders, trapped beneath a deadfall log. I observe the current and look for eddies. I decide how to hold my head and where to point my feet. And then I leap.

My face resurfaces from the frigid water as my body emits a primal wail, a backward gasp that echoes through the canyon. It is late November in central Oregon, and the riverbank is edged with frost. But the cold reaches much deeper into me. It separates me from myself.

Floating on my back under the graying sky, I let my gaze consider one world while the rest of me is concealed in another. The water laces icy fingers through my hair. I slide my hands up my legs to find goose bumps. I stroke my soft belly. The bitterness of the cold heightens my senses and calms my nerves, bringing awareness back into my body as I absorb a chill so deep it reads like heat against my stinging skin. When I finally swim to the shore and crawl out along its slimy rocks, I am overwhelmed with the familiar, unbearable weight of being wet on dry land. I know this feeling well. I dread it. Yet it has never stopped my return to the water.

I know how to push away fear.

There are people who stare at the river and never leave the shore. There are those of us who jump in repeatedly, taking risks some call reckless, choosing to be consumed. Though jumping makes me look bold, I've been afraid for as long as I can remember. River or no river, I see danger everywhere I go.

When I was a child, I thought I knew exactly what it was that scared me. I was afraid of the things grown-ups told me to be afraid of, like being kidnapped from the park, running with scissors, and getting caught in a lie. I was also afraid of the things grown-ups told me not to be afraid of, like being abducted from my bed at night, eating poisoned candy, and getting sucked into the drain at the bottom of the pool.

Nighttime was the worst. Raised on a ridge between the Ozarks and the Great Plains, hemmed in on one side by forest as far as the eye could see and on the other by fields rolling out toward the Missouri River, I learned early that it was up to me to solve my own problems. I cowered in my room, forbidden to disturb my parents or my siblings as they slept. Brewing thunderclouds hovered outside the windows of our plantation-style home through the humid, buggy summers. Intricate patterns on my wallpaper morphed into haunting faces that glared down, while my curtains, animated by the vents of the air conditioner, performed an eerie dance. When I closed my eyes, my anxiety took shape under the bed as a malevolent troll that would devour me if I touched the wall exactly three times. I gathered my tangled hair on the pillow and curled my toes along the fluffy feather bed, resolving not to let my feet stray. An accidental kick and my breath caught as my eyes snapped open.

One. I was still safe, but I needed to be more careful. I needed to stay awake. Inevitably, I would begin to doze off and be thrust into peril as my leg carelessly stretched out.

TWO! I knew the rules. I had made them. I tapped two more times in quick succession to reset my count.

THREE-one. I could never get back to zero, but the hypervigilance demanded by the first touch was better than the abject terror of the second. I could trick myself into finding comfort where there was none. If the horror were realized, it would be my own fault.

As a girl, I was convinced that so many things were my fault. It was my fault that I wasn't blonde enough. Since the summer I was six, my mother had been lightening my hair with peroxide. It was my fault that I wasn't thin enough. By eight, I knew I should restrict calories to avoid becoming overweight, even though I wasn't heavy at all. It was my fault that I wasn't smart enough. Throughout my childhood, I was told that my mind wasn't made for math and science but that I had a gift for art, like all the women in our family who had come before me.

The same observant and intuitive nature that drove my artistic talents assured me an identity within my family. My worth came from attuning myself to other people's emotions, then absorbing them, deflecting them, or reflecting them back. More than anything, I wanted to please my mother. I shut down my crying when she told me I was too sensitive. I turned on the praise when she looked to me for the reassurance and nurturing she had never found in her relationship with her own mother, who was distant and unstable. I grimaced through hugs, willing my body to relax while worrying that, if I did it wrong, I might make her sadder still. The contradiction of finding pride in feeling chosen and discomfort in feeling smothered confused me. So I sorted my world into things I could change and things I couldn't change. Then I tried to change them all.

I felt constantly compelled to control my appearance, falling into a pattern of self-loathing that my mother and her mother and her mother before her had modeled over years. I learned to believe I was imperfect. Ugly. Unworthy. Flawed. Distorted by my family's judgment, my mind shamed me into becoming who others wanted me to be, and I was eager to comply.

As a teenager, I kept dyeing my hair. I set out outfits every night, smoothing them across my bed, studying each piece carefully to anticipate anything my peers might criticize. I started skipping lunch, then eating only every other day, then making myself vomit after my boyfriend suggested it. My only peace came from art, from sculpting clay, from coaxing beauty out of mud with the flow of water and the pressure of hands. I learned to control my body in the same way. I could make it lose weight. I could make it stop crying. I could make it relax even when sex was too rough or too scary. I understood implicitly that my body's pleasures were for someone else. My body's faults were mine.

As I grew into adulthood, moving away for college and art school and marrying a wonderful man who loved my body and my mind, I carried these beliefs with me. At twenty-nine, pregnant with my own daughter, I submitted my body to her needs. I immersed myself in prenatal yoga. I tried to limit my diet to healthy whole foods. Finding myself sitting in front of a half-eaten bacon cheeseburger, I suddenly panicked that I might be causing my baby harm. I ran to the bathroom to purge, convinced I was doing it only for her, and felt a momentary relief from the anxiety.

At my next checkup, I asked my doctor if I could just gain no weight in pregnancy. In the pitiful pause before she gently told me,

"No, that wouldn't be good for the baby," I had already decided to flip the switch from restriction to abandon. As I leapt into the unknown of allowing myself to gain, I decided that getting fat was better than starving my child.

Nothing in me understood how to navigate between extremes.

Leading up to my daughter's birth, I managed my anxiety with this same sense of surrender. My plan was to have no plan, to maintain control by asserting that I had no expectations, by making every decision in the moment based on what experts said was best for the baby. I willed my body to relax for each doctor's invasive touch. I relinquished my fear to the unchoreographed dance of labor. I tried to focus on my husband's steadying hand in mine, the friends and family in birthday hats joyfully surrounding us, and the cake they'd prepared with a festive *0* candle on top. I welcomed Sarasvati Se into my arms as she wailed out her first breath.

As soon as Se was born, I started having moments of feeling intensely detached from her. At night, while she slept beside me in the shadows of the bedroom, I plunged into a fog of disorientation that muffled light and sound and left only disbelief. Everything felt wrong. I didn't belong here. When I stared down at her ten tapered fingers, too long for any mortal baby, I knew she couldn't possibly be of this world. When she opened her giant alien eyes, black as the darkest depths of the river, they hardly seemed to fit into her tiny face. I could see that she was wondrous. I could see that she was vulnerable. But even when her needs compelled me to hold her close, I felt a strain in our connection. I forced myself to act loving and prayed that it would be enough.

As soon as Se was born, I started having visions of her death, graphic, gory, and quite exaggerated—and always caused by me. In these waking dreams, I hold my newborn close to my chest as we walk along our city sidewalk. The sun is shining, and I'm wearing an elegant silk sundress printed with gold and black diamonds. I trip. With my arms around the baby, I can't break our fall. Against the slippery fabric of my dress, I can't hold her tight enough. As we crash forward, her head hits the ground, exploding under my weight like a watermelon thrown against the pavement.

As soon as Se was born, I knew I had to control the barrage of intrusive thoughts that tormented me. I pushed the images away, wrapped my baby in a soft knit carrier, and went for walks to defy them. As I focused on her warmth against my chest and her rhythmic, unburdened breathing, I felt proud of myself for hiding my struggles from those around me. I had always wanted to be a mother. I thought this was what motherhood required. I didn't think to call it brave.

But the screaming, the screaming. I hadn't expected the screaming. My beautiful daughter howled like a hot copper kettle. My husband, pained to leave us, returned to work when she was eight days old. My mother, visiting to help, watched over my shoulder as Se's enchanting eyes transformed into slits, her delicate fingers fists, her smooth fore-head a chaos of wrinkles. Her angry tongue curved upward as if to amplify the shrieks of her tiny lungs.

Before I had a child, I understood myself only in relation to my own mother. To the world, I looked like *student*. I looked like *artist*. I looked like *woman*. I looked like *wife*. But I didn't recognize myself outside of *daughter*. As I grew up, it was this identity that had both cursed and defined me. I clung tight to it, knowing that the uncomfortable bond my mother and I shared arose from her attempts to overcome painful memories from her own childhood. She loved me so desperately that she invited me far too deep into the abyss of her own insecurities. And I followed. Neither of us could tell where I ended and she began.

All I had wanted as a daughter was to make my mother happy. Now all I wanted as a mother was to make my daughter happy, especially with my own mother looking on.

When Se was screaming, it felt like she had never not been scream-ing. I would do anything to soothe her distress. I couldn't bear to see her in pain. Perched for hours at a time on a huge turquoise rubber ball, topless and ready to offer my red, cracking nipple the moment her change in pitch signaled hunger, I ached to meet her needs. When she rooted and latched, then quieted into her swallow-breathe-swallow cycle, I awaited the calm I assumed would come with silence. Instead, as her body became heavy with sleep, a familiar unease crept in, like cold fingers of river water swirling around me.

The feeling always started behind my ears. As my milk let down, my skin tightened and a chill wrapped around the back of my neck, lacing its way into my hair with an otherworldly tingle. I became aware of each follicle meeting my scalp. My jaw stiffened and my mouth went dry. My stomach soured. Sadness, fear, and shame blurred into an overpowering urge to run. I needed to kick and shove and hide away, but I contained myself. I needed to breathe, so I breathed. I took slower, deeper inhalations, pushing the monster out of my chest. I straightened my back and looked down at my baby, who had curled her beautiful fingers around a wad of my long, disheveled braid.

The most striking thing was how familiar this experience felt. I remembered noticing the same sensation many times after swimming: In second grade, in the locker room of a public pool I'd snuck into with a friend. In sixth grade, after heaving myself from lake to dock at summer camp. As an adult, the week before I'd married Rahul, while brushing damp sand from my shoulders after emerging from salty waves. Over time, I'd approached the feeling with fear, then with annoyance, and finally with acceptance, coming to understand it as a peculiar manifestation of my anxiety. Something about the water transformed me. Something about *leaving* the water transformed me. Something about the flow of wetness, a body of water, my body in water, the movement of something from me to gone—it dredged up this melancholy in me. Now, something about feeding my daughter was summoning it too.

I wanted to be strong for my baby, but there were so many things to be anxious about as a new parent: Bath toys, babysitters, choking, sleep. Feeding schedules, growth curves, dog bites, guns. Before motherhood,

I had survived by telling myself that all my fears were irrational. But now, seeing that actual dangers lurked everywhere, I didn't know what to believe. When I pushed away my anxiety, I found no instincts left to trust. I could recognize no distinction between monumental and inconsequential risks. Suddenly even the smallest decision felt filled with peril. In a desperate panic, I battle cried straight into parenting.

Connecting with other mothers brought both validation and conflict. My community chorused that baby-led weaning and cloth diapers were best. Cosleeping was a sanctioned, even sanctified, way to deal with my fear, placing my baby where I could attend to her every cry and be ready to grab her in case of a fire or home invasion. Vaccination spurred passionate debates, so I searched out stories of infants who had died of vaccine-preventable diseases to confirm my stance against the voices shouting that vaccines were poison.

By the time Se was three and her brother, Au, was one, I had done everything I thought children needed, while forgetting to notice what my actual children needed. Still, I was terrified. I knew how to fight fear, but I didn't think I could survive sadness. I spiraled down into stories of death. I became an observer, a collector, a voyeur. Televisions falling on children, face-down bodies in shallow water, a trike rider killed by his own family's minivan. I researched diligently. I memorized statistics. I studied the scenes. While Se and Au slept in the dim blue glow beside me, every story slept beside us too.

My magical thinking kicked into high gear as I convinced myself that, if I cataloged all the risks and probabilities, I could prevent these stories from becoming ours. I swam through the agony of grieving families. With the admission that every one of these parents had tried to keep their children safe, just as I did, I collapsed in the flood of their pain. In my quest to escape their fates, I had forgotten to be brave.

The patterns would have been familiar if I hadn't been too overwhelmed to see them. As my obsessions intensified, I stopped eating. I stopped sleeping. My self-hatred engaged. Each time my son began to breastfeed, I was drenched in melancholy again. Icy fingers threaded their way up the back of my neck to my ears, and hopelessness enveloped me as I curled my toes in pain. With a tightened jaw, I willed my shoulders to relax and urged myself to smile lovingly at him until the feeling subsided.

Where some people might have isolated themselves in this struggle, I had been raised to show my face and to pretend I was doing well. Exhausting as it was, I continued to try to connect with other mothers. Then I heard a friend's sister describe the overwhelming unease she experienced with breastfeeding and call it the dysphoric milk ejection reflex. I went on to learn that, although D-MER is a poorly understood phenomenon, it's reported in the medical literature, and it isn't rare. It tied clearly into my strange sensations around wetness and water. I wasn't imagining it—and I wasn't alone.

This was the moment my world opened up. The knowledge that others had experienced what I was going through filled me with hope, like color and light beckoning from a far-off entrance to a cave I'd crawled too deep inside. In the past, I'd avoided naming my struggles. Now I could start to heal, with the words for what I felt steadying me.

This was also the moment I began using the phrase *mentally ill* to describe myself. Even though accepting this label sometimes fed my self-hatred, I realized that rumination, food restriction, panic attacks, and insomnia were all manifestations of the singular problem of anxiety. And I found comfort in the idea that the words might help it all make sense—because anxiety as an experience is universal, even if anxiety as a disorder is something quite distinct. My children, like me and like my mother before me, were going to grow up with a mother who was living with mental illness. Maybe, with insight, I could do something to protect my children—to protect them in a way that my mother hadn't been able to protect me. Maybe I could learn to trust my own perceptions.

Still, every time my children would argue with each other in innocent cruelty, I would plunge back in. In the bathtub before dinner one night, their bellows grew louder and more urgent in the synchronized no-longer-a-baby voices of four and two, competing for my attention as I sat on the floor beside them.

I asked them to find a compromise so they could both play with the mermaid. I told them to use kinder words when Se called Au a poopy and declared that she'd never play with him again. I grabbed the sponge to rub mud from Au's arms and heard him begin to wail, his lungs magically, disastrously huge, as he landed a punch directly on Se's nose. Something inside me cracked.

I'm done. That's it. Am I allowed to be done?

I turned toward the ceiling and screamed too. The three of us were screaming at the heavens like three rage-filled wild things. But their screaming had changed. They were scared. Scared of me. They were crying and tired and hungry and wet and cold and scared. But I was angry. Angry that they got to be pitiful, to be helpless, to look to me for comfort. Angry that I couldn't offer it, to them or to myself. I wrestled them into towels and plunked them onto the couch and told them that I needed to take some time away. I went into the other room, but I could still hear them crying.

I'd promised I would never leave them. I was leaving them. I'd promised I would never hurt them. I was hurting them.

Working my way back from the edge, I apologized to my children. I confided in my husband. I forgave myself for not knowing all the answers. I tried to trust us all.

Guided by my therapist, I came to understand that healing would require examination of the forces outside me and the forces within me shaping my thoughts. Guided by my doctor, I opened myself to different combinations of medications and rejected the myth that mental illness unleashes the artist's creative power. I pushed forward. I got better. I got worse. I got better again.

I let myself question.

What is a mother supposed to be? Mothers are expected to keep their children safe, holding back nothing for themselves. As I began to understand my illness, I felt inadequate every time my children's anger or sadness or fear triggered my own. For years, I had directed my vigilance toward the faceless threats of the wider world. But what about the trauma of my own childhood? How could I protect my children from the legacies that had been passed down over generations? My grandmother had resented my mother and maintained a vast emotional distance. My mother had compensated by clinging to and overburdening me. I panicked. Unable to navigate between extremes, I didn't know what to do. I pledged to break the chain. I needed to find a way to build my children up so their own inner voices could save them.

What is a child supposed to be? When Se was four, she said she no longer wanted to brush her hair. I said fine. As long as she washed it, I would let her do as she pleased. When she asked to dye it pink a year later, I agreed and helped her. Her tangle of pink and brown tendrils made me ashamed and delighted. They seemed at first hideous, then gorgeous. Allowing my children to be who they wanted to be demanded a new kind of courage. I wasn't in control. I was in awe. I was fighting not only for her but for myself, trying to protect the child I had been, hoping to learn the lessons I had missed. As a child, I had feared causing my mother to withdraw her affection. I wanted Se to have the freedom to do things I didn't like. I was shouting back against the sun-bleached hair forced on me as a child—even as I kept my own hair long and blonde, through all the years.

What is a woman supposed to be? I deeply missed the hours and days I'd spent in my art studio before my children were born. I'd sacrificed my passions in the name of motherhood, when in fact modeling who I was beyond *mother* would have better served us all. I thought back on my days leaning into the soft and sensual clay, where my body had engaged my work, where my hands had become my craft. I remembered the satisfaction in sculpting forms and under-firing them, leaving the material porous, vulnerable, open. I remembered packing the clay with salt and pouring water through it, then watching crystals emerge and lace across the exterior as the salt grew and twisted around the form beyond my control or imagining. My art had been ephemeral, temporary, nonfunctional. With just a breeze, the salt would fall away. But the form would remain, offering to be rebuilt in a different incarnation once I was ready. My art had provided me a full release, let me lose myself, helped me find myself. It was the only thing that was only mine. In the days before motherhood, I had immersed myself in a body of work, my body of work, my body. I had made huge pieces that took up space. I had almost given myself permission to take up space.

I went deeper into therapy, examining my anger, confronting my past. I realized that the reason I had lost myself in motherhood was that I hadn't known who I was to begin with. I stopped bleaching my hair and felt freer. I learned to name my experiences: dissociations, derealizations, flashbacks. I accepted new diagnoses: atypical anorexia, recurrent major depression, complex post-traumatic stress disorder. I came to understand prior diagnoses more plainly: I *had* anxiety. It wasn't who I was.

For so long, I had confused my anxiety disorder for my identity, and it had blocked me from healing. But I was terrified to stop defining myself by my fears. Detachment was the only way I knew to be a person in the world. Without the disorder, who would I be? As much as I'd managed my anxiety all these years, motherhood wasn't going to heal me.

When I realized this, I grieved for the ideal mother I wouldn't become. I grieved for the innocent child I hadn't gotten to be. I grieved for all the years of my life spent hating and abusing my body. But I also started to understand that I was a person beyond how scared I was. Although I couldn't change the past, I could keep doing the work of being prepared for whatever came next.

But all the *supposed-to-be*s added up to more than I could be.

One dark and quiet autumn night, I stood above another river, looking down from the center of the bridge I'd parked beneath. Its gothic towers rose more than two hundred feet above me. Its gray water flowed more than two hundred feet below me. Its surface glowed with city lights from the shore beyond, as shivers of current blurred their reflections into blackness. I had jumped into other rivers before. I wasn't scared.

My heavy rain boots gripped the dry pavement. Would they make it hard for me to climb the railing? My red wool cloak glowed under the streetlamp. Would I soar, cascade, drift down from bridge to surface as its fabric rippled along behind me like a hero's cape? My body was compelled toward the water. Would its chill invade every crevice, mapping out the ravines of my thighs, tracing the topography of my breasts, darting into my navel to seize my core, bringing awareness back into my body as I absorbed a cold so deep it read like heat against my stinging skin?

I could almost feel the water hitting my flesh before I jumped.

I was deep inside myself, detached from reality, already submerged as I looked down at the river, when she nearly ran into me—a jogger, dodging the post I stood behind. We startled, wide-eyed. We apologized, as women are taught to do. We stared at each other for just a second before she pressed on into the night, but it was enough to rip me from my trance. I crashed back into my body. The derealization dissolved like a torrent rushing over my face, like resistance against the flow, like pressure stifling my breath.

My heart broke open. It was an hour before midnight. I had touched coldness, control, understanding, had felt a clear and straightforward resolution. I had come so close. I had wanted to die. I had been relieved. I'd spent so long pushing away fear that now, when it could have protected me, I had none left. In that alternate universe, jumping hadn't been a choice, but a need.

My heart broke open. Se and Au were just six and four, peacefully asleep at home with Rahul, who thought I was out with friends. The immeasurable love I had for my husband and children hadn't been accessible to me in the darkness. Whatever messages had gotten to me before them were still too powerful, and I was still too vulnerable. This was the bridge I drove my son to preschool across each day, but I hadn't been thinking about my family at all. I'd promised I would never hurt them. I was hurting them. I'd promised I would never leave them. I'd almost left them. This was not what a mother was supposed to be.

My heart broke open. My body wasn't mine. I had accepted its abuse for years. Where others had left off, I had taken up the task by hating it, starving it, ignoring it, belittling it. I was flooded with terror at what had almost happened, then with relief that it hadn't, then with terror again, knowing that my struggle was so far from over. I sank down on the sidewalk, lying flat beneath the tall green towers, and cried with shame until my tears ran dry. Then I stood up and walked off the bridge and drove home to my family.

I didn't think to call it brave.

But the next day, and the next day, and the next day, and the next, something started to shift, like bits of salt and shards of color crumbling away from clay as the vessel beneath emerges. Visions of my death embedded themselves in my thoughts. So did visions of my family's grief. I had glimpsed the alternate reality of my children's world without me in it, had imagined them devastated, destroyed, alone. I had looked into the future, and I had changed it. I did have power. I had chosen to spare us all.

Six months later, I dyed my long brown hair half platinum blonde and half blazing orange. Looking in the mirror afterward was shocking. At first, it scared me. Then an intense sense of freedom set in. I relished the contrast of compliance and defiance, the mix of who I had always been told to be and who I might still become. Was this how Se had felt when she'd first seen hers pink?

In the two years since that night on the bridge, I have helped Se dye her own hair many colors, pinks and blues and reds and yellows and purples and teals blurring together. Her tangled beauty reminds me that she is her own person, separate and distinct, fierce and daring, no matter what her history foretells. Maybe my healing means that she'll never have to learn the things I wish I hadn't had to.

I can clearly see the line that reaches up, from my children through me, through my mother and her mother and her mother and hers, carrying memory and unease and discomfort and fear. I wish my mother had broken the cycle before me, but I'm not angry at her anymore. She tried. I'm sorry that she didn't get help. I'm sorry that she didn't learn how to ease her pain so she could teach me how to ease my own. And I know that I'm the one who chooses what our legacy will mean for Se and Au.

Having control isn't what keeps us safe. Knowing that I have a choice is what keeps us safe.

At almost nine, Se still hasn't lost the boldness she showed as a newborn. She has never stopped screaming her needs to me. She has never stopped running toward the water, demanding what she wants from the world. I hope she can always preserve the clarity of vision of her five-year-old self that I remember from a day spent splashing in Puget Sound, near the home my parents had retired to in northern Washington.

We'd passed the afternoon prowling for treasures at the waterline as my mother walked behind us and a shroud of fog crept across the tide pools' seaweed knots. I loved finding the most scarred rocks, the irregular figures wrapped in loops of gray and black that reminded me of my work with salt and clay. My mother picked up a single rounded stone, too big to carry with just one hand. Se always chose pure white. The seaside breeze rose up, cold and damp as it grazed my legs. Before I could object, Se set down her rock collection and took off her shoes.

Countless times before, I'd had to choose: follow her in, until I had to tell her, "No, stop, too deep, come back," or let her test her own limits while I measured my increasing discomfort against her drive to explore.

This time, I was prepared. I brought Se's life jacket to the water's edge. She smiled at me as I zipped it over her thick wool sweater. I tied a rope to her back with a bowline knot I'd learned at summer camp all those years ago. She waded out until the water lapped at her knees, looking back only once to grab the rope, tug a little, and glance at me and at my mother, who was still standing on the shore behind us.

Then I held on tight as I let her go.

Marissa ~ Carry

When I finally paused to look around me, I realized that everyone I cared about was in pain. We were deep into the most wonderful, stressful, life-affirming, heartbreaking year I'd ever experienced. I was trying to carry the weight of it all—and failing.

Isabel had picked up more extra hours at work than I'd ever seen her request, while Adrien shut himself in his room, listening to angry music and punching the bed and the walls. Jada slept mostly in her portable infant car seat, where she fit her naps into everyone else's schedules of therapy appointments, job obligations, and case-worker meetings. I barely recognized myself, having sacrificed my beloved teaching career to become the stay-at-home mom I thought my children needed. My relationships—especially with my wife—were all on the verge of collapse. Even our dog seemed bedraggled and dejected.

Isabel had been one of my closest college friends long before she and I became partners. In spite of our undeniable chemistry, our bigger life visions initially seemed incompatible. I had grown up as the scrappy little tomboy on the playground, spirited and altruistic, always quick to rescue other kids who couldn't stand up for themselves. After graduation, I explored and traveled for more than a decade, taking on odd jobs in a new state each year, my desire for motion the only constant. Isabel, practical, dependable, and steady, had been raised in poverty and was the first person in her family to attend college. After graduation, she moved to Seattle and found an apartment, fully content to settle down.

Now in our thirties and both visiting our childhood homes in Indiana for the winter holidays, we met to share a beer in a smoky sports bar. Isabel, always reserved, had spent the intervening years cultivating her career behind the scenes as a diagnostic imaging specialist at a busy hospital—the less human interaction, the better. I had become a teacher in an underfunded and overcrowded elementary school in Baltimore. I spent my days talking all day long, then going to conferences to talk about how effective my talking had been.

Over bursts of raucous laughter from a pool table behind us, we leaned closer and closer to hear each other. When our arms touched, my senses flooded, reminding me of the perfect physical match we'd always been. With the maturity that the years had brought us, it seemed like we could finally appreciate rather than just tolerate our differences, like our differences might bring us complementary strengths rather than keep us apart.

After more than a year of flying back and forth across the country to spend time together, Isabel moved in with me but couldn't find work. When we heard about a job opening that sounded perfect for her in Albuquerque, we made jokes about needing to buy sun hats and get used to cooking with green chiles at every meal. Soon I'd agreed to leave a teaching job I loved in a city I knew, and we'd moved to a place we'd visited exactly once, a place that held no history for either of us, only wishes for a life together.

While Isabel commuted to the hospital, I started working with third graders as a math coach. These children brought so much to their community: rich cultures, fascinating experiences, strong beliefs, warm hearts. One boy had walked six days across the Mexican desert with his family in search of a new life. Another student's mother owned an Ethiopian restaurant and implored me, every time

I saw her at parent-teacher conferences, to come in so she could treat me to her favorite dish. I went to birthday parties, soccer games, and heritage festivals.

I also saw what was hard about their lives. My students often came to school hungry and exhausted, their schedules constantly disrupted by the comings and goings of parents and siblings working erratic shifts at multiple jobs as they strove to untangle the myths of this land of plenty. I felt a huge responsibility to advocate for my students, especially when their parents could not.

When I was offered the position of fourth-grade teacher for the following year, along with the opportunity to move up with many of these same students, I was thrilled. I requested all the so-called difficult kids, all the kids with academic and behavioral problems. Because I didn't see any of them as problems. I saw them as children. They started with my trust, and most of the time they rose to the occasion. If they didn't, the next day brought a chance to try again.

While I encouraged them to bring their true selves to the class-room, I didn't feel like I could do the same. I guarded my privacy closely as I dodged questions about boyfriends and home life. I'd heard some of my students giggling as they whispered about my asymmetrically shaved haircut and my nose ring. I knew they thought I was different. Strange. Less feminine than the other women in their lives. I never mentioned Isabel.

For all their rough edges and skepticism, these kids were really easy to fall in love with. And in my class of thirty-one students, Adrien stood out from the beginning. He'd been in and out of foster care since kindergarten, living in nine different homes over the past five years. Between placements, he'd spent a few months with his father and intellectually disabled younger half brother when his father wasn't using cocaine. There'd been talk about trying to reunite him with his mother, but that was before she'd gotten arrested again for stealing a car and setting it on fire.

Relying on a cab service coordinated by the foster care system,

Adrien often got to school late and felt self-conscious about disrupting his class or had to leave early and missed end-of-the-day gatherings. Some days he seemed really sad. But he had a way of bringing gentle humor to challenging situations, and he shared his heart with abundance. He had a beautiful, shiny soul and a spirit that lit up his face when he smiled. He thrived more each time I raised my expectations. I offered the same love to all my students, but Adrien loved back differently. Adrien needed it more.

I knew that a committed teacher was the closest thing that some of these kids had to a stable parent in their lives. Students accidentally called me Mom all the time. To me, it meant they were longing for a loving, firm, consistent presence, and I truly enjoyed being that. Working with them reinforced how much I wanted to be a mother myself. Although Isabel had never pictured herself having kids, I soon caught her lingering beside a display of animal-print booties in the mall, then looking over my shoulder at jogging strollers as I flipped through a catalog of baby gear. She said that witnessing my love for my students helped her understand why we might want a child of our own.

Ever the pragmatic one, Isabel insisted we get married first. After a simple ceremony at the end of the summer, we started talking about getting pregnant and agreed immediately that I'd be the one to carry. I was fascinated by the idea of growing a person and giving birth—and I think, having grown up feeling different for being attracted to girls and getting called a tomboy for so many years, something in me craved reassurance that the female parts of me really worked.

Choosing a sperm donor was harder than we'd expected. I couldn't imagine summing up my partner within the confines of a single typed page, and now we were trying to select the other biological half of our future child while limited to exactly that much information. As I headed into the beginning of the school year with my fourth graders, Isabel and I spent our evenings laughing over the way different registries listed their donors: Zeus was dark haired and broad shouldered, spoke three languages, and liked spicy food. 7054 was tall and thin, came from a family of architects, and had a history of mild asthma. Athletic Dancer had parents from Korea and Norway, was passionate about ballet, and had earned a prestigious tennis scholarship. After poring over hundreds of profiles, we chose someone who seemed to complement my own genetics: number 3948, a creative, artistic type to counter my mathematical mind, with Haitian and Puerto Rican roots to balance my white British heritage.

One crisp October evening after work, Isabel picked up the large canister that housed a bath of liquid nitrogen surrounding a surprisingly tiny vial of twenty million sperm. She sent me a picture of the nondescript silver vessel, then, not sure what to do, buckled it into the passenger seat of her car and drove home with it beside her like an amiable companion. Inspired by the absurdity of the situation, we took family pictures all night—holding it between us, snuggling with it, giggling together while we tickled its shiny yellow screw cap.

The next evening, wanting our conception story to be romantic, we turned on our favorite music. We poured two glasses of wine and dimmed the lights. Then we stared at the clunky tank on the bedside table. We remembered reading somewhere that the odds of conception were higher with insemination at the time of orgasm. So when we had gotten as close to the optimal moment as seemed possible, given the very unsexy context of thawing the sample and loading it into a plastic syringe, Isabel slid the tube inside me and tried to deploy the plunger. It was stuck. She pulled it out, thinking it was broken, and immediately squirted me in the face with the fluid.

She was absolutely mortified and looked like she might cry. I thought it was the most hilarious thing ever as I wondered if this happened to straight people all the time. But I was pretty confident from my memories of middle school health classes that I wasn't going to get pregnant this way. After two more unsuccessful home cycles, I told Isabel I thought we should just go on being in love and hire someone else to get the sperm to the right place.

In the spring, three things happened: I got pregnant during our third cycle at the fertility clinic. I was offered the chance to stay with my students again, including Adrien, as they moved up to fifth grade the next school year. And I heard that Adrien's plan would be changing. Because his mother was still in jail and his father, as much as he wanted to raise his boys, was still tangled in the weeds of addiction, Adrien might soon become eligible for adoption.

That was when I started having dreams that Adrien was our son. In these visions, he walked beside me, his short-sleeved plaid shirt buttoned up to the collar, his skinny jeans a little too short, his wavy shoulder-length hair braided in perfect cornrows. He shared stories about his day and asked me thoughtful questions, his wide-open smile bringing lightness to the moments when my world felt too heavy. During my waking hours, as Isabel and I built a family, it pained me to watch this lovable boy growing up without one. I began to admit to myself that, knowing how strongly Adrien identified as African American and Navajo, I might have chosen a multiracial donor subconsciously thinking about a sibling for him.

Adrien didn't know any of this. Neither did Isabel. At the end of the school year, when I mentioned to Isabel that I'd been thinking about adopting one of my students, her readiness to discuss it surprised me, especially because the rules I'd imposed on myself meant that she'd never met any of them. Like when we had first talked about trying to get pregnant, she said my excitement showed her what could be wonderful about this. She wanted to be someone who was willing to try.

By the end of June, after many consultations with the caseworker and a month of conversations ourselves, Isabel and I felt ready to move forward. We were hoping Adrien could be settled into our home before our baby, due in January, was born. But adoption isn't known for being fast or straightforward, and foster care makes it particularly slow and complex. Within this system, there are two paths to adoption: kinship, which can be expedited, and everything else, which cannot. We wondered if I might fall somewhere in between, having served as his teacher for two years with background checks already in place. We thought our process might be faster. It wasn't.

When a foster child is being considered for adoption, they're not told anything about the family considering them because there's too much potential for heartbreak in all directions. So, while I couldn't reveal our plan to Adrien, I could sign up for summer volunteer opportunities to drive him to camp and take him out for ice cream afterward, where he could meet my wife, even if I wasn't ready to tell him who she was—or allowed to tell him that she might soon be one of his mothers. While Isabel and I waited for updates, we also attended required state-sponsored parenting classes. The presentations covered topics from addressing behavior challenges to managing relationships with birth families to understanding the impacts of abuse and neglect. For two hours twice a week through the summer months, surrounded by plywood tables and wet-dog carpet smell, we sat in a basement with nine other hopeful prospective parents and smiled sheepishly as we sipped cups of instant coffee.

When I returned to my fifth graders in the fall very obviously pregnant, the students were giddy with excitement. Adrien hung back a little, nervously aware that his own plan was in flux, self-conscious that I'd been talking to his caseworker and therapist about how to best support him at school through whatever transition came next. When the music teacher asked him to leave class one day for being defiant, he sat with me, hesitantly sharing his fears: That no one would want to adopt him. That someone would, but then wouldn't like him. That his dad might feel sad about giving him up. I became more attached to him with each conversation, carrying the weight of all his uncertainty, deeply worried about the effect my absence during maternity leave would have.

Jada was born right on time at the beginning of January. Then, just two weeks later, Adrien's caseworker called to tell us that we had been chosen to foster him, with the potential for adoption if his parents

terminated rights. Isabel and I were exhausted and elated and terrified. We were head over heels in love, with Jada and with each other.
I had been hoping for—and literally dreaming about—this moment
for so long. But I also felt protective of my brand-new daughter and
our little family. I fretted about what kind of germs an eleven-year-old
boy would be tracking into the house, and whether Adrien would be
okay with having a sister, and how I would have enough time for both
my kids, and how I would have enough energy to be present in my
marriage. I wondered how I could best help Adrien and Jada connect
to the cultures that were part of their identities, even though I didn't
share these identities myself. I constantly flip-flopped between feeling
like everything was coming together exactly as I'd wanted and feeling
like I was in far over my head.

The agency advised us that Adrien's transition into our home
would begin in two months. I wished I could tell him that he didn't
have to worry because I was going to take care of him. But I had my
own worries leading up to this transition. I didn't know if Adrien
would reject me once he knew I was married to a woman, or if our
connection was something only I felt. I considered that I might have
no idea what I was getting into by intervening in this boy's life. Still,
functioning on a newborn's schedule of waking every two to three
hours around the clock, and with Isabel back at her busy hospital job
after a short parental leave, I didn't have much time for rumination.
Suddenly, the day had arrived.

On the first Monday in March, Adrien's caseworker presented him
with a family book that Isabel and I had spent many hours creating.
At first, he didn't understand why she was showing him pictures of his
teacher and her baby, and that friend she'd brought out for ice cream
after camp last summer, and this random house on the edge of town.
Once it dawned on him that we were the family who wanted to adopt
him, he was ecstatic. Together, they called me on speakerphone, and
I could almost hear that huge, beaming grin—so rare for him these
days—spreading across Adrien's face.

On Tuesday morning, he brought the book to class, thrilled to show all the other students his new family. The substitute who was filling in during my maternity leave later told me that many of them were as confused as Adrien had been. They knew I'd been home with my baby since winter break. They had noticed my wedding ring. They had made assumptions about my husband, even though my answers to their questions had always been vague and evasive. Most of them thought they didn't know any gay people, and many of their families had taught them to reject homosexuality as abhorrent to their faith. The ones who weren't upset about my sexual orientation were worried about my safety, especially with several gangs targeting the local high school's few openly gay students recently. A few of them started crying, jealous that I wasn't going to adopt them too.

Tuesday was also the day that Adrien would officially meet Isabel. Isabel had long acknowledged that while she had been advancing her career, I had been taking the lead on all things parenting. But she absolutely adored Jada and seemed genuinely excited about bringing Adrien into our family too. After work that evening, we picked Adrien up from his foster home to take him out to dinner. As we shared pizzas and sodas and laughter, I loved watching Isabel and Adrien getting to know each other.

After dinner, Isabel took Jada for a walk in her jogging stroller—recently ordered from one of those catalogs Isabel had once admired over my shoulder—while Adrien and I stopped at a nearby drugstore. He wandered the aisles, picking out a toothbrush, toothpaste, soap, shampoo, and deodorant. Then I led him to a section along the far left side of the store. He stared silently at the shelves, amazed to discover a whole industry of products specifically designed for Black skin and hair. Proudly hauling his selections, which now included cocoa butter lotion and jojoba oil spray, to the checkout, he told me he'd never chosen his own supplies before. I was happy for him, and I was grateful to provide this opportunity, but I felt conflicted about trying to teach him about a culture I didn't share.

On Wednesday, Adrien had dinner with his foster family while I spent one last day preparing for his arrival. During Jada's nap, I washed his sheets again, set a clock on his bedside table, and lined up his toiletries along the bathroom sink, hoping that our home would make him feel welcomed and loved and expected. On Thursday, Adrien came over to bake cupcakes. As they cooled, we played with Jada and read her a bedtime story. Once she was asleep, we adorned the treats with frosting and sprinkles, talking long into the night about the friends he would share them with tomorrow before he transferred to our neighborhood fifth grade next week. On Friday morning, his teacher greeted him warmly as his classmates rushed up to offer stacks of homemade cards.

On Saturday, Adrien officially moved in with us. Almost all his belongings fit into two oversized trash bags: Clothes and sneakers that were all a little too small. A worn teddy bear with its right shoulder coming unstitched. A bucket of dingy LEGO bricks mixed with marbles, paper clips, and an old pen. He carried a separate shoebox of special treasures, including letters his mother had written him from jail, the only photograph he had of himself with his father, a picture of a dragon his half brother had drawn, and, now, the cards from his classmates.

At his new school, Adrien stood out more than we'd expected. Within a few weeks, he started to show more overt signs of learning disabilities, which had been well masked in the setting of the predictable and familiar routines at his old school. Or maybe these challenges had just been overshadowed by the boundless needs of so many other kids in the community he used to be a part of, where more than one-quarter of the students were unhoused and personal, social, and academic impediments to school success were the norm. I worked closely with his teacher and counselors, spending my days in meetings and on phone calls to schedule appointments, secure evaluations and testing, review results, and draft an individualized education program for him.

At home, things were just as challenging. His ability to reason fluctuated wildly by context, and he had little concept of time. When he went into the bathroom, I heard the shower turn on and run for thirty minutes. When he emerged after another thirty, he was still dry and dirty. I realized that he'd never been taught any basic sequence of steps for washing. When he tried to figure it out, he couldn't remember which steps he had already done, so he daydreamed on the edge of the tub. I made him a shower list, to go along with his getting-ready-for-school list and his getting-ready-for-bed list, and perched on the toilet lid in the steamy bathroom, talking him through it while I breastfed three-month-old Jada.

We went over the same things every day, trying to establish new routines, but—with Adrien's combination of prenatal alcohol exposure, post-traumatic stress from physical and emotional abuse, and the ever-shifting expectations of adapting to new environments—most of it didn't stick. He wanted an adult to pay attention to him at all times, but Isabel worked long hours and I was only one person. Homework assignments intended to take twenty minutes took him three to four hours each night, with me coaching him along. Part of me relished the intensity of taking care of Adrien, and part of me knew it was all too much. The line between being loved and being needed was blurry and unsettling.

The physical demands of meeting newborn Jada's basic needs were hard enough. Becoming an instant parent to a tween was emotionally fraught on a whole different level. Isabel and I had had no time to gradually develop our styles together, and now we haltingly, chaotically, tried to figure out what kind of parents we were as Adrien looked on: How Isabel should respond when Adrien and his friends spoke disrespectfully to her. If I was the mom who gave in to my son's request for chips at the store every time, sometimes, or never. What the consequences were for lying.

Adrien needed all my attention. But so did Jada. And so did my relationship with my wife. By the end of the school year, Isabel felt like I had entirely misrepresented what we were taking on. She seemed angry and scared as she accused me of not telling her what Adrien was really like. I thought I had explained everything I knew. But I had to admit that what I had envisioned seemed naive now that we were facing the details of daily life together. I was scared too.

While Isabel burrowed deeper into her work, I tried to give Adrien a summer full of childhood pleasures. I signed him up to play for the town baseball league, a longtime wish that he hadn't been able to pursue without reliable adults to get him to practices and games, as I imagined cheering for him from the sidelines with baby Jada in my lap. Instead, by his second week, he was pouting through the whole car ride and refusing to play once we arrived. The reality was that being on a team and working toward a goal were foreign concepts to him. About to turn twelve, he was exploring his interests in activities where most kids in our district were beginners not as preteens but in preschool. Over and over, as I offered him experiences, he would get so excited to try something new, then be crushed with disappointment when it wasn't what he had expected. Nothing was ever good enough or nice enough. Nothing was ever satisfying.

One thing did go well that summer: Adrien got the hairstyle he'd always wanted. In the past, he'd had access only to options that were free. When he'd lived with his father, he'd worn his hair short and natural. When he'd moved to a home where one of the foster parents knew how to braid, he'd relished the connection to his Navajo heritage as his thick braid grew longer. But for years what he'd really wished for was dreadlocks. So I took him to a local Black-owned hair salon.

As soon as we walked in, both of us were captivated by this multi-generational space full of banter and love. Time moved differently here. Work felt unhurried as people drifted between multiple jobs, teasing each other affectionately, shouting a welcome to every new visitor, juggling one client's color treatment with another's conditioning mask and another's chemical relaxer. Watching these beautiful

Black matriarchs handle Adrien's hair so lovingly almost made up for all the uncomfortable requests we fielded at the grocery store from people who wanted to touch it. At home, I would work on his dreads while he sat on the floor in front of me. As I wove a crochet hook into the new growth, pulling it along to keep it tight and pressing the tips with oil, I longed to invest time and energy into what was important to Adrien, even as I laughed to myself about how little effort I put into my own short, spiky hairstyle.

We also kept up with therapy through the summer, as much for our own benefit as for Adrien's. So much therapy, in every configuration: Therapy for Adrien alone. Therapy that I attended with him just to listen, and some where he and I worked on problems together. Therapy for Adrien and Isabel, then for Isabel and me. Jada slept in the car as we drove across town for at least one appointment each day, missed her naps more often than not, and fussed in her carrier through countless waiting room hours.

Meanwhile, Adrien was acutely attuned to the growing fractures in my relationship with Isabel. As her frustrations rose, he sought my solitary attention even more—and he became masterful at getting between us. When he left his clothes strewn along the hallway or came home late for dinner, Isabel said he didn't respect our boundaries. I felt compelled to defend him, falling back on the excuse that he was just a kid who'd had a hard life and struggled with self-regulation. She said it was more intentional than that. That he was being manipulative and trying to push us apart. I knew she was probably right. He'd had a history of doing this in his foster families in the past. But I felt like we should be strong enough to get through it. I offered Isabel ideas about how to connect with him, and she dutifully tried, only to have him reject all her efforts. My attempts placed me squarely in line to be hit with complaints from both of them.

My response to this tension—surely the result of being raised by two unflappably stoic expat Londoners who embodied the World War II dictate to *Keep Calm and Carry On*—was to put my head down and try to meet everyone's needs while ignoring the fact that many of these needs were incompatible or even directly contradictory. When I turned inward in this way, I triggered all sorts of fears of abandonment in Isabel. But I couldn't reassure her, because she wasn't wrong to worry. I was no longer sure that I wasn't going to leave her.

By September, some things seemed broken beyond repair. Still, I scheduled another appointment with our therapist, confident she'd be able to guide Isabel toward a better understanding of what was going on with Adrien and help us all come together as a family. I was ready to receive her wise counsel when, after meeting with Isabel and Adrien, she asked Adrien to move to the waiting room and called me in to join Isabel.

As soon as she closed the door, she told me that she didn't think this was going to work out. My mind started racing. She explained why she thought the situation was unhealthy for everyone involved. My cheeks were burning as tears welled up in my eyes. She said the stress was making my wife physically ill and Adrien didn't seem happy at all. I felt a panic rise within me at the thought of choosing between my partner and my child. I just needed to try harder, to summon the strength to carry us all.

Our therapist was blunt: Adrien's life was too chaotic already. If we were considering severing the relationship, which would consign him to yet another foster placement, either he had to move out immediately or we should wait until after winter break to tell him. As I saw it—since there was no way I could agree to such a sudden change, and Isabel conceded that she didn't want to make this more disruptive than it needed to be—that gave me three months, until January, to create a deeper bond for all of us.

As hard as some days were, other days were so beautiful. I thought of Adrien and Jada sitting side by side, high chair pulled up to the dining room table as she tried her first taste of solids from his bowl of watery oatmeal. I pictured Adrien and Jada together in our old wooden rocker, her chubby legs snuggled in his lap as he read graphic novels and she chewed on a board book. I remembered Jada learning to walk and then almost immediately learning to run, with Adrien slow-chasing her until they both dissolved into giggles on the couch. They loved each other so much. In these moments, my family was just as I had pictured, just as I had hoped.

Our lives were so rich, but that didn't make them easy. Over the holidays, things got worse rather than better. Isabel and Adrien were either slamming doors on each other or sitting behind those doors stewing, and Isabel and I fought all the time. She felt pushed so far beyond what she could handle that she struggled to find any good in Adrien, while I had become so protective—yet so stuck in the middle—that I was constantly defending his actions to her and her actions to him. On the rare occasions we made time to connect with family and friends, most of them sympathized with Isabel. They couldn't understand why I hadn't given up yet. I couldn't understand how anyone could give up on a child.

Thanksgiving and Christmas and New Year's are incredibly difficult for many kids in foster care. Holidays are about tradition, but it had been impossible for Adrien to establish traditions when he was in a different house with different people every year. Holidays are about reflection, but it was painful for Adrien to remember the trauma of being removed from his dad's custody one Christmas Eve and to think back on the grief of having no gifts to unwrap. The holiday season had instead become a time of longing for things to be different, a time of sorrow about how much it hurt to revisit the past, a time of anxiety about what might come next. Through those darkest weeks of December, when he felt overwhelmed, Adrien often retreated to a small nook at the top of the stairs to thumb through his box of special things, reading and rereading the letters his mom had sent from jail. He always emerged with questions about his past that I couldn't answer.

One day over break, as Adrien and I sat with our therapist, she suggested we build our house in her play therapy sandbox. We laughed together as we outlined a living room and filled it with intricate doll-house furniture and tiny figurines: a small cat to represent Jada, drag-ons for Adrien and me, and a witchy-looking creature standing in for Isabel. Then the therapist handed Adrien a stack of feeling-words cards and asked him to choose the words he felt most often in the house and to place them where he felt them.

As I watched him sort through the words, discarding *HAPPINESS*, *JOY*, and *LOVE*, my heart sank. He placed *ANGER* on the tiny couch, *FRUSTRATION* by the bookshelf, *LONELINESS* by the front door, and *SADNESS* in the rocking chair. I realized that I was the only person who still thought we could make this work. What I had wanted to create for us all was not the experience that Adrien and Isabel were having. When I slowed down enough to reflect, it wasn't even the experience that I was having. Suddenly I understood that our home might not be the best place for Adrien to grow up after all.

A few days into January, it was time to move forward on the hor-rible, unfair, impossible decision that I'd made. I couldn't bear to tell Adrien. I asked the therapist to do it. At our next session, she sat us down and delivered the news that Adrien would be moving to a new foster placement the following week. We cried together as he begged for another chance. He offered to go somewhere else for a year and then come back and try again. He said he would do anything if I let him stay. As unhappy as he'd been lately, the tensions of our home still felt safer than the unknowns of somewhere new. He asked why he and the baby and I couldn't just live together. He asked me over and over again to pick him. The experience destroyed me.

As we went through the motions of our days, Adrien packed his things, quietly filling the large plastic bins I'd bought him to replace his plastic bags. I thought seriously about whether Isabel should be the one packing, whether I should just gather my children close to me and ask my wife to leave. She would be able to fend for herself, but I wasn't sure what was going to happen to Adrien. I couldn't think clearly through my heartbreak. I loved both of these people—

these wonderful, flawed, beautiful people—so much. I couldn't accept that they had come to hate each other.

At the end of the week, I helped Adrien move out. I thought back to the day he had arrived at our home, barely a year ago, earnestly shouldering his two tattered sacks full of outgrown possessions. Now he was leaving with six sturdy bins full of clothes that fit well, the right brand of sneakers, and books that he loved—six sturdy bins that he asked me to carry out to the car for him, a look of defeat heavy on his face.

Adrien held his special box of cards and letters as I drove us a mile down the road, where his caseworker had arranged a temporary placement. In the living room of a well-meaning first-time foster parent, we were welcomed with a huge plate of loaded nachos—Adrien's favorite food—but he refused to take a bite. He alternated between sobbing while clinging to me and sitting in a chair by the door, slouched like a limp rag. I promised him that we could still talk on the phone and meet for lunch on weekends. Then, back in the car, I leaned against the steering wheel and cried alone under the frigid winter sun.

One early spring evening a few months later, when Isabel and I were out walking in our neighborhood, I spotted Adrien on the next block, coming toward us. Isabel froze. She turned away abruptly and headed home, too pained to even say hello. Now managing Jada's stroller and the dog's leash, I approached Adrien and made excuses for Isabel's sudden departure. We walked together into the playground where we'd spent so many hours shooting hoops, setting up bike obstacle courses, and throwing tennis balls for the dog. We sat on the swings as he told me exactly how he felt: Abandoned. Lonely. Unwanted. Sad. Like maybe it had been worse for him to have spent ten months in our home than it would have been if he had never lived with us at all.

His gut-wrenching confession made me question everything

about our relationship. His suffering reinforced the connection we had, and it also made me feel even more devastated that I hadn't been able to keep us together. I had to fight the urge to try to talk him out of his feelings, to explain that this wasn't how I had meant for any of this to unfold, because the last thing I wanted to do was to invalidate his experience. I had been longing for redemption, needing to hear that he still felt the love I'd shown him and that it was steadying him through challenging times. I was hoping that out of sight meant out of pain, for all of us. Despite my best intentions, what he had taken from his time with me was exactly the opposite of what I had been trying to give him.

When Adrien called a few weeks later to tell me that he was being moved from the temporary foster home into a possible foster-to-adopt placement, I was thrilled for him. But it was in Santa Fe, more than an hour's drive away. The distance finally made our separation real, and it felt terrible. Our therapist suggested I write him a release letter. She told me that when a child in the foster system is being adopted, their birth parents—if they're still around and involved—are encouraged to write a letter giving the child permission to move on. Releasing them from one family into another is a gift, both to the child and to the parents. I loved the idea of writing this for him. I pictured him adding it to his special shoebox and carrying it with him through his life. And I tried to write it. I tried so many times. But every time I tried, I got stuck.

I didn't know how to set down the dreams I'd held for so long and back away from them. There were a million things I might have done differently, a million things I could have done better. I wanted Adrien to know how sorry I was that we couldn't make it work. How much I missed him. How important he was to me. But I didn't want to burden him with my regrets. I hadn't even made time yet to feel all my feelings myself. I was barely on the verge of admitting that my marriage wasn't going to survive either, that the family I had tried so hard to bring together couldn't withstand the weight of all that had happened. I loved being a mother, and I had loved being Adrien's mother. I felt hollowed out knowing that someone else was going to raise the boy I had thought would be my son.

In June, I drove north to Santa Fe to celebrate Adrien's birthday and meet the people who were now taking care of him. Grateful for the invitation but uncertain about how I might feel seeing them together, I showed up to the city park with a huge ice cream cake and thirteen shiny helium balloons. Here I was again, trying to layer love into his new reality, to create a joyful experience for him, to ask this other family to care about him as much as I did. Adrien hovered beside the picnic table, full of excitement, as several of his friends jumped off the stone statues they'd been climbing and made their way over to join us. His foster mom and dad lit the candles. Their two teenage daughters passed out drinks. I was relieved to see Adrien looking much happier than the last time I'd seen him.

After we sang Adrien's birthday wishes, his foster mom served the cake. Just as she went to hand him his plate, he looked away, distracted by the raucous shouting of some other kids on a nearby basketball court. The melting slice began to slip, creeping along in slow motion toward becoming a splatter in the dirt. I started to lunge for it. Then I held myself back.

This wasn't my role anymore.

Adrien needed me to let go, to trust someone else's capable hands. His new family would stumble through and figure it out with him, catching the pieces as they fell. The best way for me to love him now would be to accept both the courage and the cowardice inherent in releasing the hopes I'd carried for so long. The best way for me to love the rest of my family would be to move forward with my own life, to be present for Jada, to see if Isabel and I could heal after everything we'd been through.

And his new foster mother did step in, exactly as she should have. She grabbed the plate, stopped the cake from falling, and changed the course of the day as I could not. She took longer to reach for it than I would have. And she did it in a different way, and from a different angle.

But Adrien didn't notice any of this. He turned back toward us and took the plate, grinning at us both. Then he scooped up a big forkful of frozen vanilla clumps and chocolate cookie crumbles and eagerly downed the first bite.

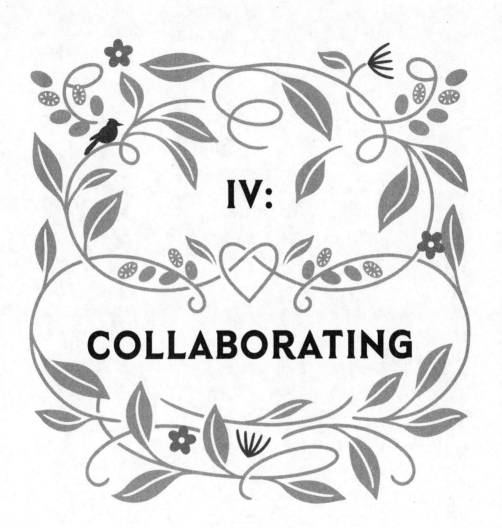

IV:

COLLABORATING

CHAPTER 8

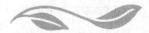

As I readjusted to residency after maternity leave, everything looked different as a parent.

My schedule was beyond challenging, with little time for reflection or self-care. The obstetrics rotation was the hardest in many ways. I had to get up by three thirty most mornings to pump and shower and drive to the hospital in time to start work at five o'clock, then work for fourteen hours. Throughout the day, I tried to carve out a few blocks of time to go to the nurses' locker room to pump again. When I traveled to an off-site clinic, I arranged my equipment under a shawl and pumped in the car en route to my destination.

But maintaining a consistent routine was difficult while attending to the unpredictable needs of laboring women and newborns. Although I'd hoped the obstetricians I worked with would be universally on board with breastfeeding, unsympathetic supervisors urged me to—in their words—*pump expeditiously*, already resenting my twenty minutes away from the unit as they glared at my black shoulder bag full of bottles and flanges.

Time with my family felt harried too. If I stayed on task through evening rounds at the hospital, I could sometimes get home to read one quick book with five-month-old Zach before his seven-thirty

bedtime. After Zach was settled, it was a race to have dinner and prepare for the next day, then a race to get to sleep after feeding him again
around ten and around one, so I could get a little rest before starting
over in a few hours. I was grateful that Ian had taken paternity leave,
so I didn't worry as much about Zach when I was gone. But I missed
them both terribly, even though we were together through most of
those half-awake nights—at least when I didn't have to work a thirty-
hour call shift at the hospital. I resigned myself to the fact that I
would never feel like I was doing anything well while I was trying to
do everything at this pace.

I wasn't alone. So many of the women I worked with seemed constantly pulled in different directions. More than once, I found myself
on a team of mothers: some pregnant, some pumping, some eager
to finish up at clinic in time to collect their children from preschool.
Still, I found satisfaction in belonging to the groups I'd distanced
myself from for so long. Now I was the one trading stories with other
pregnant residents, sharing family photos before rounds, and offering
advice and insight as we discovered common ground.

But I also remembered what it was like to be an outsider. What
it meant to be surrounded by colleagues and patients who had what
I wished for but might never have. How it felt to watch from afar. I
started to notice those who, like me, didn't take family life for granted.
When other women at work alluded to challenges in building their
own families, I didn't hesitate to share that we'd lost three pregnancies
before having our son. Having finally become a mother, I was ready
to offer whatever details of my experience might encourage others to
be persistent and help them feel less isolated.

As I opened up about my own story at work, I learned that some
of my colleagues in medicine had put off having children until their
forties to advance their careers or because of complications in their

relationships. Many were undergoing fertility treatments or struggling to manage the exhaustion of raising young children after long hours on the job. Others had been single parents in their teens and now, with their kids a little older and a little more independent, were looking to take on more responsibility at work. A few had even faced medical complications not unlike my own.

Whatever our role in caring for others, I came to see common themes running through our lives. Eriko's story of career change within medicine raised questions about how our professional identities influenced our relationships with our partners, our parents, and the families we chose and built over many years. Stacey's story as a psychologist led me to reconsider how our jobs shaped our perceptions of ourselves, especially as we faced difficult choices and compromises to become parents. Bree's story reminded me of the insights we could bring to medicine from motherhood and the strength and resilience we had as mothers thanks to our time spent in medicine.

Our professional roles and our family roles were inextricably intertwined, for better and for worse. But even on days when our jobs made our home lives harder and on days when our home lives made our jobs harder, we appreciated the privilege of having both. In the call room and the clinic, in the kitchen and the carpool, we tried to support each other as we pieced it all together. We tried to be patient with ourselves.

Eriko ~ Lines

In the ancient Japanese art of kintsugi, nothing is ever broken beyond repair. A communal serving plate, a tapering flower vase, a chopstick rest made with shards of colorful pottery—any shattered object can be mended with lines of golden lacquer. Kintsugi never tries to hide the past. Kintsugi embellishes history, bringing the fragments of the story together, until the damage and the healing become equally meaningful. It elevates the transformed object to something to be treasured rather than discarded. It celebrates the wonder of imperfection. It shapes misfortune into beauty.

My great-grandparents brought pieces of their pasts from Kyoto and Nagasaki to reassemble into new lives when they immigrated to Los Angeles at the end of the nineteenth century. Their children—my grandparents—grew up as Nisei, learning English and Japanese, embracing the opportunities of their new homeland alongside the traditions of their heritage. But in 1942, just as my grandparents were starting families of their own, the United States government issued Executive Order 9066. A response to the attack on Pearl Harbor, this decree forcibly relocated more than one hundred thousand people of Japanese ancestry over the next four years, citing concerns that anyone with sympathies toward Japan might try to subvert stateside efforts during World War II.

Entire families—nearly two-thirds of whom were American citizens—were given less than one week to leave the towns they had called home for generations. They were allowed to take with them only what they could carry. They had no idea if they would ever return. My mother, age two, and my father, age four, didn't know each other when they lined up along a curb on a hundred-degree July morning before being bussed to temporary quarters in whitewashed horse stalls and given a fabric sack to fill with straw for a mattress. Their final destination would be a concentration camp in the desert outside Death Valley. Its grounds were shadowed by tall fences of five-strand barbed wire and eight guard towers. Thirty-six lines of tarpaper barracks, with a single room allotted to each family, stretched toward the dusty horizon.

When my grandparents and their children were released after three years in confinement, they gathered up the bits of their abandoned lives, scrambling to piece together reliable shelter, adequate food, and jobs with employers willing to hire them. They spoke only

English outside their homes and didn't teach the children Japanese, hoping to avoid calling attention to their ethnicity. They prized education, holding up the toil of the hardworking student as a mark of self-discipline. Above all, they embodied the Buddhist virtue of gaman, the will to persevere with dignity in the face of all that their families had endured.

Thirty years after the war, I watched my mother serve as a nurse in our neighborhood's long-term care facility. I knew she had actually wanted to become a physician, like her father and her brother, and had been discouraged from going to medical school as a girl. But her work inspired me. As a child, I loved accompanying her to the facility and chatting with its oldest residents. I made posters for them on their birthdays, marking eighty, ninety, ninety-five years, and beyond.

By the time I was a teenager, I devoted many of my weekends to giving manicures to frail white-haired women, cutting up meat for those too weak to feed themselves, and listening to everyone's stories as the visiting piano player performed the same seven songs on a loop in the sunny common room. Although our family had abandoned many visibly Japanese traditions, a deep and abiding foundation of respect for elders was integral to our values, as was giving back to the community. When I sat with these vulnerable people, full of history and compassion but with few loved ones nearby to share it, I felt like I was making a difference in their lives.

My friends were incredulous that I wanted to spend my time at a place that, to them, felt depressing and smelled strange. My teachers, recognizing my commitment to service and my strong work ethic, told me that I should become a doctor. But my parents said it was too difficult for female physicians to have a family. My ingrained obedience meant that I followed the path they guided me along. I'd spent many hours as a child doodling pictures of wedding gowns and flower arrangements, tending to baby dolls with my sister, and having crushes on the boys in my class. If I couldn't add being a doctor to the family life I'd always dreamed of, then being a doctor wasn't an option.

After high school, I completed a college nursing-degree program and took a challenging position on a surgical ward. Five months after I'd started, my supervisor called me in for a review and told me I was doing great. She said my patients loved me and my colleagues all enjoyed working with me. But then she said that I had to change how I was charting—I had to stop including so much detail, suggesting alternative diagnoses, and overthinking possible outcomes—because I was charting like a physician.

As I worked my way through days and nights at the hospital and reflected on her words, I knew she was right. I had always wanted to learn more about the disease processes affecting my patients' lives, to understand the pathophysiology going on deep inside their cells, to explore all the treatment options and the scientific rationale behind them. I did love taking care of people's basic needs and monitoring their conditions, and I saw the value in those nursing tasks. But it wasn't enough for me. I couldn't suppress the feeling that I was constantly missing opportunities to address the underlying issues that impacted people's health. I realized that if I didn't try to go to medical school I would regret it my whole life.

So, at twenty-two, I signed up for night school science classes. I moved in to a friend's garage apartment to save money, woke up at six o'clock every morning to study, went to evening lectures and exams, got the same burrito from the same take-out window for dinner on my way home every night, and, after a quick shower, plunked back down in my chair to study until midnight. My routine was unwavering. On weekends and one weekday each week, I worked twelve-hour hospital shifts to continue my full-time nursing job.

Finding my way was both jarring and liberating. After spending my whole life meeting everyone else's expectations, I could finally see the line between what I wanted and what my family wanted for me. When I was offered admission to fourteen medical schools across the country, I felt like this success was entirely my own.

With newfound confidence and the relief of having a plan to move to New York City in three months, I relaxed into my final hospital shifts without overthinking what they might mean for my career. I hung out with friends after work instead of returning to my cramped studio to study. I even said yes to a date with the handsome young deliveryman who had recently started leaving treats for me when he brought our lunch orders to the nursing station. Knowing my departure was imminent, Azhar and I shared an understanding that I couldn't commit to anything beyond the next step of my career, and we enjoyed each other's company for what it was.

But in the tumult of moving from west to east and beginning an incredibly rigorous program in a city where I knew nobody, Azhar— even from three thousand miles away—became the most consistent presence in my life. When I returned late at night to my apartment above the subway stop, I found flowers on my doorstep. When I felt intimidated by my classmates, his nightly phone calls lifted my spirits. When I was chilled to the bone in the midst of my first northeastern winter but couldn't afford to turn up the heat, he mailed me a beautiful blue cardigan to wear while I studied. His kindness from afar reminded me that I was loved. He connected me to a piece of home.

Three months into medical school, Azhar and I got engaged, and my parents were less than thrilled. They identified strongly with their Japanese American heritage and had never considered that they might have half-Pakistani grandchildren whose father's first language was Urdu. In a reversal of their earlier admonitions, they had come to support my becoming a physician but were now concerned I might sabotage my career with marriage and family.

Azhar left his life behind to move in with me the following summer. The transition proved more difficult than starting medical school had been, as our concepts of partnership, rooted in vastly different cultures, clashed harshly. Although I was overwhelmed by the demands of intensive science classes and clinical rotations, Azhar criticized me as the laundry piled up—but he never took on washing it himself. For all his kindness, he was deeply uncomfortable having a partner who didn't subordinate her needs to men's expectations in the way that the women who'd raised him had. As we sat across from each other in silence, sharing granola bars and watered-down orange juice to stretch our breakfast budget, I thought that we could overcome our differences if we just kept loving each other fiercely enough.

We made so many wonderful memories together over the next ten years. We hosted a lavish wedding, hoping that celebrating loudly might mend the cracks in our relationship. The stately meeting hall, resplendent with dozens of pale peach roses and cascading white hydrangea swags, and the ring encircling my finger, with its unbroken line of gold and diamonds, matched every fantasy I'd had as a young girl. We toasted to the culmination of my medical training and to the innovative geriatrics program that I was about to embark on developing as a new attending physician. We talked about starting a family. We moved back to California and bought a house together, which did nothing to repair the growing rift between us. We committed to couples therapy and searched for common ground and compromise. Finally, we decided to take some time apart.

Azhar and I were always bound by love. But it wasn't enough. Our differences left us vulnerable to the wounds of our deteriorating marriage but unable to be vulnerable with each other. When we began divorce proceedings, I felt like my whole world was unraveling. Then my beloved mother was diagnosed with breast cancer, and I felt helpless possessing so much medical knowledge but having no expertise in the treatments she was receiving and no way to lessen my own fears about her uncertain prognosis. I seemed to be surrounded by misfortune, with nothing left to bind the pieces together. I poured everything into my work, hoping that my career might shield me from the colossal sense of failure that I felt.

Six months after the divorce, still devastated but somehow res-olute, I decided that I had to start building the life I wanted with intention, without letting memories of what I'd had—or longings for what I'd envisioned—crowd out the experiences I could be having now. I joined a gym to strengthen my body without the goal of look-ing a certain way for any man. I went to concerts and parties with my sister and friends and honored the amazing women in my life. I took classes in traditional Japanese arts, learning the dances of odori and the flower arrangements of ikebana, and arranged budget vacations to exotic locales I had always dreamed of visiting. As I worked my way through what sometimes felt like placeholder years, I hoped that the insights I gained about myself would become the golden lacquer to transform the shards of my experience into something that prepared me for whatever might come next.

When I met Mateo on a blind date a few months later, he seemed intimidated by my background at first. His parents had worked hard to succeed after moving to the United States from Mexico as a young couple, and they had instilled in Mateo and his siblings the values of persistence and determination, but he had never dated a woman with a professional career. Mateo's family, like mine, prized genera-tional ties and filial loyalty. We agreed that our families were the most important people in our lives. We shared an abiding respect for our elders. We both wanted to have children soon and raise them con-nected to their cousins, uncles, aunts, and grandparents. As I began to see past our superficial differences to the deeper common ground, I knew that if I chose to be in a relationship, it wouldn't be to fill a void but to share my life with a true partner.

Mateo moved in to my house four months after we met, and we eloped two months after that. He didn't want a big wedding, and I didn't want a second one. We agreed to prioritize starting our family right away. At thirty-eight, I knew I might not have a lot of time. And Mateo, at forty-four, hoped to have kids while he felt energetic enough to keep up with them. As I began to chart my cycles and learned to use ovulation predictor kits, reproductive medicine felt completely foreign to me as a geriatrician. Again I found myself thinking—as I had when I'd felt helpless to heal my mother's cancer, now mercifully in remission—that being a physician was of surprisingly little use as I stepped into this specialized field with a language and culture so far outside my area of practice.

When I wasn't pregnant after six months, Mateo and I scheduled an appointment at the fertility clinic. Soon we were riding a roller coaster of heartache and disappointment as we endured invasive tests and procedures, attended lectures about financing the costs of treatments, underwent six failed intrauterine inseminations, celebrated a spontaneous pregnancy before it turned into a devastating miscarriage, and spent hours talking with our doctors about surrogacy, preimplantation genetic screening, and other assisted reproductive technology options.

After another year that included three failed cycles of in vitro fertilization as well as a second spontaneous pregnancy and miscarriage, my doctors said it was time to consider using a donor egg and perhaps a surrogate. Although I was discouraged about spending so much time and money on fertility treatments with no success, especially while continuing to pay off debts from the missteps of my previous life, this suggestion unsettled me. It was true that I was almost forty and consumed with the desire to be a mother. I felt emptier at each family gathering, each holiday, each birthday celebrated without a child. I worried that our chance to have a family of our own might have passed. I even felt a sort of loyalty to this medical team, who had been trying to help me since the beginning. Still, my third IVF cycle had gone so smoothly. We had retrieved fourteen eggs. Thirteen had fertilized. Five had survived to transfer on their third day—but none had implanted. I felt so close. I wasn't ready to abandon the conviction that I could conceive and carry our biological child.

My mother, knowing how deeply I had always wanted a baby and having supported me through so much, reassured me that I shouldn't be afraid to try again with my own eggs. She encouraged me to change clinics if that was what my heart was telling me to do. When she told me she and my father wanted to give us their reparation money to pay for our next round of treatment, I was overwhelmed by their generosity.

These funds had come to them exactly twenty years earlier as part of a governmental attempt to offer redress to Japanese Americans for the treatment they had endured during the war. Although the payment was accompanied by a formal apology, the campaign was more about helping the next generation than it was about compensating survivors. Kodomo no tame ni—*for the sake of the children*—amends must be made for the mistakes of the past. Now my parents' reparation money might offer me the life I longed for while carrying on their own legacies through grandchildren.

Mateo and I accepted their gift with humility and gratitude and began our fourth IVF cycle, along with acupuncture and Eastern medicine, at a different fertility clinic. When we first started the new protocol, the medication doses were so much lower and the treatments so much less aggressive that I had to push away the sense that we were giving up. I was astounded that different doctors in the same specialty could have such dissimilar approaches. I couldn't imagine that this downshifted regimen could be successful.

But instead of having the diminished response that I had feared, I developed ovarian hyperstimulation syndrome. The injectable hormones we had been using to encourage egg development triggered my body to overreact. My ovaries tripled in size as their follicles swelled, leaking fluid into my hugely distended abdomen. After a startling middle-of-the-night awakening, the pain was so severe that I truly thought I might die while I gripped Mateo's hand and waited for an ambulance to arrive.

I spent much of the next several weeks in the hospital. I knew I needed to keep up my energy, but relentless nausea quashed my appetite and my bloated belly felt full after just a few bites. I wanted to move around to prevent the life-threatening clots that could develop as a complication of this condition, but the medications made me dizzy and the tangle of lines that delivered them made getting out of bed a challenge. I restlessly searched for any comfortable position, struggling to fall back asleep for hours each time a nurse woke me to check my vital signs. The three culdocentesis procedures—in which a doctor inserted the largest needle I had ever seen through my vaginal wall and removed nearly two liters of fluid each time—were excruciating, but the relief afterward was blissful.

Although my pregnancy hormones had been elevated in the hospital, I knew that could have been a lingering effect of the fertility medications I had been given. So I was beyond excited when the hormones kept rising after I was discharged. I knew this whole ordeal would be worthwhile if I got to take home a baby. At our six-week ultrasound, Mateo and I were stunned to learn that three of the embryos had implanted.

Before each of our transfers, we had fantasized about how excited we would be to have twins. We had never considered triplets. The doctor cautioned us with vague not-quite reassurances: Anything could happen. One of the embryos looked healthier than the other two. We would just have to wait and see. The next week, our follow-up ultrasound showed one bright line with a steady heartbeat, one smaller line with a slower heartbeat, and one silent line in a too-small sac. I was thrilled that one of the embryos was growing so well, but it was heartbreaking to watch the other two wither away on the ultrasound.

Two weeks later, we were down to one baby who looked healthy and strong. I had also started bleeding. Our doctors said this was common after losing a twin or triplet, but it terrified me nonetheless. Now, as I was placed on bed rest and restricted from working, my sense of what it meant to be a patient began to sink in. I had felt so helpless in the hospital, so totally dependent on the staff who took care of me, especially when they seemed harried and overworked or when I saw them furtively looking up protocols to manage a case of hyperstimulation more severe than they had previously encountered. As different as reproductive medicine was from my own area of expertise, I did understand what was happening to me most of the time. I spoke medicine. I knew how to be an advocate for myself. Navigating the fertility world, facing dangerous complications, and now sitting here hoping the bleeding would stop gave me a new appreciation for how scared and confused so many of my patients must be about their own medical care.

By ten weeks into the pregnancy, I'd been released from bed rest and was juggling a full-time clinical schedule and hospital rounds with my own long list of doctors' appointments. By thirteen weeks, all our genetic screening tests had come back reassuring. We declined amniocentesis, realizing that we couldn't imagine choosing termination at this point, no matter the results, and weren't willing to take even the tiniest risk of miscarriage from the procedure. By fifteen weeks, I'd cut back on how often I listened to the gallop of the baby's heartbeat on the portable fetal monitor I had rented to calm my lingering worry. By seventeen weeks, I'd begun to tell people at work that I was pregnant—including the longtime patient who pointed at my belly as she smirked at me and asked, "What is *that*?"

At twenty weeks, we found out that our baby was a boy. He snuggled like a little angel beside his placenta in the gold-hued three-dimensional scan that first revealed his face. I was completely surprised by how much he looked like a person with a distinct personality, sucking his thumb, rubbing his head, clasping his tiny hands together. Suddenly, he was someone I knew.

Seeing him this way made the stakes feel even higher. When my asthma flared after a respiratory infection in my thirtieth week of pregnancy, it wasn't just *the baby* whose health I fretted about, it was *my son*. It was my son I shopped for as I wandered store aisles during week thirty-four, choosing bedding and diapers. And it was my son I realized no amount of planning could ever prepare me to meet. I felt simultaneously like I should gather up every piece of baby equipment ever invented to care for this child and, in contradiction, like my gratitude for his existence should be enough alone to shelter him.

Then, during week thirty-five, my abstract worries crystallized into something more definitive. On that quiet Thursday, I spent a few hours catching up on clinic paperwork, then walked across the medical complex for my prenatal checkup in the late afternoon. A few days earlier, I had called my obstetrician with concerns that I hadn't been feeling as much fetal movement lately. Knowing how nervous I had been throughout the pregnancy, she calmly reassured me and encouraged me to keep my upcoming appointment, which would be with one of her colleagues since she would be out of town. Meanwhile, she said, I should get plenty of rest and drink more water.

But as soon as I sat on the clinic exam table and started telling this other obstetrician about the decreased movement, she looked uneasy. She rolled the bedside ultrasound up beside me. When her quick scan showed a strong heartbeat but low amniotic fluid levels, she sent me back across campus to the hospital for more thorough imaging.

The sudden escalation in events was alarming—but not as alarming as when, just a few minutes into the formal hospital scan, the ultrasound technician jumped up and left the room. I had already begun to panic when she returned with the obstetrician I had just seen in clinic. They told me that reviewing my scan together was standard protocol since the baby's heart rate had dipped briefly. We didn't need to rush Mateo here. We didn't need to transfer to a facility with a neonatal intensive care unit.

I settled in for monitoring on the labor and delivery ward, grateful for how far we had come since my hospital admission for ovarian hyperstimulation. I called Mateo, who was at work and didn't know about any of this. He sounded concerned immediately, and I found myself reassuring him that this was just a precautionary measure and that I would probably be discharged first thing in the morning. Since it was late, I encouraged him to go home to sleep. I promised to let him know if anything changed. By the time I'd had some dinner, the baby's heart rate had been stable for several hours, so I decided to get some rest too.

Just before dawn, I got up to use the restroom. As I climbed back into bed, a screeching alarm sounded and ten people sprinted into my room, shouting at each other as they rolled me onto all fours. I heard one of them say that the baby was crashing as another gave me a shot in my arm and yet another held up a clipboard, urging me to sign the consent form for an emergency cesarean delivery. I was disoriented and crying as they rolled me toward the operating room. I heard myself scream that I needed Mateo to be there. Suddenly the obstetrician from the clinic was by my side again, saying that Mateo was on his way and apologizing that they were going to have to put me under general anesthesia to get the baby out immediately.

Then she did something magical. "This is going to hurt a lot," she said, "but I need you to bear with me." With that, she pushed her whole hand into my vagina and against my cervix. My son's heart rate suddenly returned to normal.

The obstetrician's maneuvers had bought us enough time for the anesthesiologist to give me an epidural so I could be awake for the delivery. When Mateo burst into the room a few minutes later, the surgeons cut the first incision. As soon as they pulled out our son, they saw the cause of his distress. Not only did he have three tight knots in his umbilical cord, but the cord was wedged into my cervix from above, compromising his blood supply every time gravity pushed the weight of his body down against the prolapsed cord.

By some miracle, the delivery went smoothly. In spite of the cord complications, in spite of being five weeks early, in spite of whatever stress he had been under during the past few days—leading to the decreased fetal movement that, we now knew, I hadn't been imagining—baby Kai was perfect. Peeking out from his swaddle as Mateo held him close for me to kiss, our son's beautiful face looked just as I had pictured it after seeing him on all those ultrasounds. Meeting him was the best moment of my entire life.

As we both recovered in the hospital for six days, Kai proved himself tiny but mighty. The doctors said his lungs were more mature than the typical preemie's, thanks to the steroids I had been taking for my asthma exacerbations. Staring down at him, I couldn't believe he was finally here, a part of me and a part of Mateo, a real live baby with a shock of black hair and that delicious baby smell. Even his cries didn't bother me because I was so relieved to hold him in my arms.

This love was like nothing I had ever experienced. Once we were home, I slept with one eye open to keep him safe. I hesitated to have guests to the house, worried they would bring along their winter germs. We hunkered down as a family of three as friends and neighbors prepared for the end-of-year holidays. Oblivious to the festive commotion all around me, deep in the rapture of new motherhood, I felt like we were living in our own private snow globe. I couldn't believe that—after all the drama, after all the years—I had finally become a mother.

We somehow moved through those fragile newborn hours into daring toddler days and rebellious preschooler capers. When Kai was three, he started asking for a sibling. And not in a casual, occasional sort of way. Every day. Insistently, eagerly, relentlessly. What Kai didn't know was that we had gone through a fifth round of fertility treatments eight months after his birth, using our three remaining embryos. When I'd landed in the hospital with ovarian hyperstimulation again, our doctors had told us that it wouldn't be safe or wise or ethical to continue. We were done. Even as I appreciated the wonder of my son, I lamented the finality of this pronouncement. I struggled to reframe our family as complete, to accept that Kai would be an only child—and now his innocent request was rekindling my grief.

An all-too-brief surprise pregnancy when I was forty-three brought my unresolved longing even more clearly into focus. Feeling optimistic, we told Kai he was going to be a big brother. Then, after the miscarriage, Kai kept asking me what had happened to the baby in my belly. We tried to distract him with martial arts lessons, trips to amusement parks, and even a pet hamster. But he persisted, and I couldn't stop thinking about having another child either. We really did want to give Kai a sibling. As older parents, we worried about the future. Both of us had large, supportive families, and the thought of our son being alone saddened us greatly.

One morning, after Kai had spent hours crying about wanting a sibling, Mateo suggested we consider adoption. I was shocked. Through all the years of trying to get pregnant, through all the interventions, through all the obstacles, we had never discussed adoption. It wasn't that I was opposed to the idea. I just hadn't thought of it as an option. To my determined-to-get-pregnant mind, adoption had seemed to introduce so many unimaginable variables—even more than complex fertility regimens, which at least had the guise of residing in the quantifiable realm of medicine—and that scared me.

Now, several years into motherhood, the line between simple and complicated looked much less absolute. Beginning to investigate domestic adoption, we quickly learned that our chances of being chosen were low because we were in our forties and already had a biological child. Undeterred, we dug into our research and found an agency in Utah that seemed like a good fit. We especially liked that they conducted semi-open adoptions, allowing birth parents and adoptive parents to meet but requiring that all interactions go through the agency. The process reminded me of medical school applications, as we spent the better part of a year taking adoption classes, filling out background check forms, scheduling home study interviews, and creating our application portfolio, including a handmade family photo book and narrative profiles.

And we waited, trying to carry on with our lives as if we weren't waiting. We didn't tell Kai what we were doing. That turned out to be wise. Two months in a row, two different biological mothers narrowed their choices down to us and one other couple, then chose the other couple. Like in all the unsuccessful rounds of fertility treatments, we felt like we had come so close. We were heartbroken.

Then, six months later, Mateo and I flew to Salt Lake City and sat in a darkened ultrasound room that reminded me of the one where I had been examined just before Kai's birth. Beside us was a young couple named Kaylee and Robert, and in front of us was the grainy image of their twenty-four-week fetus. Robert said they had chosen us because we were a biracial couple just as they were, with Asian and Hispanic backgrounds, and they thought their son might look like us. We watched together in silence as he stretched and curled on the screen. I could barely believe it might be our turn.

Back at home, we got updates every week or two as Kaylee's pregnancy progressed through the next four months without incident, aside from what she told us was a mild case of gestational diabetes. The agency sent photos from each routine ultrasound. Mateo and I decided to name the baby Hunter. We traveled to Utah again a week before his due date to be present for the birth, while my mother-in-law stayed home with Kai. But when a scheduled induction turned into an emergency cesarean for fetal distress, I felt like I was reliving Kai's delivery from another angle, just as helpless as an adoptive mother now as I had been as a biological mother then.

After we had passed more than an hour pacing anxiously in the waiting room, Robert came in to tell us that Hunter had been taken to the neonatal intensive care unit. Eight hours later, when we finally got a detailed update about his condition, we learned that he had been born blue and unresponsive and full of fluid. He had a serious heart disease called cardiomyopathy. He was getting breathing support from a ventilator. The medical team had started him on tube feedings and powerful medications through a central line running directly into his umbilical vein. He had only one kidney, and it was failing.

The adoption agency representative, who had arrived just before

the doctors' update, sat down with Mateo and me in the family conference room as we struggled to process all this. She told us that we
could walk away if we needed to. That they'd understand if we had
changed our minds. She sounded distressingly businesslike, though
not unkind. But the idea of changing our minds made no sense to
me. Hunter was already our son. We would never abandon a child
I had given birth to who had medical issues, so why would we leave
Hunter when he needed us most?

Fortunately, Hunter was strong, and we watched him improve
slowly every day in the NICU. We rearranged our schedules to sit by
his incubator for four weeks, though we had originally planned to be
gone from home and work for only one. When the doctors suggested
extending his stay, predicting another month until discharge, we were
grateful to be able to leverage my professional training to negotiate a
complex series of accommodations so he could come home with us
sooner.

Back in California with our fragile five-week-old, we transformed
his nursery into a hospital room. A portable monitor hanging from
the crib gave a constant readout of his blood oxygen levels—when he
hadn't managed to kick the sensor off his foot. A whirring pump on a
rolling cart connected to his nutritional-support formula, delivering
calories and nutrients through his nose directly to his stomach—until
each time he dislodged the feeding tube.

As I stood guard over his healing body, restless in sleep with arms
spread wide, I knew how uncomfortable he was. Every bit of his skin
was stretched taut with swelling as his overworked heart strained to
maintain the flow of his circulation. I remembered the intense pain
of my ovarian hyperstimulation syndrome, which had caused only
localized distension in my abdomen, and the blessed relief after each
fluid removal. I felt the deepest empathy for this little boy.

Even with my experience as a nurse and a physician, I was overwhelmed by the near-constant sounding of alarms, refilling of feeds,
and flushing of lines. I didn't sleep for more than two hours at a

stretch. I requested an extended leave from work. I tried to carve out special time with Kai so he wouldn't feel ignored. I rarely had a conversation with Mateo that didn't relate to our sons' immediate needs.

But to see Kai cradle his baby brother with such tenderness made it all worthwhile. And I was in awe of Hunter's resilience. As a parade of therapists entered our home, as we bundled him up to shuttle him to endless medical appointments, as he endured yet another procedure to check his blood chemistry or scan his heart, this amazing little boy smiled through it all. His huge grin charmed everyone he met, announcing, "Hi! I'm Hunter! And I'm just happy to be here!"

Five years after Hunter's birth, our days are full of sibling bonding and bickering, of medical setbacks and triumphs, of change and consistency. Until we adopted him, I never could have imagined I would feel so close to a child who was not biologically connected to me. There really is no difference in the way I love each of my two sons. When I was young, my elders taught me to value family above all else. Now that I'm older, I still do—but adoption has opened my mind to a broader view of what a family can be. And bringing Hunter into our lives turns out to have prepared me for the biggest surprise our family has experienced yet.

Last year, Mateo and I were traveling after a work conference, where I had delivered a presentation about balancing parenthood and medicine, when he received a message from an unfamiliar person. I watched his face as he took it in, his expression cryptic. I asked him what it was about, but he didn't seem to hear. Then he turned toward me, eyes wide, saying it was from someone named Christa. She had run a commercial genetic test, trying out the new technology just for fun, and believed she was his daughter.

A flurry of photos and phone calls over the next few weeks confirmed it. She looked and sounded just like him. She had been told her whole life that another man was her father, while Mateo had been completely unaware of her existence. A poised and successful thirty-two-year-old teacher with children of her own, she wanted nothing more from Mateo than to get to know him and the rest of our family. Shocking as her sudden appearance was, it didn't take me very long to sort out my initial misgivings about what her role in our lives could be.

As I opened myself to a relationship with her, I felt so fortunate to call this thoughtful, intelligent woman my stepdaughter. I realized that, biologically, Christa was just the adult version of the child we might have had if we had followed the recommendation of our doctor ten years ago to use a donor egg with a surrogate. She is now unequivocally part of our family. Our holiday cards this winter featured all three of our children, biological, adopted, and discovered, now united through strange grace and good fortune.

Looking at my life today, I can't believe how these pieces have come together. Sometimes my memories feel like shards of countless different lives. When the medical students and residents I teach ask me how I got to where I am, I smile and think to myself, *How long do you have to listen?*

Because it's almost certainly not the path they are imagining. These trainees respect me as a professional at the pinnacle of my career but don't understand that work was one of the only things that kept me grounded when the rest of my life had shattered. They hear that I have a supportive husband but don't know that my first marriage ended in devastation. They learn that I'm close to my family but aren't aware of the connection that Kai and I have to our elders through my parents' reparation funds. They admire the photographs of two sweet little boys adorning my office desktop but don't see the three miscarriages, six failed intrauterine inseminations, five in vitro fertilization cycles, loss of two out of three triplets, and eighteen months of adoption proceedings we went through to get them—and they have no idea of the richness that Christa and her family have added to our lives.

Years ago, I put my faith in love, and it wasn't enough. Now, in this life that Mateo and I have built together, loving each other fiercely is exactly what makes us a family. The cracks that run through our stories remind us of where we've broken and where we've healed. The golden lines that bind us trace the wonder of our imperfections.

We do not try to hide the past. We have shaped these moments into beauty.

We were never beyond repair.

Stacey ~ This One Thing

Part of me must have thought that our relationship was the best I was ever going to get.

We were passionate about exploring the world together, from plunging into cold-water dive trips with the giant Pacific octopus to soaking up history lessons in the halls of fourteenth-century European cathedrals. We could shift seamlessly from a sweaty morning racing side by side on treadmills to an evening dressed in our finest for the symphony. As an established entrepreneur with a thriving landscaping business, he had the time and the money to provide for his aging parents and to shower his beloved nieces and nephews with gifts. He was one of the first men I'd dated who didn't need anyone to take care of him. Most appealing of all, his strong personality and his incredible self-assurance were balanced by a rare and genuine kindness. Having him in my life brought all these great things. But I was still missing this one thing I really wanted, this one thing I had always expected to have. Maybe this was the compromise I'd need to accept: David did not want to have kids.

We had met at the local scuba shop where I worked nights and weekends. At twenty-seven years old, I had the day job I'd always dreamed of. But my elementary school teaching salary alone couldn't fund the travel I loved, and I had visions of a trip to whitewashed hilltop villas among the Greek Isles. David, just a few years older and a friend of my coworker, had come in one day to buy a new wetsuit. After regaling me with tales from a recent adventure—the dive boat he was on had run aground on a rocky outcropping, and their group had needed an airlift rescue—he gave me his business card and smiled. His eyes were as captivating as his stories. He said he'd really like to take me out sometime. It was refreshing to be approached by someone so direct.

Our connection felt just as natural, and within a couple of months we were spending all our free time together. One weekend, as we drove home from a spectacular trip full of sunsets and beach wanderings, our conversation drifted through big questions about our pasts and our priorities. When David asked me if I'd always wanted to be a teacher, I recalled the summer just before I turned six, when my parents had brought home a secretary's desk, an oversized roll of paper, and a pile of old textbooks from a yard sale, then watched me spend hours inventing lessons for my brothers. But as much as I loved witnessing the joy of discovery in other people, I relished my quiet time at the end of the day—and I wasn't quite ready to be like my colleagues with young children, who went home to the same developmental stages and conflicts we dealt with in the classroom. David agreed, shaking his head, and said he didn't know how I could be around kids all day long. We laughed together, deciding that teaching was natural birth control.

Serving as a teacher, what I had grown to value most was being a trusted listener for my students' concerns about their lives at and beyond school. When I learned in a staff meeting that our district was down to a single counselor who visited for one day every other week to support a population of more than three hundred students, this void called to me. I came home one night and told David that I wanted to go to graduate school to become a clinical psychologist.

He encouraged me from my first mention of changing careers and was unabashedly enthusiastic about how much more money I would make once I was done with my training. The youngest of five, David had grown up in a family that was sometimes destitute from poor investment decisions, occasionally flush from transient business successes, and always financially unstable. He had learned to equate a steady salary with worth and achievement.

He suggested that, while I was in training, I could manage the office side of his company to sharpen my business skills, to bring in some extra wages, and to feel better about contributing to our shared aspirations. He was right that I needed all those things. Having already quit my job at the scuba shop to have more time to spend with David, I was very concerned that I would become financially dependent on him.

If we were going to take this huge leap together, I also needed much more clarity on how he envisioned our future. I knew that exotic travel and intellectual conversations wouldn't be enough to sustain me. I told him I needed to know if he wanted children. David made the point—and I didn't disagree—that I wouldn't want to have a baby while I was in school or trying to launch a new career, which would probably take several years. He convinced me that it was too soon to have the conversation. So we waited. We waited to talk about it more, we waited to think about the decision, and we waited to confront it more intentionally.

I was excited—and, admittedly, distracted—by the thrill of jumping into a new professional field with so much to learn. But as I moved into my psychology training, I was unnerved by how much of our coursework required deep self-reflection. As the months went by, I learned to acknowledge struggles that were lingering in the back of my mind, to draw them forward, to explore their origins, to confront them. I started being more observant about my own relationships. I noticed that every time I mentioned children to David, I felt a resistance I couldn't explain. This felt bigger than I'd hoped it would be. I decided I just wasn't ready to poke that bear.

Instead, I turned my attention toward other things that had

contributed to making me the person I was. I wrote papers reevaluating my relationship with my mother, the impact of my inspiring second-grade teacher, and the influence of a questionable high school boyfriend. But I avoided thinking about whether David and I were headed toward having a family—because this single question was too important to me to risk uncovering an answer I couldn't accept. In every other aspect, our relationship seemed so close to perfect that I feared jeopardizing what we had together. But I was starting to notice that this was true only as long as I stayed to the agreed-upon topics and within the range of agreed-upon behavior. As long as I didn't force this one thing.

Like all psychology students, toward the end of my training I was required to go through individual counseling. As I worked with a truly gifted therapist to explore the parallels between my childhood family dynamics and my partnership with David, any misgivings I held about whether therapy would actually prove useful to me—seeing myself as fairly content and eminently well adjusted, and having never undergone any sort of therapy before—were quickly dashed. I came to see that, as much as I avoided confrontation, David was masterful at deflection. He was manipulative in such a loving way that I had never realized just how manipulative he was. With newfound resolve, I tried to be honest with David—and myself—about how much I wanted children. While our relationship had previously seemed so carefree, so compatible, our discussions now more and more often led to fights.

Still, I felt like I had a little more sympathy for his hesitation after he confided in me about a memory that had hardly faded in twenty years: the feeling of walking into his girlfriend's room one afternoon when they were both just sixteen and seeing pieces of pastel fabric laid out in a neat line across her bed. Realizing that he was looking at a collection of tiny one-piece jammies and booties, he felt the course of his life suddenly and irreparably wrenched out of his control. Even though the pregnancy had ended in a first-trimester miscarriage, being railroaded into fatherhood still loomed as a terrifying prospect for him.

Several months later, we stood beside the Space Needle on New Year's Eve, surrounded by a sea of strangers, huddled together and looking up as we waited for the ball to drop over the skies of Seattle. With his chest pressed against my back, David whispered that he loved me—and that he wanted to marry me. I turned toward him, and we kissed as the first firework lit up the night. The crowd around us realized what was going on and started cheering. In their reverie, they missed the startlingly unromantic clause that followed as he locked eyes with me: "But before we get married," he said, "we'll need to do some counseling around whether we're going to have a family."

My hold on him loosened. Our timeless moment began to tarnish immediately, as I realized just how conditional David's love for me was. I held back my tears as the fireworks kept crashing overhead.

Over the next three months in couples counseling, we explored my assumptions about motherhood and the identity I envisioned for myself in a marriage. We considered the impact of David's family's humiliating excommunication from the Church of Jesus Christ of Latter-day Saints when he was a teenager on his views of fatherhood and family traditions. We went in circles trying to understand the roots of how we each felt about parenthood. Week after week, even our therapist seemed unable to pin David down.

Finally she told him that she needed to understand—right now—what he was thinking. David replied clearly and immediately that he was not ready to have children. That he did not want them. Then he skipped a beat and added that that might change once he got closer to forty. So I heard him saying, at thirty-five, that he just needed more time. I finally had my answer, and it was the one I'd wanted to hear.

Bolstered by the counseling we'd done, our early years of marriage were blissful. I felt confident we were finally on the same page about having a family eventually. I just needed to be patient, and part of me was grateful to have a respite from revisiting the topic constantly. Deep into my counseling internship and pursuing a second master's in marriage and family therapy, I was consumed enough by my work to suppress any insights into my own life that I might be gaining. Putting aside self-reflection was a welcome relief as I focused on counseling others through their troubled relationships instead.

But a couple of years into our marriage, I started to feel the pull of motherhood more intensely. My practice was growing steadily, my days felt predictable again, and, at thirty-four, I was ready to reassess my goals in life. David was almost thirty-eight, which certainly sounded closer to forty to me. Still, every time I brought up the topic of starting a family, he would reiterate that we'd had this discussion already, that I knew what his answer was. He may have been thinking *No*, but I was still hearing *You just need to give me more time.*

On Christmas Eve, when I unwrapped a huge box covered in dancing snowmen, I discovered seven layers of tissue paper surrounding a note on a scrap of white paper. *Your gift,* it read in David's tiny, precise script, *is a big adventure.* Thrilled, I followed clues on a scavenger hunt and solved each riddle. I wandered around the house, finding one clue under the bathroom sink tucked into a spare roll of toilet paper, one nestled by the forks in a kitchen drawer, one hanging from my key chain.

When I pulled the last clue out from behind the picture frame on the mantel, I was giddy with anticipation. David stopped me. In the light of the fire, back where we had started beside our tree, he held up a second envelope and told me I had a choice to make. The gift I had found, he said, taking it in his right hand, was for someone who wanted to have a family. But the gift he was holding, he said, raising it steadily higher in his left, was the one I would get if I wanted to continue our adventures by ourselves. I could open the second envelope only if I would promise to stop talking about having kids for the next six months.

I was speechless—and furious. All this work, all the thought that had gone into this special occasion, and this was the message he wanted to give me? It was just like his misguided wedding proposal.

Another holiday, another utterly romantic idea ruined in the cruelest way. I grabbed both envelopes out of his hands and tossed them into the fire.

Later, when he told me that the gift in the no-children envelope had been the trip to the Greek Isles I'd been dreaming of for years, I barely cared. He'd taken something that I'd always wished for and turned it into something that highlighted what I longed for but didn't have. But his ploy worked, in a way. I was so frustrated by the scavenger hunt that our communication all but shut down for the rest of the winter and well into the spring.

Then, in June, Savannah came into our life. But this precious baby wasn't ours, so we had her only for a day or two a week, while her mom—one of my best friends—needed to work. For eight months, I felt like we were practicing being a family as my husband and I took care of this beautiful dark-haired creature. David was so nurturing with her. He loved to take her to sing-alongs and art classes and the zoo. He talked about her when we weren't with her and always wanted to hold her when we were. He even took up photography—researching and buying all the best, most expensive equipment—specifically to take her milestone pictures and family portraits. It felt like David was finally warming up to parenthood now that he had a real child to spend time with. I could see our future. It was thrilling.

Being with Savannah filled my heart with love, but it was also incredibly painful. Even though we were in the thick of it, carting around her stroller and washing her sippy cups and changing her diapers, we were still just pretending. I loved my friend so much and I loved that baby so much and I wanted to be there for them. But giving her back and walking away—and reminding myself that this life wasn't really mine—was disorienting every time. I was getting less effective at distracting myself from what I really wanted. So many things that I'd used to enjoy felt hollow: hiking with friends, redecorating our home, even connecting with my patients. I started getting terrible headaches and nausea. I felt constantly off-balance, both literally and figuratively, like the room was spinning and I didn't know what to do to make it stop.

That's when David surprised me with the sports car I'd wanted for years. Looking out the window, I saw the shiny silver coupe with a huge red bow in the driveway below our bedroom, just like in a commercial. But as we strolled through the neighborhood with Savannah a few days later, with me still swept away by the generosity and thoughtfulness of this incredible gift and rambling on about how amazing our life together was and how I couldn't wait to have a baby of our own too, he stopped suddenly and turned to face me.

Didn't I see? He didn't want to be a father. Didn't I understand? The car he'd bought me—it was a two-seater. By accepting it, he said, I was agreeing that we didn't need children in our life.

I was completely shocked. I felt betrayed and misled, devastated that he hadn't moved any closer to wanting a family while I'd given him the time I thought he'd needed. We went back into counseling. The therapist guided us through discussion after discussion, seeking compassion, seeking solutions. It quickly became clear that, for David, there was no option. Nothing had changed for him.

I began to realize that our struggles were rooted in the vast difference in how David and I understood compromise. I saw compromise as a mutual seeking of balance, a graceful negotiation, a coming together in a place of agreement. He saw compromise as a sacrifice without gain, a weakening to others' demands, a negative to which he was unwilling to succumb. I heard it as a noun: *I'm sure we can work together to find a compromise.* He heard it as a verb: *She's asking me to compromise myself and all that I believe in.* Would I end up fulfilling his definition, compromising myself entirely to suit David and losing myself in the process, while he never changed a bit? I had promised to make our partnership work, but was I willing—or even able—to alter the foundations of who I thought I was?

My headaches kept getting worse, and news of friends' new babies kept arriving, with each announcement setting me off-balance again. Couple by couple, they started declining evening cocktails and spontaneous nights at the movies. The annual summer houseboat trip we'd all taken together in the past was now—with sheepish apologies—open only to families. I'd been warning David for years that as our friends had children their priorities were going to change, and we were going to be left behind. We would only have each other. As I saw the future unfolding, I didn't think that was going to be enough. But as painful as it was to be in this increasingly lonely marriage, I was too afraid of the unknown to leave.

In an effort to rekindle our connection, we were planning a trip to Costa Rica. One humid August night, we sat down with maps and itineraries spread out on the table before us. I asked David if he wanted to spend more time in the nature reserves or the cities. He paused, looking at me as if the question didn't quite make sense.

He answered flatly that he wanted a divorce.

I was blindsided. I started sobbing. Then it dawned on me: for the past six months, he'd been separating shared accounts, itemizing our individual purchases, and training an office assistant to take over my job responsibilities. While I'd been trying to reconcile our differences and looking deeper into myself to seek common ground, David had been carving me out of his life so delicately that I hadn't even noticed.

Over the weeks that followed, I tried to talk to him. I begged and I pleaded, but he was unmovable. I said things that I'm glad I can't quite remember, because they would be far too humiliating to revisit. He grew mean-spirited and callous, making hurtful comments as if solidifying the bad parts of our relationship might make it easier for me to let go. It didn't.

My head was spinning, both emotionally with the sudden changes in my life and physically with the headaches and vertigo that seemed to get worse with each day. I was certainly under enough stress to explain away these symptoms, but when I started losing the hearing in my left ear, I finally sought medical advice. In October, on my thirty-sixth birthday, in the midst of a divorce, and while living on my own with no idea what my future would hold, I received my diagnosis: a brain tumor on my seventh cranial nerve, right around my ear.

After so many years straining to hear the meanings behind David's words, hearing only what I wanted and needed to hear, my hearing was literally failing me. I was told I needed immediate surgery. I didn't know if I'd need chemotherapy or radiation—or if the treatment would spare my fertility. Getting out of this bad marriage certainly didn't guarantee I was ever going to have the family I longed for.

Fortunately, my surgery went smoothly and my physical prognosis was excellent, with no need for further medical treatment. I was left feeling both incredibly grateful and completely lost as I headed into the cold of winter. December was not my favorite month, reminiscent as it was of clumsy proposals and misguided scavenger hunts. As I began to recover on the other side of this ordeal, I started going on blind dates and exploring dating services. I wasn't sure I was ready to be dating again. But the last nine years of my life blurred behind me, and I was not willing to risk wasting any more time. I couldn't sit around feeling sorry for myself that there was one man out there who didn't love me.

I was disarmingly honest with everyone I met. I would open each conversation with questions about whether he wanted to have kids. Anyone who was intimidated by my forwardness wasn't worth my energy. For all its heartbreak, my time with David had shown me that bringing a child into the world was so much more than just one thing. To me, it meant being open to love, embracing hope and optimism, and wanting to shape the future. It proclaimed a shared purpose and a vision that was greater than two people. It embraced the messiness and complexity and change that define love itself. It was the one thing that meant *everything*. And I could build a life only with someone who understood that and felt the same way.

Keith and I met up at a restaurant less than six months after

David had asked me for a divorce. Whereas the dates I'd been on before this had felt like job interviews, our time together immediately felt like reconnecting with a friend. We spent hours lingering over a five-course dinner as we recounted stories of our travels, our families, our careers—and the disappointments of our past relationships. He had recently broken up with a woman who had strung him along for more than three years before admitting that she never wanted to have kids.

Keith had always wanted to be a father. Now in his early forties, he was struggling to meet single women who wanted children and were still physically able to have them. Many of the women he met who wanted families were too young for him and felt too immature or in-experienced. The ones who were more confident and interesting were usually—by their own assessments—too old to have children. He had never been married, but he had dated many people and had learned a lot about himself in the process. Keith felt like he'd spent most of his adult life trying to find someone who shared his values and his vision of family. When the restaurant closed, we walked to his car so I could meet his regal gray Weimaraner, who licked me all over and then leapt out of the car and galloped down the street. Keith chased after him and I laughed, feeling hopeful again for the first time in as long as I could remember.

Keith asked me to marry him six months after we met, and we were married six months after that, on the one-year anniversary of our first date. We had a lot of serious discussions very early, which was not very romantic. Then again, maybe it was, because communicating openly was important to both of us, and we cared enough to be sure we were committed to building a life that reflected our shared values. I was still really skeptical about love. I constantly worried: *Am I doing this all too fast? If I pushed through doubts I should have had last time, should I be having more doubts now? What am I missing this time around?*

Five years have passed since that first date. This morning, I dropped off our three-year-old son at preschool and went for a walk in the woods. Twenty-five weeks pregnant with our daughter, I did all I could to keep up as our nineteen-month-old son toddled off the path and played among the ferns. Reflecting on the past makes me deeply grateful for what I have and who I am today. Still, I can't help but remember a blur of mistakes and misinterpretations. Did this all happen because I didn't wait for the right person? Or was David the right person for that time in my life because he got me to where I am now?

Emotionally, I wish I had been able to end my relationship with David sooner, to take back all the years I lost. But intellectually, I can see that the steps I took with David, and on my own during our years together, prepared me for this life. Without that time with David, I wouldn't be here, now, with these kids, with this family, with my beloved husband.

Now, even as we're happily into marriage and parenthood together, I vividly remember how much reassurance I needed to let Keith into my life, to trust love again. Whenever I got nervous about how quickly things were moving, Keith would say the words that healed me a little more each time I heard them, reminding me patiently that this wasn't fast. That we'd waited a long time for each other. That this love was the one thing we'd been searching for all our lives.

Bree ~ Maker

They had planned the celebratory dinner for weeks. Charlotte had layered a hearty lasagna and tossed a bowl of the freshest greens. James had baked crisp cannoli and selected the perfect red wine to complement the menu. Now, unable to reconcile the long-imagined event with the reality, they left it all in the fridge and called in an order for takeout. The guest of honor would not be attending. Charlotte and James asked us to come anyway.

Mark and I sat in our car in their driveway and talked about what had happened. I knew that this couple, both dear friends of his since middle school, had started trying to have a child when they were first married fifteen years ago. They had been through a merciless series of expensive and painful fertility tests, medical procedures, and adoption applications, but none of their efforts had led to parenthood. Today was the day their luck was supposed to turn around. Today was supposed to be their first day at home with their new son.

But yesterday, as Charlotte and James were leaving the hospital with the three-day-old baby they were about to adopt, the three-day-old baby they had already named, a security guard had run down the hallway to catch up with them. Given a seventy-two-hour window to call off the adoption, the baby's birth mother had changed her mind at hour seventy-one. They'd had to carry the little boy back into the hospital and walk away without him.

On the phone last night, James had described the experience to Mark, and now Mark described it to me: Driving five hours home, silent and heartbroken. Removing the blue plaid car seat. Dropping the diaper bag in a corner of the dinosaur-themed nursery they had prepared when they had been matched four months ago.

"It just makes me so sad," I said, staring blankly at the windshield. "I could totally have their baby."

At twenty-two, I had already had two uncomplicated full-term pregnancies. Vivian, my two-and-a-half-year-old daughter, had been an accident, conceived when I was eighteen and still in high school. Her brother, Nolan, just sixteen months younger, wasn't exactly planned either. But they were both healthy, and so was I, and I loved them more than anything. Being a mother, becoming their mother, was a defining part of what had made me who I was.

Vivi and Nolan's father wasn't someone I wanted in any of our lives. Jake seemed to come around only when he was courting a new woman he hoped to impress by acting the part of a doting dad. He was nearly impossible to pin down for child support. In the ten months we'd been dating, Mark had already proven himself a far better parent to my kids than Jake had ever been. Something in me still longed to have another baby with a father who wanted to be involved. Mark, now in his mid-thirties, had had testicular cancer twelve years earlier. Because of the surgeries and treatments he'd been through, we knew he would never be able to have biological children.

Maybe this is my chance to give a child to a father who wants to be in that child's life, I thought, as we sat in front of the house. But if I were to make such a personal offer, would they be offended? Would they think I was good enough to carry their baby? As I told Mark what I was thinking—and how strange I knew it sounded—he said he could help me talk to them if that was something I really wanted. Knowing that I tended to be anxious and a little shy, Mark suggested that I go pick up the takeout while he went inside to raise the idea that I might be open to trying to help them.

Within half an hour, we were eating together in awkward silence, clustered at one end of their massive dining room table as six extra chairs sat unoccupied, calling out to be filled with large family gatherings. Then I saw Charlotte reach for James across the table. Her knuckles blanched as she squeezed his hand in hers. They looked at each other nervously. "Charlotte and I would like to talk to you about what you told Mark," James finally said, both of them now turning to look at me. Their expressions were at once expectant and doubting, like a child who has been promised a gift that seems too good to be true—like a couple who has glimpsed one final opportunity to fulfill a dream they had been about to give up forever.

The longing in their eyes stirred something in me akin to the feelings I'd had when Mark and I had visited an animal shelter a few months earlier. As we'd left the building, I'd looked back over my shoulder and thought to myself, *I could adopt all these dogs.* Mark and I shared a soft spot for downtrodden creatures, and we had brought one dog home that day. She was a wild gray rescue mutt, a beautiful, exotic girl that we named Dakota. I think I was drawn to her guarded, wolflike glare and her history of abuse because I'd grown up feeling a little broken. Loved, for sure, and not neglected, but cautious and wary, eager to be a loving companion yet somehow defined by the instability I'd endured in my own young life. Had Charlotte's experience with infertility left her feeling damaged too? Could I do anything to make another woman feel more whole?

Within weeks, the idea that I might be able to help James and Charlotte had transformed from a heartfelt but abstract notion into a real possibility. When we met again to talk more about how we each envisioned the situation working, I realized that I was also drawn to their story because I was part of a pieced-together and chosen family of sorts myself. Since my mother had worked long and irregular hours at the local grocery store to provide for me, her only child, I'd grown up living mostly with my best friend and her parents. Now, I was trying to raise two children myself, with a little help from my mom and Mark and a lot of help from one very accommodating day care provider. Striving to keep us financially stable, as my mother had done for me, I cleaned houses for a living while putting myself through school to become an emergency medical technician.

I couldn't tell James and Charlotte much about my family medical history. I'd always thought of myself as healthy, but I hadn't been to the doctor too often growing up. My mother didn't have extra time or money to spend on medical care for me or for herself, and I didn't know anything about my father's health, other than the fact that he was still alive. Struggling with his temper and his drinking, he had been in and out of prison—mostly in—since I was a toddler. Automated messages updated me about the smallest changes in his status and his location within the system. Getting a notification that he'd just moved cell blocks could be jarring in the middle of an ordinary day, but having more information also helped me feel safer. I couldn't dig for details about him, because I knew that past inquiries had made him feel threatened. If he thought I wanted something from him, he might come looking for me when he got out, jeopardizing my family's safety. I had to keep as much distance as I could.

I understood that, although I was only in my early twenties, I'd already lived a hard life. Because of this, I also saw myself as independent, adaptable, and self-made. My go-to coping mechanism was to cobble together whatever resources I could and look for the humor in any situation. With this strategy, I'd never found something I couldn't handle. Now, when I witnessed the void in James and Charlotte's life created by their yearning for a child, I felt like all their reserves had been depleted and there was no brighter side. That was difficult for me to process and even more difficult for me to accept. I felt like if I might be able to help them, I needed to offer to try.

James and Charlotte had attempted to become parents in so many ways over so many years that everything was already in place. In the wake of their failed adoption, they had connections to a legal team who knew them well and were eager to assist. They had completed home studies and psychological evaluations and financial counseling sessions. They were established patients at the local fertility clinic. They had looked into surrogacy several times in the past but had never felt they could afford the tens of thousands of dollars the surrogates charged in addition to the costs of the medical procedures.

I didn't want compensation. If James and Charlotte had any savings left in the bank after all the expenses of their previous efforts, I just wanted them to use those funds to take care of their future child. I did understand why many surrogates would welcome payment. In gestational surrogacy, the surrogate carries an embryo that's been created via an in vitro fertilization procedure and has no genetic relationship to her. In our traditional surrogacy arrangement, we'd be using insemination to try to combine James's sperm with my egg when I ovulated, since Charlotte had recently been advised to consider using a donor egg anyway. With either method, all the steps of the procedures and the prenatal appointments took time, involved risk, and created plenty of inconvenience. But surrogacy also presented an opportunity to help make a family like no other. I couldn't imagine placing a monetary value on what I was doing. We agreed that James and Charlotte would cover all my medical bills, and would reimburse my wages if I had to cancel work clients due to complications, but would give me no personal stipend or other form of payment.

Their lawyer's office, with its sage green carpet, warm brown curtains, and abundance of houseplants, was much more welcoming than I'd expected. I sat down as the lawyer brought me a cup of tea and a stack of what looked like five hundred documents. She smiled, reflecting on how much she enjoyed the rare days like these when she got to contribute to a happy story. Over the next several hours, I confirmed financial agreements and initialed the pages of something entitled *Intent to Terminate Parental Rights*. In spite of its coldly impersonal language, which made it sound like I was selling them a used car, this document was the hardest to sign. *Termination* felt so harsh and violent, like such a contrast to this tender situation. Knowing the primal love I had for my children, I found it surreal to promise to relinquish a baby even before conception.

I think James and Charlotte must have believed, since I had volunteered, that I understood what the process would entail. I didn't really. I was quite naive to all the things that might happen next—medically, logistically, emotionally. But we jumped in, managing hormone shots and ultrasound appointments and notary signatures as they came, all of us glossing over the details in our excitement to move forward with the vision we shared to make their family.

On the day of the insemination, I drove into downtown Sacramento and arrived early at the clinic, then spent half an hour flipping through outdated parenting magazines in the waiting room. It was strange to be looking at ads for formula and diapers while thinking about a not-yet-existent baby who I wouldn't be buying any of those supplies for. My gaze drifted absently to the window as I took in the view of the Sierra foothills, and I began to realize how scared I was of the insemination procedure itself. I considered how far into the open lands beyond the city I might be able to get before anyone noticed, if I started walking now. Then the nurse called my name.

Four huge lamps illuminated the room as I lay back and found the stirrups with my feet. I listened to the doctor and her assistant speaking in unfamiliar acronyms as they went through the procedure, their tones clinical but not unkind. When the tube to transfer the sperm went in through my cervix, viselike cramps seized my lower abdomen and I squeezed my eyes closed tight. Though I thought I'd been paying close attention to everything the doctors had explained ahead of time, and I'd agreed to all of it, I guess I hadn't really anticipated what was about to happen to me. The pain was so much worse than I had expected, like being dropped into the middle of labor with no buildup. So dull, but so central and intense, straight through to my core. I thought of the many procedures Charlotte had undergone, including seven insemination attempts and four rounds of IVF, and wondered what she'd done to cope with all the kinds of hurt they must have caused.

Twelve days later, in the middle of a Wednesday afternoon, I found myself trying to study at our neighborhood coffee shop. It was my favorite place to retreat to when my mom had the kids and I wasn't at a job, when I could get away to catch up on some reading for my emergency medicine program. I loved learning about the workings of the human body. I was intrigued by the foreign language of medical terminology. I was fascinated by science and felt driven to use my curiosity to help others. I was determined to use this certification to create new opportunities for my family and make something bigger of my life.

But on that day, I couldn't concentrate. I wandered across the street to the pharmacy and bought a pregnancy test. In the store's small bathroom, I stared at two pink lines as they emerged. I blinked hard, awash in gratitude and terror and relief and uncertainty. What had I done?

As soon as the doctor stepped into the clinic room on Friday and officially congratulated us on the results of my blood tests, Charlotte squealed and gave me a big hug, and James joked about being careful not to squeeze me too hard. At our six-week appointment, James and

Charlotte gazed in rapture as a tiny pulsating heartbeat appeared on the bedside ultrasound. At the twelve-week development scan, they held hands as we watched the shadow of a foot move across the screen. At the twenty-week anatomy evaluation, we all cried with happiness when the ultrasound technician told us that everything looked reassuring and that the baby was a boy.

While we celebrated these milestones together, we also kept very much to ourselves. Privacy was important to all of us. James and Charlotte hadn't yet decided how open they planned to be about their history as their child grew up. They wanted to be honest with him, but they also wanted to be certain he would never doubt their commitment. They wanted to live their lives as an ordinary family, avoiding the assumptions and judgments of others. As the intended parents, they wanted to be sure this child would feel completely theirs.

I had agreed to maintain an ongoing relationship with them, to an extent, and I had signed a medical release specifically authorizing contact for health information in the future. If he ever needed a kidney and they thought I might be a match, I said, I hoped they wouldn't hesitate to reach out. But I also felt like it wasn't my place to be too involved. I would be content with observing from afar and grateful to receive any updates they wanted to share with me. I didn't want to pursue an active connection. To me, the gift was in helping make this family and then stepping aside.

I wanted to minimize calling attention to our unusual situation just as much as James and Charlotte did. It makes me incredibly uncomfortable when people fuss over me or scrutinize my motivations, and I chafed at the idea that someone might think I was doing this for money. My mother was one of the only people I had told, and she'd freaked out immediately. As much as I loved my mother, I didn't feel like my decision to be a surrogate was any of her business. My body and my reasons were my own. I would rather most of our family and friends not know what was going on at all—and this seemed possible because all my pregnancies had been easy enough.

Fortunately, I didn't start showing too obviously until seven to eight months in. With the baby's April due date, most of the duration of this pregnancy was easily disguised by the cozy sweatshirts and yoga pants of mild California winters.

Mark, in contrast to my mother, had been unwaveringly supportive from the beginning. But there were a few awkward moments in the third trimester when well-meaning strangers would gesture toward my belly and congratulate us, or him, as we walked our dog through the neighborhood. Even more uncomfortable were the days when Charlotte and James met us at the park to visit while we played fetch with Dakota and pushed Vivi and Nolan on the swings. While Mark was chatting with Charlotte and facing away from us, I would sometimes notice James watching me for a beat too long. It was unsettling—and even more so when he commented in a hushed voice on how much my bump had grown since the last time he saw me, or how radiant I looked. His attention didn't exactly feel sexual. But it did feel intimate in a way that made me fear that his boundaries might not be as clear as mine and that Charlotte might feel pain or envy when he looked at me with any hint of admiration.

As we approached the end of the pregnancy, my sense of vulnerability lingered in other ways too. Even though we'd gone over all the legal papers in great detail, I couldn't shake the feeling that I might have missed some loophole or technicality. Was I protected if the intended parents changed their minds? If they split up? If this baby had an unforeseen disability or significant complications at birth? The territory we were in was so unfamiliar, the volume of the documents I'd signed so vast, and the language so complex and beyond my understanding. A few times, I felt a panic rise in me when I thought about the possibility that I could end up left with this baby that I wasn't prepared to raise as my own—especially as the delivery approached. We were no longer on some abstract, faraway timeline. It was six weeks until he was expected, then two weeks, then one.

My contractions began early in the morning, three days before my due date. In the delivery room, Charlotte and James and the nurses and obstetrician hovered over me as I pushed, a bizarre circus of spectators cheering on the progress of my vagina. Although I'd been through this twice before, it was very different to be surrounded by people who weren't my own family. But the labor was short and manageable, and baby Jackson came out pink and screaming and perfect. Seeing James gather him up and lean him against Charlotte's bare chest was one of the most beautiful moments I've ever experienced.

The next day, I was ready to go home. Mark came to pick me up, so I was surprised when the ward clerk insisted on escorting us out to our car. I knew what it was like to leave the hospital with a newborn, but I didn't know what it was supposed to be like to leave without one. Had the nurses flagged concerns about my mental health? I had admittedly been a little tearful since Jackson was born, but even with the swirl of hormones and emotions after such an intense experience, I was feeling completely at peace with my choices. Was everyone being extra attentive because they found it unnatural for me to be coping so well in this unusual situation? Or because they thought I might not be coping well at all?

The hardest part of separating from my pregnancy actually came the following week, when I went back to school. Over lectures on managing gastrointestinal emergencies and at workshops on inserting artificial airways, I noticed some of my classmates staring at me like they were trying to figure something out. Since I hadn't shared details of my situation with other students or with my instructors—I thought I had concealed my physical changes well enough through the winter, and I was still dressing in oversized clothing—I was a little surprised each time someone stopped me between classes to ask how my baby was doing. But I stuck to my plan of pretending they meant Nolan and just said, "Oh, he's almost two now, but he's doing well!"

That always brought a quizzical look. I think people assumed that my baby had died and that this was how I was dealing with the loss. A few months of this left me feeling oddly isolated. I squirmed beneath the presumptuousness of others looking at me and thinking they knew my story. I wished I could say to them, *You have no idea what is guarded by this little heart.* But I still preferred to just say nothing. I preferred to separate myself from the experience and move on, compartmentalizing that time as a blip that sat outside my actual life. I ended up switching to a different school across town to evade the unwarranted pity I imagined trailing along behind me.

About a year after Jackson's birth, as I completed the last semester of my training and considered looking for a job at a local urgent care center or with an ambulance company, I started to wonder if staying in Sacramento was the right choice. I'd likely end up working with people from school, as well as from the program I'd left behind, and questions about my last pregnancy could surface again. Catching glimpses of James and Charlotte walking down the street with Jackson left me feeling like an accidental intruder, appreciating the visible reassurance that they seemed to be doing well but also hoping they wouldn't notice me—and wishing I hadn't seen them at all. Separating from him, I had felt an absence I didn't like to be reminded of, but it wasn't because I wanted Jackson to myself. My mother, although she kept helping with Vivi and Nolan, always seemed irritated at me and made frequent comments about how she didn't understand how I could just have a baby and then give him away. I felt lots of complicated emotions, but regret wasn't one of them.

Too many people here thought they knew me. But they were wrong. When Mark said he was ready for a fresh start too, I shifted my focus from looking for work nearby to researching opportunities in smaller towns all over the country. Having always valued self-sufficiency, I was drawn to the idea of getting some acreage in a rural setting, but near enough to a town that would have steady employment for me. Mark had taken a few college classes in agribusiness management. He was excited about applying for positions where he could use those skills. And Vivi and Nolan, now four and a half and three, were getting old enough that they'd be in school soon, so we wouldn't have to rely on my mom for childcare.

The most affordable communities were scattered throughout the Midwest, and we quickly identified a cozy homestead for sale in northeastern Ohio, about an hour from Cleveland's modern medical centers. We were excited to be moving to a place with no history for either of us, where we hoped to find ourselves among widely dispersed neighbors and unpretentious farmers and verdant fields as far as the eye could see.

Before we left, we planned a casual wedding. Festive and fun and lighthearted, something between a celebration of marriage and a going-away party with a small group of family and friends, our event took over the sports bar that Mark's stepbrother had owned for years. My floor-length dress was layered with lace and chiffon that I'd pieced together myself on the sewing machine I'd gotten for my fourteenth birthday. With dancing and games and a carnival-worthy cotton candy machine, it was the perfect send-off to our new lives.

We arrived in Ohio in early spring, as eager as we were exhausted. It had taken us ten months to complete the purchase of our new home and coordinate our move, but everything was finally coming together. I'd taken Mark's last name. I'd secured a job as an emergency room technician, where I'd be monitoring patients' vital signs, assisting with procedures, and calling loved ones to give updates. I'd left Jackson's family behind, with the mutual understanding that we knew how to find each other but were all ready to put some distance between us. I was relieved to be farther away from any threat of my dad, who was still in prison in Nevada, tracking me down if he got out on parole.

As our little farm awakened from its thaw, I loved watching Vivi's and Nolan's constant discoveries. They scoured the pond's edge for frogs, gathered buttercups while running through the fields with Dakota, and tended to the chickens we'd inherited from the property's last owner. But the first year learning to take care of the land wasn't easy. In the summer, we harvested delicious heirloom tomatoes but bungled our entire crop of lettuce in the heat. In the fall, we ran out of time to use all our zucchini, so we learned about canning to be ready to preserve the next crop. In the winter, we gathered rain and snow in barrels to water the beets and turnips sheltered within our makeshift greenhouse. We had almost made it through every season, and we were starting to find our stride.

That was when the pandemic struck. The first time I registered the gravity of the new coronavirus, I had just clocked out from a long night in the emergency department. Retrieving my jacket to brave the February winds, I found several nurses gathered around the break room coffee maker, nervously talking about a mysterious new pneumonia-like illness that had started in China and now had cases popping up all over the world. Within weeks, cruise ships full of infected passengers were quarantined off the coast of Japan, Italy had instituted a national lockdown, and our evening news was broadcasting images of the huge white refrigerated trucks that lined the streets of New York City to house an overflow of bodies since the local morgues had reached capacity.

As case numbers rose, local restaurants converted to takeout, park rangers wrapped playgrounds in caution tape, and our department meetings migrated to virtual platforms. We wiped down our groceries and postponed birthday parties. I pulled out my sewing machine again, for the first time since I'd finished my wedding dress, and began making masks out of old clothes while the kids, with schools and preschools shuttered, asked me for constant snacks and screen time.

Even as we canceled almost everything, those of us who staffed the hospital had to keep the facility running. On the front lines, we managed heart attacks, dog bites, abdominal pain, drug overdoses, farm injuries, and everything else that rolled through the doors, just as we'd always done. But now we were also managing the ventilator settings of our friends and colleagues who'd been most unlucky in their brushes with this terrible virus, and sometimes, devastatingly, our efforts weren't enough to save them. Our days were filled with uncertainty. Too often, we felt like we were trying to build a plane while flying it. Along the city streets each night, neighbors leaned out their windows to bang pots and pans together in appreciation for essential workers. But a noisy show of gratitude didn't keep us safe.

I've blocked a lot of my memories from those brutal early days. For nearly four years now, our family has weathered the ups and downs of these unprecedented times—and I have come to hate that phrase for all that it recalls. Millions of people worldwide have died of COVID-19, and many more have lost their lives or livelihoods as a result of the broader impacts it's had on community resources. So many of the healthcare workers that I know are utterly burned out. The pandemic brought out the best and the worst in humanity, unifying some groups while laying bare the irreconcilable differences among others. It ushered forth an age of hope and despair, of science and skepticism, of good enough and making do, of too much and too little all at once.

Some things have gone back to normal and some things, I think, never will. The schools are open again, and the kids take turns with their friends on the swings at the park while Dakota parades proudly with her favorite stick. But my life feels like it's been cleaved in two—or maybe three. The pandemic split time into *before* and *after* for so many of us, just as moving to the farm had done for our family, just as becoming a mother had ended my childhood. I've lived these monumental shifts and their divisions. But I also hold a third piece, separate and distinct.

Carrying and giving birth to a baby for another family is an experience I've carved out from the rest of my history. I think about it more often than I let on, but I almost never talk about it. I keep it as hidden as the tattoos I have under my clothes, and I don't think I should have to explain myself to anyone. Mark keeps in touch with James and Charlotte a little through mutual friends. He tells me Jackson is thriving, but he also respects my boundaries and doesn't say much more. Vivi and Nolan don't seem to remember. No one else where we live now knows, and that mostly brings me peace.

I still question why I decided to become a surrogate. I tell myself that I saw another person hurting and I saw a way that I could make things better. But really, *why?* What was it about me that led me to respond with this act, when so many others would just express superficial sympathy and move on? Going through the process made me into someone who could go through the process. It's kind of an explanation and a nonanswer all at once. At each moment, I changed in imperceptible ways to become the person who was needed, never quite examining who that really was. I haven't made sense of the whole thing yet. Maybe I never will. Maybe I don't talk about it because I don't know how to tell a story that I've never even told myself.

I don't think I could be a surrogate again. I don't think I could agree to walk away, knowing what it's like to walk away. I'm not exactly saying that I wish I hadn't done it. I'm glad I did. There's a difference between acknowledging that I wouldn't take on the role a second time and asserting that I wouldn't choose it in the first place if I were starting over. I didn't realize how much Jackson would remain a part of me even as our lives diverged. I didn't realize how often I would wonder what was happening to him but have no way of knowing, and how empty that would feel.

Some days, as I watch my children grow, it's enough to know that another little boy is growing up in a loving family too. When I'm having a rough go of things, just the fact of his existence can bring me comfort. There are days I burn everything I cook, and no one can find their socks, and even the smallest transition leads to a tantrum—for myself and for the kids. There are days that I crawl into bed feeling pretty defeated. But when I think about what I've been able to do for Charlotte, it makes me feel like I haven't failed so hard. I've given another woman a chance to win at the day, to be a good mom, to have a child to share her love with. My day isn't all about me.

Sometimes we're very alone as parents, and sometimes we need to rely on one another. At the beginning of the pandemic, hand-painted signs sprang up in every store window, at every medical clinic, on every street corner: *We're all in this together!* It's a sentiment that changed and morphed and finally faded as the stresses of the pandemic brought the many fractures in our culture to the fore. But for me, its echoes will always ring through motherhood, pure and true and universal.

I guess, in the end, that's the answer. That's why I became a surrogate. To be part of something bigger. I did it for the same reasons that I moved my family, that I trained in medicine, and that I've done everything else I've done: To seek a better future that might take us further from our pain. To bring more love and connection into the world. To give what I can give by creating something out of nothing. To make the best of this one life.

CHAPTER 9

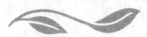

We didn't know how long it might take us to have a second child—or if we'd have to go through as much as we'd endured to get Zach, or if I'd be able to get pregnant again at all—but we knew that we wanted to try. And we also knew that we didn't want to do any of it again during residency.

We didn't want to wait too long either. I was thirty-six, solidly in the advanced maternal age category, and it had taken more than two years to have our first. If we put off trying, we could miss our chance, or find ourselves dealing with an entirely different set of obstacles— obstacles that I'd seen too many of my colleagues in medicine face after delaying getting pregnant themselves.

As I gained more experience and confidence as a physician, other healthcare professionals had begun to come to me as patients. Through their struggles with infertility, pregnancy loss, and devastating diagnoses in much-wanted babies, I felt honored to support them. Through medical crises in their parents, their children, and themselves, I drew on my memories of being a scared and overwhelmed patient as I watched them grapple with becoming vulnerable in ways they'd never expected. I had felt it myself and I saw it again in every one of them: it's incredibly difficult to accept help as a healer in need.

But soon I came to feel that helping wasn't precisely the goal. Helping seemed to imply an imbalance of power, an authority that drew unnecessarily harsh lines between giver and receiver. Helping created distance. As a physician caring for my colleagues, I watched our boundaries blur and shift. And I accepted this ambiguity. I tried to care for them as I would have wanted had our situations been reversed—just as Devorah had done for me.

My intention to collaborate as equals when I took care of my colleagues soon spilled into how I saw all my patients. Rather than helping, I understood that I wanted to serve: To stand beside families rather than above them. To be an advocate, adviser, and witness. To guide and to comfort them as they tried to make sense of their stories.

When my fifth pregnancy came easily in the second month we tried, Ian and I were grateful and relieved. Our six-week clinic ultrasound confirmed my due date, which was ten weeks after I was scheduled to finish residency. My blood tests looked good. I felt reassuringly queasy all day long. I hadn't had a single hint of spotting or of pain. Juggling the exhaustion of mothering a two-year-old at home and working as a senior resident on call, I opted for coffee a little more often to get through morning rounds but felt otherwise the same as I had during my pregnancy with Zach.

But at eleven weeks, when the ultrasound technician went quiet during our first formal scan, I was convinced that we were about to plummet back into a pit of complications and loss. The radiologist was next, joining us in the dark room to glide her smooth wand silently across my abdomen, mapping out fetal cross sections, profiles, back views, and structures of the skull from above.

Finally, she told us that the baby had no visible nasal bone. This finding was present in approximately one percent of pregnancies with typical chromosomes but up to seventy-five percent of pregnancies with trisomies such as Down syndrome, Edwards syndrome, and

Patau syndrome, which could cause profound intellectual disability, problems with nearly every organ system in the body, and a painful death in infancy or early childhood—or which could result in a relatively healthy child with mild to moderate learning delays.

She emphasized that everything else looked fine. Reviewing the printed pages that outlined our ultrasound results, blood tests, demographics, and prenatal history—just as we had done when Zach's cardiac marker had been discovered—she advised that the probability of this being an incidental finding rather than a clue to something more ominous was in the ninety-some percent range. But the absent nasal bone did increase our risk of a chromosomal disorder by fiftyfold. Definitive answers could come only from the kind of analysis available through invasive tissue collection, such as chorionic villus sampling or amniocentesis, both of which carried a small but nonzero risk of harming the fetus.

We scheduled a follow-up scan in one week and hoped that the nasal bone might grow big enough to visualize by then. While we waited, nearly unable to focus on anything else, Ian and I talked about how much information we wanted. Declining invasive testing with Zach had been a fairly straightforward matter. Before he was born, we hadn't wanted to take even the smallest risk of a procedure causing a miscarriage. We had felt confident, or at least confident enough, that the odds were relatively low that he would have a major medical problem. And we'd believed that, even if he did, we could handle it.

Now, chasing our toddler around, the question of whether to do the testing seemed much more fraught. It wasn't because I was clear about what we'd do with the results. I just knew that the calculations were more complicated, the stakes different. We had to consider not just how this baby's health would affect the baby's life and our experience as parents, but how this baby's health might affect our family as a whole. What losses—and gains—might each of us experience if we knowingly brought a child into our family whose time with us was expected to be short and painful, requiring vast amounts of medical attention? What would our days look like with our emotional and financial resources concentrated on the needs of one child, dramatically impacting our ability to care for their sibling? Given the chance to learn more, how much uncertainty would we choose to tolerate?

We didn't realize it yet, but we were facing a pivotal moment that I would watch many of my friends and colleagues confront over the next few years, including some of them as my patients. Before Zach's birth, our story had felt like Rachel's, enduring the desperation of recurrent loss, then Erin's, waiting to meet her son with lingering doubts about his health. After Zach's birth, I had boundless empathy for Anna's NICU ordeal and Maya's devastating neonatal loss. Now, my story had shifted again, becoming much more about questions of predicting and waiting and deciding exactly how much I wanted to know—like the stories I would soon hear from fellow physicians Olivia and Lia.

When nothing had changed at our twelve-week scan, we agreed to invasive testing.

Olivia ~ Anticipation

Scott and I held hands as the last few minutes of waiting expanded to rival the anticipation of the days that had already passed. Two weeks ago at this same medical center, our perinatologist had performed a chorionic villus sampling, the procedure to collect the fragment of placenta that would determine our course. I had been tested for Huntington's disease myself almost ten years earlier, and, after an equally long two-week wait, my results had been confirmed: *Positive.* I was a carrier of the genetic mutation that would almost certainly lead me to develop this incurable and fatal disorder. Now I was waiting to learn if my baby had the mutation too.

At fourteen weeks pregnant and thirty-five years old, I was not invested in this baby—or, more honestly, I had been using every emotional reserve I could summon to avoid becoming invested. The blandness of the beige walls in the geneticist's office and the nondescript mountain-sunset painting hanging over her desk matched the attitude I'd been striving for.

It was unsettling to be looking at mountains in this context, with such detachment. The mountains had always been a place of comfort for me. When I first received my Huntington's diagnosis, I was splitting my time between San Francisco's urban bustle and Northern California's untamable wilderness. During the week, I balanced an uninspiring day job in the hotel industry with rewarding volunteer work advocating for healthcare for HIV-positive people. But my true home was in the backcountry. I spent many evenings climbing at local crags and nearly every weekend on expeditions in Yosemite with an incredible group of mountaineering friends, challenging ourselves and supporting each other as we explored the world. I was in the best physical and mental shape I'd ever been in. I loved my life.

Still, when I had learned about a nearby clinic that offered anonymous Huntington's testing, I felt compelled to find out what might lie ahead for me. In her late forties, my mother's mother had started suffering from a constellation of mysterious symptoms, including repeated episodes of stumbling on flat ground, sudden swings between rage and depression that were completely out of character, and gradually worsening memory loss after having always been renowned for keeping track of every birthday and every anniversary in our family. Countless lab tests and clinic visits finally led her doctors to diagnose what was causing her deteriorating health after more than a decade of observation. I had witnessed the insidious progression of my grandmother's disease since I was six years old, and I'd had a name for it since I was seventeen.

Huntington's is a scary disorder precisely because it disrupts brain function in otherwise healthy young people, progressively eating away at the abilities that make us human. It causes uncontrolled muscle movements, disorienting emotional problems, and loss of the ability to think clearly, typically starting in a person's thirties or forties. Some have compared it to having Parkinson's, Alzheimer's, and amyotrophic lateral sclerosis—also known as ALS or Lou Gehrig's disease—all at the same time. In its late stages, typically ten to twenty-five years after the onset of symptoms, a person with Huntington's becomes trapped inside her body, unable to walk or speak. Although she still understands much of what is going on around her, she is completely dependent on others for care.

The explanation for my grandmother's condition probably eluded her doctors for so long because most of her twelve siblings had lived into their seventies with minimal medical problems. Huntington's disease is a classic genetic condition. It is passed down through families in an autosomal dominant pattern, meaning that its inheritance has nothing to do with being male or female and that each child of a parent with Huntington's has a fifty percent chance of inheriting the mutation. Because of the dominance of the gene, those who carry it have a one hundred percent chance of developing the disorder, assuming they live long enough to do so. The decision about whether to undergo testing for Huntington's is complex and difficult and intensely personal. Family members often disagree strongly about how to handle the situation—and whether to be tested themselves. Some people prefer to find peace with the ambiguity of not knowing.

I am not one of those people. Even if I didn't get the answer I wanted, I believed that having knowledge was always preferable to living in fear of the unknown. I'd been worrying enough already, convinced that the test would be positive. If I took the test, at least there was a chance I could be proven wrong. Throughout my life, I had tended to plan for the worst even while hoping for the best. I called the neurology clinic and enrolled in their Huntington's program.

At my first visit, I sat in the waiting room wondering what to expect. To my left, a tired-looking woman was tending to a freckled, dark-haired boy. I guessed that he was her son and that he was about thirteen years old. As I filled out questionnaires about my family and health history, the writhing movements of the teenager's slender body brought him into and out of my peripheral vision. He furrowed his brow in concentration, trying to contain himself in his narrow chair, but he began to slide down when his abdominal muscles went involuntarily rigid. His right arm jerked at the shoulder. The back of his hand wiped his chin then grazed upward to hit the tip of his nose. His mother repositioned him gently, chatting casually about where they might stop for lunch after his appointment. He leaned sideways against her and smiled. His trembling fingers reached for her hand in a movement both painfully erratic and eerily fluid, as he mumbled something I couldn't understand. I averted my eyes, pressing my pen hard against the stack of clinic paperwork. At twenty-six years old, I swore to myself that I would never knowingly bring a child into this world who would have to endure what I was witnessing that morning.

Over the course of the next year, I followed the prescribed visit schedule. The practice's policy was to run definitive genetic testing only after I'd undergone a twelve-month series of neurologic examinations, psychological evaluations, and genetic counseling sessions—and only if I remained steadfast in my desire to discover my status at the end of that time. A positive test can sway people away from having children or pursuing careers. It can make them ineligible for health insurance or life insurance. It can cause them to withdraw from friends and family when they most need support. Getting tested for Huntington's is not a decision to be taken lightly. I never doubted my need to know.

My mother, in contrast, adamantly refused to get tested. Though I didn't understand her decision, I respected it. Because a positive result for me would mean that she had a one hundred percent chance of carrying the mutation, I didn't tell her that I had sought out the clinic. I told only a few close friends and my sister, who was twenty-one years old and in the process of deciding whether to get tested herself. My brother, only sixteen, wouldn't be eligible for testing until he turned eighteen.

Throughout that year, walking into the waiting room, which usually contained at least one or two severely affected young people, was always the hardest part of the visit—until the day that my blood was collected for testing. Before that moment, I had been able to protect myself by lingering in denial. Maybe Huntington's would begin and end with my grandmother, a random mutation rather than a genetic legacy to be passed on through generations. Now the two-week countdown to receive my results began, and the anticipation was agonizing.

As if to remind me how unfair life could be, my best friend called a few days later to tell me that her mother had developed complications from severe multiple sclerosis. I flew to Australia to be with them. I sat with my friend at her mother's bedside in the intensive care unit for a week, and we cried together as friends and family cycled through the airless room. I watched this beloved forty-four-year-old woman become confused and incontinent and unable to speak. I felt like I was seeing my grandmother's years of decline condensed into a few days, like I was observing one of my own life's possibilities played out before me at hyperspeed. She died on my birthday, and I flew back across the ocean the next day, numb and sleep-deprived and utterly miserable.

After a fitful five hours of rest, I awoke disoriented to find myself home in my San Francisco walk-up. I must have gotten dressed and made my way to the Huntington's clinic for the appointment I'd scheduled two weeks prior, because soon I was being escorted from the waiting area into the counseling room. Mercifully, the doctor didn't stall. She looked right at me, not unkindly, and told me that my result was positive. I know I cried, but I'd already been crying all week. Everything in the universe seemed wrong. I almost didn't care.

For many months, the diagnosis floated loose in my mind. It jostled every other thought, looking for a place to land. Carrying the Huntington's mutation seemed so significant in one sense. Yet, at the moment, it changed nothing. I had no idea how—or even if—this new knowledge should guide my choices, my goals, my self-imposed limitations. I'd thought I'd prepared for this possibility by expecting the result to be positive all along, but I still felt completely ungrounded as I faced its confirmation. I continued to work in the city and visit Yosemite for a few more months, then decided I needed more distance to process everything. To seek refuge deeper in the wilderness, I moved to Nepal. I volunteered at a mountainside medical clinic. I trekked through lands of terraced river bluffs. I tried to get away from everything that reminded me of anything.

A year after my diagnosis, when my mother started manifesting Huntington's symptoms in her early fifties and was forced to take an early retirement from teaching, I left the mountains and moved home to Minnesota. She must have known what her emerging difficulties with balance and speech portended. But she was still opposed to being tested, so I never spoke about my results around her. I didn't want her to know I'd been consigned to the fate that I already knew for myself.

I also didn't want her to realize that, whatever she was going through, my course would likely be more severe. Although the gene responsible for Huntington's disease exists in everyone, in those with the mutation it contains extra copies—known as repeats—of part of its code. The repeats prompt cells to manufacture a protein that's too long. The body tries to compensate by chopping the oversized proteins into smaller fragments. But these fragments bind together, clogging neurons and disrupting the functions of these brain cells, ultimately leading to cell death.

Because of a cruel phenomenon known as genetic anticipation, the number of these damaging repeats often increases as the altered gene is passed from generation to generation. A larger number of repeats is associated with an earlier onset of symptoms. In so much of life, anticipation is a slippery thing. Sometimes what we fear is much worse than what actually comes to pass. But with Huntington's, the fear is justified. Because its symptoms manifest in the prime of life, many people realize that they're carriers only after they've had children. And because of genetic anticipation, all children with Huntington's have a worse prognosis than their affected parent.

Watching my mother's slow decline, I felt an increasing urgency to make active choices about my life. More than even my own family's tribulations, my work with communities of people living with HIV had shown me how interested I was in clinical medicine. As I explored healthcare professions—doctor, nurse practitioner, physical therapist—I realized that my desire to be in control of my own decisions, as well as my tendency to take charge in groups, made me much better suited to being a doctor than to any other role. Since working at a local bakery filled my early-morning hours and helping my mother consumed my afternoons, I signed up for night school science classes.

The year I moved back to my hometown was also the year I started dating Scott, who'd been a close friend in college. Every bit as avid an outdoorsperson as I was, Scott volunteered on the local search and rescue team and worked as a firefighter. We reconnected over memories of wilderness trips we'd taken together in school, from frigid winter weekends snowshoeing along the edge of Lake Superior to one surprisingly slushy late-spring expedition canoeing the Boundary Waters with a group of classmates. For our first date, we took a whitewater kayaking trip on Sand Creek that left us undeterred even after Scott flipped his boat twice and I dropped my lunch overboard.

Even while I was embarking on a new relationship, balancing all my obligations reminded me how much I valued self-sufficiency. I had grown up watching my friends' parents get divorced and suddenly found myself part of the first generation for whom this was almost as common as having parents who stayed together. Even more distressing were the terrible marriages in which women felt trapped because, after years invested in raising their families, they didn't know how to reenter the workforce. As much as I trusted Scott, I needed to be able to take care of myself.

Scott understood this impulse all too well. He'd seen my family's story unfold all through college and had known since we'd first reconnected that I carried the Huntington's mutation. He'd watched his own mother worry about whether she would develop early-onset

Alzheimer's since her mother had died of it at fifty-two. He respected the calling that I felt to serve families in times of health crises, and he understood why I felt compelled to do something useful and measurable with my life.

Scott and I got married in our early thirties, right before I began medical school. We both wanted kids, but having a baby felt like too much to even think about as I moved through the rigorous basic science curriculum and into clinical rotations. Even after we decided to start trying, realizing that things weren't going to get easier in residency, it took us more than a year and a half to get pregnant. As two busy professionals working incredibly taxing and irregularly aligning overnight shifts, we couldn't have had more than seven or eight chances to conceive during a true fertile window over those twenty-some cycles.

But there we sat, finally, in the geneticist's office, six years after our whitewater fiasco, four years married, and more than three years into my medical training. We had barely let ourselves accept the possibility of my pregnancy yet. Friends had questioned why I was so terrified of having a child who would have the same condition that I did, arguing that I was living a rewarding and full life unhindered by my diagnosis. But I had seen the possibilities for juvenile Huntington's. I knew about genetic anticipation, so I knew that my child, if affected, would likely not be as fortunate as I had been. The vulnerability of parenthood brings with it enough pain and doubt. I felt no need to invite more. Planning for the worst, I had already scheduled an appointment for termination the next morning.

Our geneticist walked into the office, sat down, and looked straight at me. "Negative," she said softly. We would be having a boy, and his chromosomes were normal. The ordeal I had envisioned had not come to pass. I shook with sobs of relief. Even the mountain-sunset painting on the wall now looked more peaceful than bland. Next came a flicker of generous envy. The flood of joy for my son was coupled with a wish that I'd had his good fortune when I'd been conceived. He wouldn't grow up with the specter of Huntington's, or even some mysterious ill-defined condition, hanging over him as I had. We canceled our appointment at the abortion clinic and called my sister, who was even more relieved to hear the results once I was able to speak, since I had started sobbing again when she'd picked up the phone.

As Scott and I moved through the pregnancy thinking grateful thoughts about our healthy son, I recalled a story about another firefighter years ago. On one searingly hot day in August 1949, a lightning strike on dry brush had sparked a wildfire in Montana's Mann Gulch. Fifteen smokejumpers parachuted in to join the lone nearby ranger in an effort to control the fire. But sudden wind turbulence sent the blazes raging up the ravine, expanding to more than three thousand acres in ten minutes and trapping all sixteen men in the narrow chasm of loose scree and boulders. The crew's foreman had the presence of mind to light a smaller fire nearby and to step into the parched area once no combustible material remained. He huddled in safety among the smoldering embers of this escape fire, with flames licking the sky all around him. He called out to his fifteen compatriots, trying to convince them to do the same. None of them would follow. They couldn't believe that, once it ran out of fuel, the fire could extinguish itself. They couldn't accept that there was safety to be found at the heart of the crisis. But he did survive, nearly unscathed. Thirteen others perished.

I was keenly aware of my own relative good fortune amid so many things going wrong around me. In my training, I witnessed diagnoses of developmental delays and reported cases of suspected child abuse. In my family life, I watched my mother and her mother deteriorate, while I remained in excellent health beyond the years that the genetic anticipation of Huntington's would have predicted. I'd sat with my best friend beside her mother, through all those days and nights in intensive care, as multiple sclerosis stole her from us. Among my other close friends, I had recently seen one lose a desperately longed-for baby to severe anatomical anomalies, another make the heartbreaking choice to sacrifice one of her triplets in the second trimester to give the other two a chance at survival, and still another terminate four pregnancies in a row because of a recurring fatal genetic syndrome. Now, at this tiny but monumental point of inflection, my life had pivoted toward one outcome when it could have just as easily turned toward another. How had I ended up here, crouched among these embers, clinging to the good news of my son's normal chromosomes?

Rourke was born shortly after his due date, bright-eyed and vigorous and defiantly healthy. Fifteen weeks later, I started my pediatrics residency. Suddenly I shifted from the erratic and sleepless schedule of newborn parenthood to the erratic and sleepless schedule of internship. Since I was required to be in the hospital and clinics for eighty to ninety hours most weeks, Scott arranged his work around my obligations, spending his days with Rourke and keeping up with most of the responsibilities of our domestic lives. But he was also a wage earner for our family, leaving for his twice-weekly overnight shifts as a firefighter as I drifted off to sleep with Rourke in the crib beside our bed.

The next three years were a blur. I was always tired, but I knew I had to keep up a facade of strength. I'd seen how the attendings had treated my coresident, hugely pregnant, who had taken a seat on morning rounds and been chided for being unable to keep up with the work. In my first few months back, my mind was constantly calculating how long it had been since I had last pumped and how many more chart notes I had to write before I could go home to see my baby. Having a family at home made residency both much easier and much, much harder. I didn't have any trouble maintaining my perspective on the importance of life outside work. But it physically pained me to imagine the time I'd be missing with Scott and Rourke as I said goodbye to them each morning. Achieving any semblance of balance was impossible. Both my work life and my family life were all-consuming, and there weren't two of me to give.

After residency training, I felt ready to think further ahead than the day-by-day survival mode I'd been in for so long. Scott and I began to consider having a second child. As the oldest of three, I loved my younger siblings. As a pediatrician, I was devoted to babies and children. As a parent, I recognized how fortunate we had been that Rourke was so easygoing and funny and engaging—and healthy. We had flipped a coin, and we had won.

If I didn't carry the Huntington's mutation, or maybe if we'd had our first child earlier, I think I would have wanted a bigger family. At the low-income clinic where I had just started my first job out of residency, I thoroughly enjoyed the ebullient chaos of the well-child checks where multiple babies and toddlers tumbled around the room as I tried to examine each brother and sister in turn. Several of the parents and children in these families were living with HIV. Their stories gave me hope. Since my days volunteering in San Francisco ten years earlier, I'd watched HIV evolve from a uniformly fatal infection to a chronic disease that could often be managed with oral medication and attentive clinical care. Maybe Huntington's would get there too.

But, at almost forty, I wasn't sure I had enough time to get my hopes up only to have them crushed, then summon the will to try again. I knew that I would never force a child to carry the weight of Huntington's. I was more comfortable with the finality of termination than with the ambiguity of the future of this disorder. So many people let things unfold as they will without intention or commitment. They open themselves and see what the world brings them. I can see the beauty in that. But I didn't feel like I had that luxury. I wanted to know that Scott and I had made a choice rather than settled for a default.

I thought of the incredible bond that Scott and Rourke had built during all the time they'd spent together while I was a resident. They were so devoted to each other. I wondered if Scott could love a second child as deeply and what effect it would have on Rourke to have to share his father's love. I thought about Scott and Rourke without me after I was gone. I could picture the two of them as a father-son team, taking care of each other, just as they'd gotten through those first three years together. I couldn't picture another person in the mix.

I also worried about Scott. Seasonal wildfire patterns had escalated dramatically throughout the country in recent years. Burns on a scale once unheard of had become disturbingly common, and Scott received frequent requests to assist overwhelmed communities as lives and property went up in flames. Cautious though he was, he did put his life at risk to help others. We knew that other professions were even more dangerous—farming, fishing, logging—and that firefighters protected themselves with disciplined training regimens and thoughtful response protocols. Still, now that we had a child, I saw his job differently. I worried more about how long I would be around to take care of my son, especially if something happened to Scott. I had no idea how and when I was going to tell Rourke about my own diagnosis. I wasn't ready to imagine him taking care of me.

Women often feel like we can't say no, as we join committees at work and school and then struggle to balance our jobs with our families. We try to be the ones—like my grandmother so many years ago—who witness and chronicle all the birthdays and anniversaries and meanings within our progression of days. A colleague that I deeply admire, one of my mentors through medical training and a mother of two young children herself, gave me some advice that really struck me. She warned me that people are always going to expect a lot of me but that I don't have to come through on all of it. When I completed residency, she urged me to give myself permission to say no to everything for a year.

This spoke to me even more than she could have guessed, not knowing my story. I didn't know how many good years I had left. Whatever time we had together, I wanted to travel with Rourke to Yosemite and Nepal and the Boundary Waters, to reclaim the wonder of the rivers and forests and ridges and peaks of the wider world with my husband and son. Caring for another baby, I would have to put off these dreams for several more years. For me, maybe saying no included saying no to a second child.

As I was settling into our decision to remain a family of three, I got a call from one of my closest friends from my Northern California days. Lana and I had first connected over our love of travel and adventure, often escaping together from our city jobs to the sanctuary of the mountains on weekends. She had worked as a backcountry ranger in Yosemite for several summers during college and knew its meadows and peaks better than anyone else I'd ever met had known a place. We had both gone on to become pediatricians. Nearly eight months pregnant with her first child, she was almost done with residency. We hadn't talked in several weeks, and I wondered if she was calling to announce that her son had come early or that she'd had to take a leave from her program because of some sort of complication.

As soon as she spoke, the flatness in her voice foretold much graver news. Her husband, Brent, climbing in our old haunts with another good friend from our mountaineering days, had been killed by a freak rockfall accident. He had died among the talus ledges and craggy spires that once were our cathedrals. He had left her just when they were both so full of hope and anticipation for the future they had spent a decade building together.

Lana has always been an inspiration to me. For all the years I've known her, she's been mindful of living an intentional life, a life both true to herself and enriching to the world—and it's an attitude that's rare among physicians. During medical school several years ago, well before any of us had become parents, our old crew had gotten together for a climbing reunion. Scott and Brent and Lana and I had crowded around a table in a poorly lit cabin, playing cards, drinking beer, and reminiscing long into the night. As we recalled the blissful simplicity of our mountaineering days, Brent had teased us that medical training had warped our expectations.

"You're all just happy if you're not working," I remember him declaring with a laugh, shaking his head incredulously at what we allowed as a passable quality of life. He urged us to define our goals around what we actively wanted, to choose the positive rather than to be satisfied with an absence of the negative. "You don't even know what you want to be doing—except not working," he insisted. "Don't let yourself accept that anything is better than that."

Five years after that reunion, these were our truths: Brent was dead and we were alive. The strongest among us, the persistent optimist, the seizer of life, had been ripped away, leaving his wife to make the huge leaps of becoming a mother and starting her first job as a supervising physician all on her own. My husband, in a profession that continually tasked him to risk his own safety to help others, and I, harboring an incurable and fatal disorder, were doing fine. Scientists were inching closer to a gene editing technology that might cure Huntington's. When my brother tested positive for the mutation, he and his wife used in vitro fertilization to select embryos that would not carry Huntington's, and were eagerly awaiting the birth of their daughter. My sister tested negative, and now had a healthy infant son. My siblings and I had stopped our family's Huntington's at our generation.

Sometimes risk is an illusion. I thought back to the escape fire of Mann Gulch, which had created a brand-new solution—one that could be imagined only by embracing the crisis itself. I realized that I had been worrying about the wrong things. It was time to question my perception that the safest place was where the fire had never been. It was time to have faith that I could preserve myself even as chaos swirled around me. It was time to walk directly into the smoldering embers of uncertainty that I had feared for so long—and sometimes even spark new fires—trusting that uncertainty was really nothing less than possibility. It was time to step into my moment with confidence, even as the world was burning.

So much of fear is simply love. Fear signals that we value something deeply enough that it would break our hearts to lose it. When I worry about my time being cut short by Huntington's, it's too easy to forget what I do have. Today is another opportunity to celebrate my love for Scott and Rourke. To watch my son grow. To see my husband father him more tenderly than I could have imagined. To care for my patients with the insight of all I've witnessed and withstood. Brent's intense and beautiful life, and too-soon death, reminded us again that worrying that a known threat would end our days was every bit as naive as expecting a certain amount of time out of life just because we were young and vibrant.

Anticipation, too, has two sides. Knowing about genetic anticipation leaves me with apprehension over the worsening of Huntington's with each generation, and even allowing too much ordinary anticipation into life can let the future steal joy from the present. But sometimes anticipation is a blessing. When I have the freedom to consider possibilities and make a choice, I feel powerful. When I think ahead to the promise of medical breakthroughs, I feel hopeful. When I acknowledge that—although I will not be here forever—I am here now and can look forward to the moments I will have, I embrace what is to come. I am learning to find comfort in the realization that the fears I most anticipate rarely come to pass. Other fires will ignite instead, and I will endure. I hold my loves close to my chest, step into the charred embers, and call out for others to follow me to safety.

Lia ~ Third Child

Last December, we were trying to simplify our lives. Tyler and I had spent many hours over many months talking about strategies to balance our two careers with our two kids' schedules, and I had decided to step back from my work as a family medicine doctor to be more present for my own family. Dylan was seven, in second grade, and on a busy soccer team with several practices and games each week. Josie was five, in kindergarten, and thrilled to finally join her brother at the big kids' school. My days were filled with mornings volunteering in their classrooms, afternoons coaching soccer, and weekends enjoying playdates with neighborhood friends. Our little family was growing up.

My sense that I needed to be around more for Dylan and Josie—that they needed a parent's help to navigate the complexities of school and activities, both logistical and social—had been steadily increasing. Meanwhile, Tyler's construction business had been getting more demanding and less flexible, requiring him to travel for two to three days each week. Both of us believed that it was crucial to be consistently available for the kids during these early years, to be there for after-school transitions and car rides and to hear about their days. Their brains were changing so fast. They were so impressionable. Besides, they were so much fun to be around. We wanted at least one of us to be a steady presence for them.

In only a week, I'd be leaving a practice I'd joined right out of residency more than six years prior. As I sorted through files and cleaned out my office, I grew nostalgic about how I'd miss so many of the patients and families I'd cared for while I'd been there. Digging deep in my desk drawers, I unearthed layers of thank-you notes. From along the windowsill, I gathered up my collection of keepsakes gifted by patients—a flowering cactus, a silver paperweight, a small knitted red bird ornament that had watched over me as I'd charted office visits and shared difficult news over the phone. I loaded everything into a cardboard box and thought about how I'd have to find new places for these memories at home. But I was excited and relieved to take a break for a little while, to have the time and the mental space to reflect more deeply on how I wanted to shape my personal and professional life going forward.

To celebrate the winter holidays and to mark the beginning of this new era, Tyler and Dylan and Josie and I took a trip to Hawaii, where I'd grown up and gone to medical school. We joined my parents for a week on Kauai, spending time at their home and on the beach where Tyler and I had gotten married. One day, I remembered that my period was due to start so I bought a pack of pads at the grocery store. In their crinkly plastic bag, they drifted down to the bottom of my suitcase day by day as we snorkeled with turtles, hiked through forests, and ate fresh fish and macadamia nut ice cream. Toward the end of the trip, I had the fleeting thought that my period still hadn't come, but I hadn't been paying much attention to the calendar. Maybe I'd miscalculated somehow. Maybe the stresses of recent transitions had disrupted my cycle.

By the time we got home to Oregon a few days later, I'd realized that I really could be pregnant. Exhausted, jet-lagged, and incredulous, I sent Tyler out to the pharmacy while I helped the kids get ready for bed. Once they were settled for the night, Tyler and I huddled in the bathroom together as we watched the positive result appear. Tyler was immediately excited about the news. In the backs of our minds—maybe Tyler's more than mine—we had long been considering having another child. He jumped right to imagining a new baby in the house, talking about how much Dylan and Josie would love having a little brother or sister. He was okay with being outnumbered. He reassured me that the love was in the chaos. He was ready to start again.

But I wasn't so sure. The best word I could come up with to describe my feelings was *indefinite*. *Indefinite*: not clearly defined, vague. *Indefinite*: undetermined, unspecified, unsettled. *Indefinite*: lasting for an unknown or unstated length of time, immeasurable, infinite.

I remembered how sick I had been with both of my other pregnancies. I remembered throwing up every day through all nine months, unable to focus on the words to read a book without overpowering nausea, struggling through long clinic days, and falling asleep on the couch at seven o'clock before dragging myself to bed for the night a few hours later. Right now I was feeling physically strong, and I relished having reclaimed my body as the kids had gotten older. I had started to intensify my training as a competitive distance runner. I was disappointed that being pregnant would eliminate me from many upcoming races after I'd been a solid competitor last year.

Looking at starting over with diapers, baby care, and sleepless nights troubled me too. My goal in taking a leave from work had been to focus on Dylan and Josie. Now I feared I would be stretched in too many directions again. I wasn't sure our family could adjust to the demands of a newborn. Dylan would be so much older than this sibling. Would he be able to connect with a baby? Josie loved the attention she got from being the youngest in the family and the only girl, just as I had been, growing up with my three older brothers. Would she be able to embrace being in the middle? I had to admit that this pregnancy felt like an imposition. I didn't know if there was space in our lives for a third child.

One by one, my doubts fell away. The days that Dylan and Josie were born had been the best days of my life so far, and the most rewarding experiences I'd ever had came from watching them grow and blossom. I knew I'd feel the same about this baby. I gradually shifted into a place where I was ready to make the sacrifice of cutting back on the intensity of my exercise routine, and I started to fantasize about the joy of having a tiny baby in the house again. Soon, I had become completely committed to and honestly thrilled about this unplanned new path. When we told the big kids about the little sibling we were expecting, they were beyond excited.

When I was seven weeks pregnant, the nausea hit hard, dominating my thoughts at all times of day. Then I woke up on a Sunday morning with an excruciating pain wrapped from my lower back around to my abdomen. Since it was the weekend, I found myself in the emergency department, with no cause for my symptoms identified after many hours of ultrasounds and blood tests. The doctors offered me strong prescription pain medications.

Reluctant but desperate for relief, I accepted the treatment. I was immediately consumed by an overwhelming sense of guilt about being too weak to handle what was probably just a muscle strain from the workout I'd done the day before. I had barely even used pain medication for childbirth and recovery, including after one cesarean delivery. Suddenly I couldn't sit upright for a car ride or get off the couch without assistance. Tyler's mom flew in from Pennsylvania to take care of Dylan and Josie. I felt helpless. I didn't want to use the amount of medication I needed to function as a mother because I was so concerned about possible effects on the baby, but the pain and the guilt both grew so unbearable that sometimes I wished the pregnancy would end. Many nights I would lie awake in bed, tearful and cringing, trying to squelch those thoughts, trying to visualize surviving this crisis and having it all be worthwhile.

Gradually, the nausea, the fatigue, and the pain all began to lighten enough for me to imagine getting through the next few months. I still didn't feel quite myself, but I'd finally had some almost normal days again when we went in for our twelve-week appointment. Since I was thirty-six years old, our doctor recommended screening for chromosomal anomalies. A new form of noninvasive prenatal testing could check my blood for genetic markers of the baby's health and had the advantage of being highly accurate with no risk to the baby. Our doctor encouraged it, and he talked about his observation that people with more information—even if the test detected a concern and they continued the pregnancy—seemed to feel better about their situation once the baby was born.

Tyler was easily convinced, and I was fine with it. I understood the statistics, had counseled plenty of people about them as a doctor myself, and knew I was unlikely to be that textbook older mom who ends up having a pregnancy with a chromosomal difference. On the other hand, we felt so fortunate to have two healthy children that having a third felt like pushing our luck. It would be nice to have some reassurance, to be able to enjoy the pregnancy more without this worry hanging over us. The test seemed like the right thing to do.

We didn't give it much thought after the blood draw, just went about our school and work and family routines. On Monday morning one week after the test, I was at home alone combing through shelves and looking under couches for a missing library book when my phone rang. The clinic number appeared on its display, and I answered immediately, excited to get our result. But when I heard my own doctor's voice on the other end rather than his nurse's, my heart dropped. He wouldn't be calling me himself with good news.

He told me quickly but gently that the test was positive for an extra chromosome 21. The baby was a girl, and she had a very high likelihood of having Down syndrome. I sank heavily to the floor. Time stood still as my life took a sudden and sharp turn off the path I thought I had been following. I asked questions about odds and percentages and what we should do next, grasping for any ray of hope. I knew that his estimate of a few percent chance of the test being wrong was overly generous, but he was trying to soften the blow.

Rationally, I understood that this test, when it shows the marker of concern, is wrong far less than one percent of the time. But I wasn't ready to accept that reality. I told myself that, as accurate as the blood test was, it was still considered screening rather than diagnostic. The next step would be one final invasive test. He mentioned amniocentesis, and I asked if we could do chorionic villus sampling. CVS, which collects tissue from the placenta, could be performed now, whereas for an amnio, which collects fluid from around the baby, we would have to delay the procedure to minimize its risks.

I couldn't imagine not knowing for another month. I wanted as many answers as anyone could give me as soon as possible. We'd shared our news with a few close family members and friends, but I wasn't obviously pregnant to anyone else—or even to myself in some ways, since I wasn't feeling the baby move yet. It was still easy to remain a little detached, but I knew that would change once I felt those first rolling flutters from inside. I scheduled the CVS for Wednesday, two days later.

I hung up the phone and started to dial Tyler at work, then hesitated. I knew how upset he would be. But I couldn't have waited more than a minute. He needed to know too.

He came home, and we sat on the couch and cried together. We kept reminding ourselves that there was every possibility that ours was one of those false positives I'd warned my own patients about. Something this big couldn't be wrong now, after we had begun to reshape our lives around this new person. Tyler and I had started budgeting for a remodel to make room for another family member in our quaint but cramped craftsman home. I'd agreed to work a few shifts, filling in temporarily for another physician's leave at a nearby clinic to earn some extra money. I'd scheduled volunteer hours at the kids' school for the coming months, knowing how much harder it would be to stay involved once the baby arrived. Dylan and Josie had gotten so excited about having a little sibling. When we picked them up together after school that day and—just as we had shared the news of the pregnancy with them from the beginning—we told them there might be a problem with the baby, they were sad and scared and worried too.

Two long days later, on Wednesday morning, Tyler and I made our way to the high-risk obstetrician's office. The procedure started with an ultrasound to assess the baby and the placenta, then to find the landmarks that would allow the perinatologist to collect the sample safely. The baby showed no visible abnormalities and had a normal neck-fold thickness, without the increase that's common in babies with chromosomal differences. She was moving all over the place. I kept closing my eyes, wincing as I glanced away. She looked so much more like a baby than she had at the earlier ultrasound. The doctor gave us lots of hope, saying that if we had done first-trimester screening without the newer technology our results would have come back normal. We allowed ourselves the luxury of imagining that the blood test could still be wrong.

To get our minds off having to wait several days to learn more, we spent a rainy weekend at the coast, in a small oceanside bungalow that our family had started visiting before Josie was born. I can still remember the feeling of not knowing what was going to happen, of uncertainty tempered by the optimism of denial. It was comforting to be in a different place, away from where things were being decided about our lives. Away from our usual environment, but still at home in a different way. Familiar, but separate. I tried to enjoy the ordinariness of lingering over meals, watching rain drip down the large picture windows, and playing with my children on the foggy beach.

Still, I think I was beginning to come to terms with the reality that we weren't—she wasn't—going to be one of those rare false positives. I think I knew in my gut what I would do before we even got the results. On Monday, with Tyler by my side, I called the clinic early in the morning. The genetic counselor was so kind and patient when she broke the news and waited for our reactions. Tyler's eyes welled up with tears while I stayed on the phone, numb and composed, to schedule an appointment at the abortion clinic for two days later. By the time I hung up, we were both crying.

We leaned together and hugged each other tightly, reluctant to face the day of work ahead of each of us. I was grateful, at least, that no one at the primary care clinic where I was filling in knew I was pregnant, so no one had cheerful questions for me about baby names or any reason to suspect why I seemed distracted. When I needed to, I could retreat into the back office and cry for a few minutes. I could give myself the space to let the sadness flow through me before gathering my thoughts and stepping back into my patients' lives. My schedule was just busy enough to keep my attention on something productive, to be soothing in its routine without being overwhelming in its demands. Making my way through some semblance of a typical day—carrying on in my usual role and connecting with others who knew nothing of my grief—made me feel like there would be life beyond this.

Somehow the time passed. As much as I didn't want to believe that any of this was happening to me, to Tyler, to the baby herself, my decision to end the pregnancy never wavered. I thought back to times when I had sat with women in clinic, feeling removed and somewhat distant, to counsel them about abortion, adoption, and parenting options. While I felt compassion toward my patients and their families, reproductive challenges had never resonated with me on a personal level. Even as I had watched controversy about abortion swirl through mainstream media and political debates over the years, I had found myself passing very little judgment.

Now, confronting this choice for myself, I understood what it felt like to know that there would be many people who would condemn my decision to have an abortion as selfish and wrong. But I also knew that the decision came from a place of deep unselfishness. I needed to do what I felt was best for this baby and for our other children, what would bring our daughter the least suffering and our family the most peace. Tyler and I were heartbroken that we would never experience her birth, would never hear her laughter, would never witness her growth. We knew we had to choose to let her go. We knew she would always be part of our lives.

On the day of the procedure, we tried to keep our family routines as normal as possible. My mom, who had flown in from Hawaii to help, got Dylan and Josie up and dressed. We kissed them goodbye as they sat at the kitchen table eating breakfast. I didn't cry until we got into the car. As we drove across town, I felt so sad. Just so, so sad. Very soon, this small being inside me would be no longer. My brothers and my sister-in-law sent us messages to say how much our family loved us and that they all supported us completely. Through stoplights, bridge crossings, and an ordinary jumble of commuter traffic, the world moved on. Tyler and I didn't need to say much to each other. We had made our decision together, and we both found some comfort in that. I struggled to reconcile how awful I felt about the choices we'd had to face with how fortunate I was to live somewhere that I could make the choice I knew was best, no matter how heart-wrenching it was.

When we arrived at the clinic, I was immensely grateful that no protesters stood outside to obstruct our walk up the dingy concrete staircase. After checking me in, a nurse recorded my weight and measured my blood pressure. She smiled sympathetically as she held out misoprostol—the same medication commonly used for pregnancy inductions—to place between my lower lip and gum. I put on a thin blue gown and moved to a bed in a room with three other women. These anonymous women and I were separated by rows of curtains that hung just long enough for me to make out a pair of brown shoes here, a crumpled pink shirt on the floor there, one foot swaying nervously as it dangled off the bed a few curtains down. But we were joined in a common experience that day, and knowing I wasn't alone made the whole thing a little more bearable.

The staff kept me moving along, and soon it was my turn. The procedure itself was mercifully easy—no bleeding, no cramping, no memory of anything between asking the anesthesiologist a few questions and waking up tired but relieved in the post-op area. I looked down at the gray baseboard and cracked tiles beside my IV pole. The facilities seemed old and worn, carrying the weight of all that had passed through the clinic over the years. But every person I met that day was kind and professional, dedicated without reservation to providing healing and compassion to the women they served.

After the abortion, my physical discomfort vanished almost immediately. The back pain was completely gone. The nausea faded over the next few days. I never vomited again. I felt lucky that my body recovered quickly and that I had the unflagging support of my family and friends.

I spent time over the next few months with a skilled therapist recommended by the genetic counselor. Drawing on the wisdom she'd gleaned from working with so many women before me who'd experienced a loss, she guided me gently through the grieving process. I learned that my feelings were normal and that someday I'd be able to reflect on these moments and understand how important it was to honor my grief as I healed. I kept to myself a lot. I carved out the space to turn inward. I felt even more grateful for my two living children.

Dylan and Josie seemed to handle the loss appropriately. Tyler and I kept our words to them simple and straightforward, telling them the baby wasn't healthy and wasn't going to make it. Josie was sad that she wasn't going to have a little sister to cuddle with and teach to sing the alphabet song. With Dylan, explaining things was a little harder, since he understood more. I did tell him a little about the baby's medical condition and difficulties she would have been likely to have, and he said bravely that it would have been all right, that he could have helped her. He had a friend whose mom was exactly as far along as I had been, so he had to watch her continue through the pregnancy and see his friend get a new little brother. But he was also very protective of my health. He felt a lot of stress when I was sick, took on a lot of worry about me, and kept trying to reassure me that we were happy as a family of four and that I didn't need to go through all this.

Tyler, for his part, coped with the whole experience astoundingly well. When I got angry and questioned *Why us?* his attitude was *Why not us?* It was just one experience that was part of our lives, he insisted. And it would remain part of our lives, as individuals and as a family. He helped me keep my balance, helped me avoid feeling like a victim. He didn't believe it had happened to us for any grander reason or that it was inherently good or bad. I drew great comfort from learning to let that part of it go.

When we had gotten married ten years earlier, Tyler and I had exchanged those classic vows about being together for better or for worse. Visions of the good times ahead were easy to imagine when we were starting out as a young couple. But I understood, at least abstractly, that each family's difficulties are uniquely its own, even if I couldn't foresee what ours would turn out to be. Since then, struggles have been just as important as celebrations in defining who we are and who we might become together. As we worked through the grief of losing our daughter, I felt an even stronger sense of partnership with Tyler, an even deeper connection to our little family of four, and an even greater appreciation for the wonderful people we had in our lives. Acknowledging all of that felt good too, even under the weight of our sadness.

As those painful days now begin to recede into the distance, I think this was the hardest thing our family has ever gone through. I'm continually amazed that we did it, that we're doing it. And who knows what harder things may come? Last week, I was talking with a friend who had a healthy pregnancy, then several miscarriages, then another healthy pregnancy. Her older son, like Dylan, had struggled with watching his parents suffer through these losses. She said it was a really difficult time for all of them. But then she said she thought it was good for children to have experiences of things not going well sometimes.

Her words resonated with me immediately. As a mother, I thought of myself as my children's shelter from all kinds of harm. I had spent years catching sudden falls, scanning streets for traffic, brushing away tears after callous playground insults. I was always alert for dangers and vulnerabilities. Now, suddenly, I appreciated the awareness and the growth that this loss might bring them as individuals. I knew that they would get through this, that we would get through this, that we would all come out stronger on the other side.

To say that this experience has made me more mindful of what I do have almost cheapens the feelings—or at the very least doesn't do the whole ordeal justice. I found myself in a situation I had never, ever thought I'd find myself in, facing decisions I'd never imagined having to face. I realized that it was possible to come to some sort of peace with this loss, even though I know I'll never get over it.

Today, I'm happy and anxious and relieved to be pregnant again. Tomorrow I'll be at fourteen weeks and two days, the exact point where I was when we went through the termination more than six months ago. Tomorrow will be hard for me, and I'll try to make it as ordinary a day as possible. Tomorrow will be hard, even though we've already had the genetic tests and everything looks reassuring. Tomorrow will be hard, even though this baby is a boy, and for that simple fact I am grateful. There's just no haziness between him and our third child, no ambiguity of where the vision of one baby stops and the next one begins. He will be our fourth child, even when people look at our family and see only three. He will be his own being, imagined and wanted and not yet known.

At the beginning of my third pregnancy, I had worried that our family couldn't fit a newborn. But losing her taught me that the opposite was true. I'd opened up a desire, a readiness to love, and her absence left an empty place in me that called out to be filled with another child. I knew that if we didn't try I would look back years later and wish I'd been brave enough to face the unknown. But I was so scared that the same thing might happen again. I didn't know if I could survive it.

Because even though I chose to end that third pregnancy, I loved that baby deeply too, in her own way, in my own way. For a month after the procedure, I kept her ashes at my bedside. I had become so attached to her that I couldn't bear to separate myself from her yet, and keeping her close brought me some small comfort. Each night, I cracked the drawer and looked at the unexpectedly tiny square tin that held her ashes. In the dark, I lifted it up and opened it, smelling the faintest hints of earth and bone. I wasn't ready to look inside.

Then, one clear and windy day, Tyler and I drove to the coast, to a spot where our children have always loved to play. We waded into the water together. Waves lapped at our ankles while families flew kites and chased dogs on the beach all around us. We opened the tin. I saw our daughter's ashes for the first time as we scattered them in the vast blue expanse. Then I reached down and scooped up the seawater in my hands, drinking it in, splashing my face, mixing its salt with the salt of my tears. The surf rolled and crashed and foamed and settled, in this beautiful place that our family will return to again and again.

V:

RECONSIDERING

CHAPTER 10

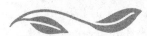

The plane was about to take off. I stared at my phone and willed it to ring as Zach bounced on the seat beside me, his toddler energy uncontainable by narrow gray pleather. Several flight attendants were chatting up front. Though I sensed some urgency in their voices, my only concern was if the call would come before we were asked to turn off our electronics for the flight.

Zach and I were on our way to meet Ian in California, where he'd traveled for work and where we would join him to visit family and attend a good friend's wedding. It was also the day the hospital geneticist was expecting to get the results of our chorionic villus sampling, one week after we'd undergone the procedure. She'd promised to call as soon as she had any news.

But instead of a ringing phone, I heard my name on an overhead page. With my hand in the air and a look of confusion on the flight attendants' faces, I realized that the commotion at the front door had been about me. The scanner had registered Zach's ticket but not mine at check-in, and the crew was getting alerts about an unaccompanied—and exceedingly young—minor. Finding me, they were relieved at the misunderstanding and went to secure the doors, beginning their preflight announcements.

I reached for my phone to turn it off just as it rang. When I answered, the geneticist shouted, "Normal chromosomes!"

I scrambled to thank her and asked her to call back to leave a message about the sex of the baby as we'd planned, so Ian and I could find out together later, then I left a quick message for Ian, who would be in meetings all day. How strange and incredible, I thought, that it was confusion over my own ticket that had delayed our flight just long enough to get her call. Zach sat happily distracted, latching and unlatching his tray table as he chattered away about forklifts and bucket trucks. Other passengers, just as unconcerned all around me, cinched down their seat belts, thumbed through glossy magazines, and pulled snacks from their carry-ons.

I leaned back and closed my eyes. Anonymous again among this sea of people, I marveled at how monumental a thing had just happened to me without causing a ripple in any of their days, how easily this moment could have pivoted in such a different direction. As this fresh relief washed over me, I knew that I couldn't begin to imagine all the stories the passengers around me were living.

From the moment we landed, our trip was a whirlwind. We shared home-cooked meals and late-night conversations with Ian's aunt and uncle. We danced with Zach at the wedding, dapper as he was in his tiny blue suit and tie, spinning and dipping around the parquet tile floor on a beautiful spring afternoon among the redwoods. We caught up with old friends we hadn't seen in years, including Tess and Khenan, who had come to town with their girls to join in the festivities too. We found out that Zach's little sibling would be a sister.

As our weekend of gatherings and celebrations came to a close on Sunday morning, Tess and I watched two-year-old Zach and three-year-old Elena playing together on the edge of the hotel bed, adorably out of sync as they shouted, "Go boing!" then tumbled backward in fits of laughter. Baby Cecilia babbled her approval as Khenan and Ian sat with her on a small couch nearby. Just before Zach was born, I'd told Tess the whole ordeal of what Ian and I had been through to get him. I'd admitted how painful it had been for me to hear her complaints about her routine pregnancy discomforts and Elena's difficult infancy while I hadn't even been able to stay pregnant. With that conversation, the rift in our friendship that had opened two years earlier had finally begun to close. Having gained so much empathy from her struggles with Elena, Tess was truly able to listen to my story. And I was ready to explain my experience and appreciate hers in a way I hadn't been able to when I'd been mired in my own pain.

On this blissfully ordinary morning, with this rare opportunity to be together in person, Tess and I both understood how fortunate we were to be the mothers of these giggly, happy children. We had forgiven each other and ourselves for being unable to offer support through our dark and lonely hours. We were better friends now because of our vulnerabilities. On that day, we shared something like exhilaration—but something quieter, calmer, steadier—at making it to the other side together.

FORTY-SIX XX declared the boldface lettering on the official report we received the following week: *Normal female karyotype.* Although we already knew the results, staring down at a paper with my daughter's chromosomal makeup typed out in precise, technical language was vastly reassuring.

After arriving in California, we'd waited to listen to the geneticist's message until we were all together, Ian and Zach and I, curled up in bed to read picture books on an unrushed vacation morning. We'd actually waited two days, choosing to learn the news on Friday the thirteenth, since thirteen is a lucky number on both sides of our family.

As a physician and a scientist, I considered myself a believer in evidence and logic. But as a person who acknowledged that the complexity of the world was far greater than my ability to comprehend it, I held fast to superstition too. Even having been told that our results were normal, some part of me was conditioned to seek any advantage, any coincidence that might imply that we were not being unreasonable to continue to hope for the best.

I didn't see any contradiction in this.

Parenthood—and, in my experience, everything along the way to becoming a parent—is full of opposing conditions. After my ectopic surgery, I was devastated and optimistic. When I remembered Zach's birth, I was grateful and full of regrets. When he took his first steps, I cheered him on, even knowing that as he grew up I'd miss those baby days.

The further we moved into parenthood, the more we discovered that two things could be true at once. In conversations with friends about how our challenges had widened our perspectives, I began to notice common threads that ran through the most divergent of experiences. Before motherhood, Nancy had turned to science each time she sought bright lines and unambiguous boundaries. Tina had shied away from unknowns, relying on rationality to define who she was. Eileen had looked to technology to build her family and had found comfort in calculations. Now, in becoming parents, all of them had come to value uncertainties and explorations as much as facts and data.

And I wondered: What are we left with when the frameworks we once depended on no longer make sense of the lives we are living? What shifts within each of us when we discover the central, irreconcilable calculus of motherhood, that it is a constant process of losing something in order to gain something else? What magic might our days reveal when we accept that logic and reason can coexist with hope and faith, and sometimes even with a little mystery?

Nancy ~ Remotely

I stepped from daylight into darkness. There were no windows in the ultrasound room, a detail that might have seemed soothing and private to some but, to me, felt like a renunciation of something scarce and precious. In October in central Alaska, each stretch of sunlight is seven minutes shorter than the previous one as the subarctic autumn descends swiftly into winter.

The technician ran her wand over my lower abdomen and peered at her screen. In this alien space, its glow drew my gaze too, with the promise of data and facts—but it was turned away from me, its images invisible from where I lay on the examining table. The technician scanned. She clicked. She furrowed her brow. Then she started giggling.

I had first suspected I was pregnant six weeks earlier, when my breasts—body parts that had always felt awkward to me, even at their modest size—began to inflate. My husband, Jay, seemed flummoxed, but not displeased. "Are they supposed to do that?" he asked me with a grin. After confirming my suspicions with a test at home, I contacted my doctor, a stalwart outdoorswoman whose down-to-earth optimism and scientific mind seemed to match my own outlook perfectly. She calmly advised me to start taking prenatal vitamins and make an appointment to see her in a few weeks. As the days went by, I observed my body with the fascination of the geeky biologist that I am. I was curious. I was intrigued. I can't say I was awash in maternal joy.

It wasn't that I didn't want offspring. I did—with a vehemence that surprised me, because I hadn't felt particularly strongly about it for most of the previous thirty-three years of my life. When I was six, parenthood had seemed like a side note to the more pressing business of being an inventor or an engineer or an astronaut. Even at sixteen and at twenty-six, being a scientist was an immediate reality, whereas having a child was something that would happen eventually. But *eventually* had crept up on me and become, with the emotional surety of crossing a line, *now*.

Jay and I had discussed our views on parenthood from many angles. We considered how creating a new human would impact the resources of the planet, an issue that was all too pressing to me as a climate change researcher. How it would influence our choices, our finances, our schedules. How it would affect our freedom.

Until now, we'd been in the habit of roaming into remote wilderness as often and as deeply as we could, not only in the endless daylight of mosquito-infested June, but also in the somber chill of January. We lived not quite in the middle of nowhere, because we had a comfortably short commute to our university jobs, but certainly somewhere near its edges. We were still putting the finishing touches on the nine-hundred-square-foot cabin we'd been building outside Fairbanks. Over the past four years, we'd measured and calculated and cut and sawed, installing triple-paned argon-filled windows, twelve-inch-thick roof insulation, floor-to-ceiling bookshelves, and a dedicated closet for camping gear. We'd constructed an outhouse. We'd even built shelters for the three sled dogs that helped us haul materials to our site, a quarter mile from the end of the road. But we hadn't made space for a kid.

At the same time, our lives did have space for a kid, in myriad ways. Our home, however wild, was welcoming. While it lacked some amenities, including indoor plumbing, it was nestled in a spindly, moose-rich forest with five other cabins. With a small cadre of close friends, we'd purchased eighty acres of marginal swampland and built a community. We co-owned a cozy shared building where families took turns cooking dinner and hung out playing games, ranting about politics, rifling through magazines, and watching movies together. Every other week, a tanker truck lumbered down our long gravel driveway to fill the central tank with a thousand gallons of the precious fresh water needed to hand-wash our dishes, run our high-efficiency clothes washer, and enjoy our low-flow shower. We knew any child of ours—though most likely an only child—would be born into a prefabricated family of sorts, with an assortment of overly intellectual adults and chatty school-aged playmates to adulate, mimic, and annoy.

Once we'd decided we wanted a baby, I'd gotten pregnant almost instantly. I understood I should be happy, yet somehow I felt uncertain in a way I couldn't explain. Then I started bleeding.

Now, here I was, in this room that smelled of medical procedure, more invested than I'd expected to be. I was in the dark, both figuratively and literally, as the technician giggled at me. Much as I enjoy mirth, it was unnerving to be the punch line of a joke I didn't understand while half-undressed and smeared with viscous jelly. The technician wasn't allowed to comment or diagnose. She wasn't allowed to say anything at all. But she made some adjustments and turned her screen toward me.

Light. Dark. Patterns of light and dark. And then I realized what I was looking at. Not one blob of light, but two. Not a single dark fluid-filled sac, but a pair. Paired lights in paired darkness. Twins.

A few minutes later, I sat down to call Jay from an antiquated courtesy phone in the waiting room. When he answered, still under the impression that we were going to have a baby—as in precisely *one* baby—I stumbled over words and emotions. This felt like wonderful news, and also terrible news. It felt scary and special, incredibly daunting and undeniably exciting. It was most definitely not what we'd planned.

When she reviewed the results, my doctor confirmed that the embryos looked fine and appeared to be about nine weeks along. We'd never know what had caused the bleeding, which had already resolved, but one likely possibility was that I had miscarried. That is, I might have lost a triplet.

Triplets. My mind spun. I felt not loss, but relief.

Even expecting twins had doubled—or perhaps squared?—the

doubts I was already confronting. I wasn't sure I could articulate the source of my ambivalence. My hesitancy wasn't rooted in anything as simple as the universally accepted truth that being a parent is hard work. I could handle challenges. I felt, in many ways, ready to be a parent. What I wasn't sure about was if I was ready to be a *mother*.

Being female seemed to me not so much a biological fact as a heavily freighted set of stereotypes, expectations, and assumptions. Many of these I was in the habit of studiously ignoring. As a kid, I had liked wrestling with friends and building construction-set masterpieces. But I'd also adored playing hopscotch and cuddling my baby-faced doll. I climbed every available tree with a degree of enthusiasm that horrified adults, but I couldn't hurl a snowball the width of my residential New York street. On the weekends, I dissected old appliances with a screwdriver, then, with equal enthusiasm, sewed myself a quilt using scraps from my grandfather's upholstery business. Sometimes I wished I were a boy. More often, I simply wished adults would stop drawing the gender lines so starkly.

Gender felt like a skill I didn't have, and my disregard for its norms became more zealous as I grew up. The closest I ever came to style in middle school, when many of the other girls were experimenting with eyeshadow and curling irons, was matching my shirt color with my sock color. In college, I slouched around wearing baggy overalls and oversized hoodies, hiding from ideals of beauty and all its foreign trappings as I sighed longingly over science fiction and higher mathematics. I did like boys, though I had very little success in finding any who wanted to date someone who spent less energy selecting her wardrobe than maintaining the axe and crowbar she used in her summer job building hiking trails.

I didn't entirely recognize what a heavy burden gender was until that burden subsided. When I moved to Fairbanks in my twenties, I suddenly felt almost normal. I traveled comfortably in social and professional circles in which work boots passed effortlessly as evening wear. My utilitarian grooming habits didn't set me apart in a crowd.

My penchants for minimalism and do-it-yourselfery were admired and put to use on expeditions far and wide. *Pretty* no longer felt like an important currency.

Jay and I spent our first dates in rugged backcountry locales with names like Granite Tors, Bison Gulch, and Wickersham Dome. During our courtship, Jay gifted me skis instead of flowers. On the morning of our wedding, he inquired, with some consternation, if I was going to wear makeup. I wasn't, and I didn't. I didn't own any. But I did brush out my thick braid and don a blue dress I'd sewn myself. I didn't quite feel like a bride, but I did feel like a thrilled-to-be-getting-married person.

Now I was a pregnant person. I was a slightly nauseated and bloated person. And I was a person who really wanted this kid—make that *these kids*. But I was realizing that having children was going to change me into someone very different from who I'd always been.

For a short time, I thought I could untangle my uncertainties with research. During my first trimester, I browsed the local used bookstore and found books with contradictory opinions about the best way to get babies to sleep, eat, burp, and do whatever babies were supposed to do, as well as articles whose main intent was to caution me that I might do it all wrong. Most of the information I found about multiples focused on pregnancy and delivery risks I'd never thought to consider. Some of what I learned was useful. Some of it was alarming. None of it assuaged my fears, which I could barely articulate myself.

Turning to mother-specific sources left me feeling even more alone. Cheery lists outlined steps for coloring hair safely in pregnancy and ranked designer diaper bags. No one offered a perspective on how long I could continue mountain biking through the snow to my makeshift trailer office at the university. Although everyone wanted to sell me matching bedding and curtains for my babies' nursery—which, in our case, was a half-built extension that Jay and I were rushing to complete in the bitter darkness—no one was advertising a double-wide kid carrier for hiking.

By the time I had stopped feeling nauseated and started feeling round, I'd gotten better at ignoring irrelevant advice. But I was actively floundering with how to reconcile becoming a parent with remaining a devoted outdoorsperson. Jay and I consulted our likeminded friends. Could we raise a family while still living in our simple cabin in the woods? Could we take the babies hiking? Dogsledding? Cross-country skiing? Even when it was forty degrees below zero? The exposed beams in our cabin were always draped with gear in various stages of airing out or drying, never to be put away before being packed for the next adventure. This wasn't a matter of compromising on my hobbies. This was who I was, and who I wanted to be.

Not sure how to solve my identity crisis before the babies were born, I found myself becoming concerned instead by a potential identity crisis I foresaw for the twins themselves. What if we couldn't tell them apart? I really, really hoped they'd be fraternal. I deeply wanted these kids to have unequivocally distinct personhoods from their earliest days.

Jay assured me that our children would be different, even if they were identical, and I started to almost believe him. I have friends who have identical twins and friends who are identical twins. I didn't have trouble seeing them as individuals. But I'd never bothered to ask any of those people exactly how they'd forged their identities or whether it had been a fraught process. When I worried that we'd mix up the babies, Jay suggested that we could label them. I wasn't sure if he was thinking of string, or duct tape, or perhaps permanent markers.

Throughout the winter, I continued to expand until my body had become a caricature of pregnancy. I craved minestrone soup, so I ate it by the gallon. I passed all the milestones with the sugar solutions, the blood tests sent to labs, and the machines that went beep. I attended numerous follow-up ultrasounds, though my little blobs remained coy at each one. Part of me was relieved by this—I didn't want to think about gender. I continued biking everywhere, with the permission of my doctor and the help of my studded snow tires. As the sun crawled along the horizon into spring, my body seemed to know exactly what it was doing. I was, by all accounts, a delightfully healthy pregnant person. I was busy. I was happy. I still harbored worries about adventure, individuality, and the expectations of motherhood.

And then I had two daughters.

From the moment the girls were born and were so clearly not identical, one of my fears fell away. Admittedly, all the other babies boxed up in the nursery looked kind of the same to us. The hospital staff had enthusiastically marked every infant with a veritable luggage department of scribbled plastic labels, which felt like further endorsement of their homogenous babyness. But to us, Baby A—Elizabeth—and Baby B—Molly—each had an appearance and an awesome newborn style all her own.

Still, there were plenty of strands of my own uncertainty to unravel. When Lizzy and Molly were fourteen days old, I dutifully brought them, via an awkward car seat in the crook of each elbow, to their two-week checkup. My doctor asked how we were all doing.

"We hiked Angel Rocks yesterday," I told her.

She stared at me for a moment. Then she laughed.

In retrospect, it seems obvious that I had something to prove. At the time, my only conscious rationale was that the twins were born at the end of May, just when Fairbanks was bursting into the greenness of summer with an ardor fueled by the almost-midnight sun. So Jay and I had set off with friends for a favorite trailhead, hauling two newborns, two baby carriers, a stash of extra diapers and wipes and itty-bitty spare clothes, and my not-yet-fully-healed cesarean incision.

This was, I knew, a ridiculous thing to do. Although the three-mile Angel Rocks loop is considered an easy hike by local consensus, it's not without some degree of challenge, given its steep switchbacks and rocky outcroppings. It's often recommended for novices or families with young children. It is not often recommended for adults recovering from major abdominal surgery or for children who still have umbilical stumps.

The venture had been a success by most objective standards. I'd herniated nothing, ruptured nothing, and dropped nothing off a precipice. It had been sunny. It had been warm. It had been, in short, a beautiful day for a picnic. And now, apparently convinced by my gurgling babies and in-one-piece self, our doctor gave us a pass. She had known me long enough not to be too surprised by our outing. I was vindicated. I should have felt victorious.

But I had to acknowledge that I had also felt different from everyone else on that mountainside, and not quite equal. My tiny new people were helplessly voracious. They could barely last a whole hour without sustenance, and that sustenance came only from me. Jay and I juggled the two of them back and forth, back and forth. Each time one squawked, I put her to my breast. I was glad to feed them. I was amazed that my body, which had so recently done one astonishing thing, could also do this other astonishing thing. Biologically, I was fascinated. Generally, I was grateful. But dishearteningly, I was aware that I was no longer the same as Jay. I was no longer just myself. I was the mom.

A few months later, a friend who'd known me since I was seven watched with a mixture of amusement and concern as I plunged a stack of pink onesies into a bucket of forest green dye.

"You won't be able to escape it in a few years, you know," she said. The utility sink in our communal laundry room was covered with dark splatters. I felt a twinge of defensiveness and wondered if rejection of pink was a sign of some deep-rooted self-hatred. Maybe it meant I'd absorbed the males-are-better assertions of the patriarchy. I rationalized my actions as being driven by logic. Pale pink, I reasoned, looked particularly hideous with strained-carrot stains. Lace and ruffles collected chunks and curds of the various substances that oozed out of babies. Bows glued to children's bald heads must've been as uncomfortable as they were ludicrous. But I knew my arguments were also masking a deeper and more complicated frustration.

Gendered infancy was so ubiquitous that I was having a hard time finding clothes, toys, crib mattresses, or really anything that wasn't gender specific. Girls' products featured stitched-on princess crowns, pastel rainbows, and sparkle ponies with humongous eyes. Boys' gear came emblazoned with modes of transportation, camouflage print, and bigger, fiercer animals—dinosaurs, dogs, snarling saber-toothed tigers. Boys' clothes hung on different racks than girls', sometimes many aisles away, presumably to avoid cross contamination. As I lugged our two grayish third-hand car seats around town, I discovered that everyone I talked to—which was fairly close to everyone, given the magnetic qualities of infant twins—expected me to adhere to social norms on behalf of my three-month-olds. Even in independent-thinking, no-nonsense-tolerating Alaska, strangers seemed quite annoyed that I had not decorated these small humans in a manner that correlated with the genitalia under their diapers.

When I stood at that laundry sink turning pink onesies green, I knew that my drive had something to do with who I was, and something to do with who I wasn't. It had something to do with who my daughters were, and who they might become. Yes, they were twins, and yes, they had both been assigned female at birth, but they were also two separate, unique, self-determining individuals.

From their earliest days, Molly and Lizzy did everything differently. Molly insisted on walking at ten months, repeatedly crashing into the perilous edges of cabinets and shelves, while Lizzy waited until she could cruise smoothly at thirteen months. When they were three, Molly spent an entire afternoon learning to tie her own shoes, yelling in frustration and turning away all help, but Lizzy wanted nothing to do with any shoes with laces. At four, Molly begged me to take the training wheels off her bike. She wobbled, then tumbled, then rode. Three months later, Lizzy still wanted me running alongside her with one hand as symbolic support, even though she was perfectly balanced. On the playground, in the pool, at the library, Molly's eyes were always observing the other kids—especially the bigger kids—while Lizzy was content to spend hours alone making a cardboard mushing sled for her stuffed dogs, unconcerned with keeping up with anyone else.

The girls soon had their own opinions about clothes too—four-year-olds' opinions as individual as their four-year-old selves—and I knew it was no longer my role to dictate or dye their choices. Molly had taken note of which clothes were preferred by which gender, and she gravitated toward items intended for girls but not girly: *NO* to princess dresses, to frills, to all items deemed excessively pink, but a resounding *YES* to stretch pants and to anything with a puppy motif. Lizzy also had strong preferences for her wardrobe—so strong that I sometimes had to wrestle clothes off her body to wash them—but her tastes were quirkier and gender-oblivious. Her three favorite pairs of pants were navy leggings with a skull and crossbones pattern, olive drab overalls with pockets and hammer loops, and too-short brown corduroys with patches on both knees.

Fraternal twins have no more in common genetically than any other siblings, which Molly was eager to explain as soon as she could speak in complete sentences. "We came from two eggs and two sperms!" she informed a friendly store cashier who had engaged her in conversation, while Lizzy sat silent and wide-eyed beside her in the grocery cart. I shrugged and smiled at this kid-of-a-scientist overshare.

A scientist: that part of my identity, at least, I was sure of.

But my biology research career wasn't the whole of my identity, any more than biological sex is the only determinant of gender. As I grew into parenthood, I found that the world around me kept trying to draw more bright lines even as true opposites felt rarer. Yes, becoming a mother was forcing me to wrangle with society about gender expectations. But it was also prompting me to consider the harsh—and false—dichotomy imposed between childhood and adulthood.

By preschool, Lizzy and Molly had started to notice that the separation of kid stuff from grown-up stuff meant a raw deal for the big people. They offered me heartfelt sympathy when I received nothing from the Easter Bunny. They puzzled over why my underwear came only in sad solid colors when theirs was covered with animals and superheroes. Immersed in the sticky, illogical, fantastical gleefulness of childhood's every discovery, they didn't want me to miss out just because I was so ancient.

But nowhere was the sorting of young from old more blatant than on the neighborhood playground.

"Hey, you're a good climber!" The speaker, a tousle-headed boy of about eight, was staring at me. So was a tiny girl in purple glitter rain boots. So were seven other kids on the jungle gym and merry-go-round. Every adult at the playground was diligently not staring at me.

Adults have learned that staring is rude. Children understand that staring is justified when a so-called grown-up is perched atop the twelve-foot-high pole of a swing set, with her feet hooked around its end supports, her belly stretched along its ridgeline, and her right hand firmly anchoring her to its crossbar while her left untangles the chains of one swing, then another. I love this about children. I'm a sucker for the charm of a person whose honest curiosity has not yet been buried in forced politeness.

The chains rattled and crashed as the black rubber seats descended. With a flush of pride, I realized I could manage the tasks of pole shimmying and swing unwrapping just as well as in the days when the playground aides tooted their whistles at younger me in consternation, exasperation, and possibly genuine fear.

But my exhilaration was tinged with misgivings. The other grown-ups were working really hard to ignore me, which reminded me that parents just didn't do this stuff. Moms *especially* didn't do this stuff. Dads might sometimes mock-wrestle and throw kids over their shoulders, but I always felt the awkward sidelong glances when I did the same. Once again, I was the mother who didn't know how to act like a mother. Who was prone to hiding in tree houses and licking ketchup off her fingers. Who relished muddy snail ponds and even muddier trails. I was obviously getting it all wrong.

And yet, as the twins leapt onto the two newly freed swings and pumped their legs skyward, I felt triumphant in my rebellion. I wouldn't give up all the pleasures of childhood just because I wasn't a child, or apologize for doing adventurous things just because I wasn't a dad. I wanted to model living in the in-betweens for my children. I grabbed a third swing and joined them. Some rules were unwritten, and easily ignored.

Some rules, on the other hand, were plainly outlined in black and white. *This hike is not recommended for young children*, noted Parks Canada in its guide to navigating the thirty-three-mile Chilkoot Trail. The Chilkoot traces the route of Klondike gold rush pioneers from the 1890s as they trudged through cool coastal rainforest, scrambled over a notoriously steep mountain pass, and descended into the unforgiving landscape of British Columbia. Jay had spent a good part of his own childhood on this trail along Alaska's southeast panhandle, where his dad had once been a ranger. I had never been there before, but as soon as we arrived I felt at home. It was precisely the kind of place where I wanted my four-year-olds to feel at home too.

Nonetheless, I worried about breaking rules, about being judged, and about whether such judgment might prove to be well-founded. Long before we set out on the trail—in fact, ever since Jay and I had first casually mentioned the destination for our end-of-summer family trip—I'd seen eyebrows skyrocketing. Even our hardiest friends questioned the wisdom of our plan.

Spurred on by their doubts, some of my own had crept in. How could we cover such rough terrain carrying all our own gear along with all the gear of our preschoolers—including the requisite stuffed animals, bedtime books, and footy pajamas—and sometimes the preschoolers themselves? What about gale-force winds, bird-sized bugs, grizzly bears, and unceasing rain? What if we ran out of chocolate?

On the trail, these doubts redoubled. Strangers gawked. Park employees were dubious. The one at the ranger station had reminded us, just before we'd started out, that the day ascending the notorious Golden Staircase takes the average hiker ten hours. Then he'd stared at us meaningfully. No one actually called me the most irresponsible mom they'd ever met, but the subtext was clear.

Chastened and slightly anxious, I urged my family onto the trail early on our summit day. A long, steep scree field rose to a barren pass at the border, with the red peaks and hanging snow fields of the Yukon beckoning in the distance, as we climbed up and up.

And it was incredible. As it turned out, our girls loved to hike, and scrambling over rocks was fun. Despite a thick and chilly fog, there was plenty to see along the way. Especially big, exciting, rusty stuff. Lizzy announced, with righteous indignation, that the gold rushers were litterbugs. If children are chastised for dropping paper scraps and candy wrappers, how did these miners get away with leaving piles of cans, the soles of worn-out shoes, and all these contraptions involving pulleys, winches, levers, and gears? This was not trash, I explained solemnly. These were artifacts. *Artifacts!* That sounded important. "Look, another artifact!" Lizzy informed me, every three feet, as we walked.

At the top, the Canadian border agent appeared from a one-room cabin perched on the wild edge of nothing. News of our group had preceded us by radio. He peered at Lizzy and Molly, searching for open sores, fresh blood, and signs of extreme emotional distress. Instead, the girls regaled him, through mouthfuls of peanut butter crackers, with observations about artifacts. "We don't usually get 'em below eight," he grunted. But I thought I saw a hint of a smile as he waved us on our way, down into another country.

That afternoon, I searched our campsite's scattered wooden platforms for mom-judging eyes. Instead I just saw fellow travelers, fatigued and footsore, working together to set up tents. A motley assortment of cookstoves roared and hissed. A few clouds had rolled in across the nearby lake. It was starting to drizzle.

Lizzy and Molly were unfazed, and still full of energy. They were jumping. And stomping.

"See the red lights?" Molly asked our neighbor enthusiastically, pointing to her sneakers. "They blink!"

He smiled. "Did you hike over the pass in those?"

"These are my train sneakers!" chirped Molly, as if that explained everything.

My little girls had summited the pass in their playground shoes. In fact, in the course of four days, they walked well over half the trail on their own strong feet and happily climbed their thirty-something-pound selves into their backpack carriers every so often to half nap while enjoying the ride. Like most of the hopeful miners before us, our family had failed to find our fortunes. What I'd discovered instead was something more valuable: a surprised relief at how much I'd enjoyed recalibrating my expectations of outdoor adventure to match the abilities, interests, and attention spans of my children. Their little feet didn't cover ground quickly. Their legs were half the length of mine. They challenged me and delighted me and stretched my patience nearly to the breaking point with their compulsion to fill their pockets with crumbling chunks of damp moss, and their constant stream of requests for songs and games. My mom pace was very different from my pre-parenthood pace. To reconcile the two, I'd had to open myself up to who I could become. But I was also exactly who I'd always been.

When I'd been pregnant, I had told my doctor, with some anxiety, that although I liked children, I'd never been a big fan of babies. I didn't ache to hold them, to dress them, to rock them, to fawn and to coo over them the way so many women did. I was frustrated and intimidated by their inability to communicate, their proclivity for screaming, and their sheer helpless fragility.

My doctor, ever unflappable, had reassured me that I didn't have to adore babies. That I'd feel different when they were mine. There was something teasingly familiar about this pronouncement, but it wasn't until the twins were well past babyhood that it struck me. This was advice for a dad. *Don't worry, young man, you'll love your own bundle of joy! And when the bundle grows to a more interesting and interactive age, you'll be stoked to teach your kiddo to ride a bicycle and build a snow fort. You'll go camping and light fires and roast stuff together. You'll look at bugs under a magnifying glass. In short, you'll be an excellent father!*

As my daughters have grown into young adults, the rigid lines of gender have been stretching, blurring, flipping, and blending—driven in large part by their generation. Thankfully, my parent friends are embracing these shifts, and embracing their kids, whoever they turn out to be. When I do hear discontented mutterings or outright hatred directed toward those who don't fit neatly into binary gender identities, my hackles rise.

None of this is a fad. I know transgender and nonbinary people of all ages, and history attests to struggles throughout decades, centuries, millennia. I know other middle-aged people like me—people who have managed to slide through life with our original pronouns but who feel over-categorized by or conflicted about our assigned labels. For those who need medical treatment to align their appearance with their understanding of self, greater support and acceptance are emerging, desperately needed and long overdue. The constraints are loosening around us all, creating a larger space for me to be who I am, a larger space for my children to become who they are becoming, a larger space for everyone to inhabit together. I've always wanted to create a better world for my daughters' generation. I never considered that their generation would create a better world for me.

Identifying with gender-fluid norms and living in a down-to-earth frontier state have helped me find myself without reinventing myself. I still don't spend time or effort working toward my culture's standard of feminine beauty or fashion. I still wear straight-cut men's jeans and T-shirts that only sometimes match my socks. When I go to professional meetings, I step it up a notch by putting on clean black slacks, dress oxfords, and a button-down shirt—but I trust that colleagues, elected officials, and university deans will be more concerned with what I am saying than how I look.

I want my daughters to believe that this is how things should be. I want to reassure them that humans aren't binary beings to be assigned to only two categories, or static works of art to be presented like carefully composed photographs. All humans look weird if you catch them eating a mouthful of spaghetti or bending over to scratch an itch. Real people get ingrown hairs, ill-timed zits, and period-stained underwear.

At the same time, I want my daughters to know that rejecting stereotypes doesn't have to mean rejecting their gender—or rejecting beauty. Despite my predilections for accessorizing with bandanas and decorating with duct tape, I've always appreciated beauty even while I dismiss rigid definitions of it. I see it in the laughter that fills the room after a coworker's clever story, the twinkle in my husband's glance as we share an inside joke, the languid stretch of our cat rising from his nap beside the crackling woodstove. Sometimes it takes my breath away when I glimpse it in low-angled sunlight scattering through yellow birch leaves, in distant white-topped crags of mountains set against a cerulean sky, in the lithe energy of my children in motion. It is not masculine or feminine. It isn't something that can be measured scientifically. It's something that every person, every creature, can participate in, can attain, in certain transcendent moments, captured in a mood, in a moment, in a memory, in the eye of the right beholder.

I still care about the messages I give my girls, but I've let go of some of my fears about how they navigate the world. I still seek the forests, the trails, and the mountains, but in sharing their intangible joys with my kids, I've been given the opportunity to reimagine what these places mean to me. I still skip in public occasionally, even though my kids are old enough to be embarrassed. I can lower my defenses as I watch my daughters grow stronger, making their own choices about which beliefs to accept and which to reject.

Life as a mother has been an entirely new kind of adventure. It's not remotely like anything I've done before, while also being an extension of exactly what I have been doing my whole life. My daughters and I have sewed and sawed and shoveled together, creating skirts and sheds and snow caves. We've cooked and skied and painted and run and climbed and shrieked with glee. We've ventured into forty-below-zero darkness in pursuit of the aurora borealis. We've biked the high passes of the Denali Park Road and the windswept coast of Iceland. We still live as a family of four in our unplumbed cabin on a patch of wooded swampland in central Alaska, traversing from light to darkness as the seasons mark our days.

And I could not possibly love my kids any more than I do.

More than once, Molly and Lizzy have told me I'm not like most other moms—not even remotely. I have reminded them, in return, that no person is quite like any other person. No two individuals are alike. No two moms are the same. There are no stark lines.

They accede to these truisms, while hedging that I might be just a little weirder than average. Then they say that they like me this way.

Tina ~ Solving for Unknowns

There are things that I may never know: What Kevin was thinking when he wrote the letters. Why he looked so strange in that photo on the guesthouse stairs. What Justin saw from his car seat as I sped down the road, knowing that it didn't really matter how fast we got there. Why the rainbows appear on such ordinary days.

But this, at least, is certain: I knew from the moment I met Kevin that he was going to be an amazing father.

Actually, it would be much more accurate to say that I knew this the third time we met. The first time, on a blind date arranged by a mutual friend, our night was an unmitigated disaster that left me holding a bag of ice to my swelling lip and eye. The second time was the next morning, when I walked out of a calculus lecture and saw Kevin sprinting up the stairs with an overflowing bouquet of orange and yellow wildflowers. As he stumbled over his feet and his words, rushing to apologize for the injuries that a malfunctioning umbrella had inflicted on me the night before, I saw that this was a guy who deserved another chance.

Our second date—our third meeting—felt absolutely charmed. Both lifelong Midwesterners raised to be polite and straightforward, we settled into an easy rapport as we strolled along the sidewalks of our university town. Kevin was such a great listener and such a natural storyteller that I barely remember what we said. He may have told me about his jobs nannying for one of his chemistry professors and teaching at a preschool. We probably discovered our common love of music. We likely commiserated about the pressures of our high-stress science majors. As the early-fall evening grew darker, he bought me a single red rose from a street vendor, and I twirled it by its long green stem as we walked, laughing to myself about the painfully obvious cliché of his romantic gesture. I didn't really like roses, but I did really like Kevin.

At a gathering with my extended family a few months later, he made conversation just as easily with everyone. But as soon as he could excuse himself from grown-up small talk, he found his way to my little cousins and spent hours inventing games with them. The kids flocked to him. They told him knock-knock jokes, and he chuckled. They begged for piggyback rides, and he obliged. They crowded onto our checkered plaid blanket as he read a picture book aloud, and they hung on his every word.

Kevin's playful side had drawn me to him just as surely. In my own life, I'd long valued rationality above all else, treating emotions as a distraction as I approached every problem with logic. Kevin was much better than I was about not judging each moment for whether it was useful or productive, and I came to love him for this.

We got married five years later and began to think about when we might want to have kids. Being a father was an extremely big deal to Kevin, but I didn't feel quite the same enthusiasm about starting a family. I had always believed that it made sense to establish myself professionally first, to reach some idealized midpoint of adult life when I'd be deep enough into my career that I'd be willing to step back a bit and make the sacrifices that raising children would require. An engineer to the core, I was deliberate and methodical in my decision-making. Considering motherhood was no exception.

I also prioritized pursuing adventures as a couple before we settled down. As we followed job opportunities after college, leaving the Midwest and buying a house far away in Colorado had felt antithetical to the traditions of both our families, but Kevin and I were ready to push beyond the limitations set by their expectations. After work and on weekends, we camped in the foothills of the Rockies, biked through golden aspen trees, and tried to climb fourteen-thousand-footers—though we didn't always make it to their summits.

Kevin didn't share my concerns about the ways having kids might change us. He was convinced that he would weave his children seamlessly into his life as he taught them to do the things he loved, and that having a family would only make our travels together better. Gradually, Kevin's eagerness convinced me that maybe I could have it all—maybe not all at once, and maybe not in the way I'd been envisioning. But he helped me believe that our lives would be richer and fuller as parents. As I calculated the benefits and drawbacks of different timelines, I kept coming back to one central thought: Kevin would be a great dad. I had every confidence that he'd be fully involved in our children's lives, and I was excited to move forward together. I decided that I was ready for our next adventure.

Justin was born when I was twenty-nine, five years after our wedding, eleven years after the incident with the errant umbrella, precisely forty weeks into a very difficult pregnancy. From the moment Kevin held Justin and kissed his tiny nose, he was overwhelmed by the intensity of his love for this little boy. So when Kevin was laid off from his technical marketing position six weeks later, neither of us hesitated to decide that he would be a stay-at-home dad for a stint. After one of the most dramatic periods of economic growth ever seen, the whole country was plummeting into a historic recession triggered by the bursting of the dot-com bubble, and our industries were at the heart of it all. Then, when we relocated to California shortly before Justin's second birthday to complete on-site requirements for a graduate degree I'd been working toward, it made more sense for Kevin to continue caring for Justin than to try to advance his career in a place where we planned to stay for only a year.

That's not to say that every moment of fatherhood was easy or fun for Kevin. He was quick to admit that he had underestimated the challenges of taking care of a young child. Lovable as Justin might be, he was such a little bundle of need. But by the time he'd turned three, the boys were exploring trails through the woods, splashing in the campus fountains, and playing with other families in the shared courtyard behind our student housing. An inseparable father-son team, Justin and Kevin spent the spring and summer adventuring together, exactly as Kevin had always dreamed of doing.

We moved back to Fort Collins at the end of August. When Kevin and I were invited to present and consult at prestigious industry events in Europe in early September, my dad and my grandmother drove out from Wisconsin to stay with Justin so Kevin and I could also make a couples vacation out of our business trip before Kevin embarked on his job search.

From the moment we landed in Frankfurt, Kevin was eager to connect with people. A seasoned traveler, he had a gift for discovering what was interesting in everyone he talked to, and he immersed himself in the local culture wherever we went. When we spoke English, we felt self-conscious and presumptuous, like we were expecting everyone else to accommodate us. When we attempted even our most rudimentary German, we were welcomed wholeheartedly. By the end of one particularly memorable dinner party—after having recovered from our initial shock at the menu's offering of horse meat—we had invitations to stay with new friends in four countries.

Once the work events were done, we spent days riding the rail lines to link up relics of thousand-year-old history through Germany,

France, Italy, and Switzerland. The castles of southern Switzerland truly enchanted us. Many had weaving staircases that connected to extensive systems of trails through the surrounding hillside towns. Kevin, in his favorite lace-up dress shoes—the only footwear he'd thought to bring, being so focused on the formal functions we'd be attending—struggled to manage the endless steps. His legs cramped with fatigue each day after less than an hour of walking. He kept bumping his toes into the old stone risers as he lifted his feet to climb.

We both laughed about how uncharacteristically tired and un-coordinated he seemed, especially as a gifted athlete who competed in several hockey and soccer leagues, spent his weekends biking, ski-ing, golfing, and playing tennis, and ran long-distance races without training, talking all the way to encourage the less fit friends he ac-companied. I teased him mercilessly about forgetting his sneakers. A meticulous packer myself, I found it amusing that his dedication to adventure did not grant him an ability to foresee the proper equip-ment to enjoy it.

The vacation was idyllic, despite this minor inconvenience. We celebrated our wedding anniversary with a candlelit meal in an ele-gant Swiss restaurant. Temporarily liberated from the responsibilities of home, we finally delved into conversations that had been hard to make time for while juggling work and studies and parenthood—especially conversations about parenthood itself. By the time our trip was over, we'd realized we were both ready to start trying for our second child.

We returned home on a Wednesday night. I spent the next two days catching up at work while Kevin and Justin visited with my dad and grandma before their trip back home on Friday. When the weekend arrived, Kevin and I were happy to reconnect with Justin on our own and settle in as a family of three, chatting about the new preschool Justin would be starting next week, as we unpacked boxes from our still-recent move alongside suitcases from our trip.

But as Saturday afternoon turned into evening, my initial good

feelings of resettling were replaced by agitation. I had no explanation for it, and I had no idea what it was. Justin was asleep in the
next room. Kevin was playing video games on the couch nearby. As
I fidgeted with a stack of books on the coffee table, he asked me if
I was mad at him for some reason, but that wasn't it at all. It was
just me, completely unmoored and getting worse by the minute. I
remembered that I'd felt the same way the night my mother's mother
had died a few years earlier, and I'd only learned the next morning
that she'd been found slumped in her recliner, tablets of emergency
heart medication still clutched in her palm. Distressed at feeling so
inexplicably out of sorts, unable to find a way of centering myself as I
recalled this premonition, I finally went to bed.

After breakfast on Sunday, when Kevin left to play soccer, Justin
and I drove to Denver to pick up a secondhand kitchen table and
chairs. I maneuvered them like puzzle pieces into the back of our
truck, thinking about how glad I was to have our errand done as I
watched clouds gather over the mountains. The sky was uncharacteristically gray and ominous for a late-September Colorado day, and I
was intent on getting home before it started pouring.

We were halfway back when my phone rang. It was Kevin's mom,
telling me that she'd gotten a message that Kevin had hurt himself
playing soccer. From his car seat behind me, Justin happily made up
words as he pretended to sing along with the radio. Kevin's mom and
I agreed to check in with each other once either of us learned more.

Less than a minute later, my phone rang again. An unfamiliar-
sounding woman introduced herself and told me that she was calling
from the hospital. She asked if I was Kevin's wife. I turned off the
music to listen.

"Where are you?" she asked calmly. "Who are you with?" I heard
her telling me in an unnaturally measured voice not to hurry but to
come in as soon as I could.

With those words, I knew something horrible was going on. I
knew that Kevin was dead.

I hung up the phone and picked up speed. Justin, strapped in behind the driver's seat, couldn't see my face, but he sensed my rising panic. He started crying and asking me where we were going. I tried to concentrate on the road. I understood that whatever had happened had already happened. I couldn't get there fast enough to change the past. But still I made the thirty-minute drive in twenty.

As Justin and I pushed through the swinging emergency room doors, two social workers met us. One reached out for Justin's hand, asking if they could play for a little while, then walked away with him as I stammered my agreement. The second led me into a windowless room with a tiny couch where she introduced me to two other people whose roles I didn't catch. Doctor? Nurse? Police officer? It didn't matter. She motioned for me to sit down, then positioned herself in a chair and looked directly at me.

"Kevin collapsed on the soccer field an hour ago," she began. I remembered hugging him that morning as we'd parted ways, our argument over how to balance recreation—like his soccer game—with responsibilities—like procuring furniture for our home—mostly resolved but still stinging.

"His teammates tried to help him. They started rescue breathing and chest compressions right away, but they couldn't get a pulse." I pictured Kevin surrounded by other players on the turf the last time I'd watched him play, high fives all around to celebrate a hard-earned goal.

"When the paramedics arrived, they shocked his chest with the defibrillator as they rushed him to the hospital." I saw Kevin kneeling down on the airport carpet as Justin ran to welcome us home, just three days ago, giggling and throwing himself into Kevin's open arms.

"But the doctors were not able to revive him." Nothing. I saw nothing.

She said that she was so, so sorry for my loss. She paused. I breathed. I looked at the ceiling, at my hands, at her eyes again. Then, gently but methodically, she moved into a series of questions: *Did*

Kevin have any illnesses? Take any medications? Use any drugs? In my bewilderment, the only response I could think to offer was that he'd recently tried a new allergy pill.

I asked to see Kevin. We walked along a hallway and she gestured me through a door, where I found myself numbly staring down at a disconnected breathing tube and a tangle of wires overshadowing this unmoving figure that was no longer him. I could barely comprehend what was happening. As I stood alone beside his body for several long, empty minutes, my mind was awash not with an urge to say goodbye but with the crush of plans unrealized: traveling the world, growing old together, having a sibling for Justin. All of it was gone.

I must have offered a name and a phone number when the social worker stepped back into the room behind me and quietly asked if I had anyone we could call for a ride, because soon a good friend's arm around my shoulders steadied me as we loaded my now-dozing son into the back seat of her car.

By the time we got home, a few other close friends she'd called had come by too. They milled about, speaking in hushed tones as they tried to come up with something helpful to do. They brought me blankets and snacks and glasses of water. They ordered takeout and tucked Justin into bed with his favorite stuffed animals. They tried to convince me to do things like eat and shower and lie down to rest.

But I just didn't have it in me. I didn't know what to do with myself now that I'd seen how fast the world could crumble. Nothing about this made sense, and nothing could soften the blow. Thirty-four-year-olds weren't supposed to die on soccer fields. Their hearts didn't suddenly stop beating. Kevin had no medical problems, never used drugs, and took impeccable care of himself. He was the healthiest person I knew.

I wandered from room to room aimlessly. My mind replayed the terrible call I had made to Kevin's parents from the hospital. Again I heard myself tell them that Kevin had died, using the same words the social worker had used with me, then cringing as his mother

sobbed and shouted and fell apart in all the ways that I hadn't allowed myself to.

I was restless through the night while Justin slept, tired out by the
attentions of doting adults and undisturbed by Kevin's absence. By
midmorning on Monday, our friends had headed off to tend to their
jobs and care for their own families. With the emptiness of the house
echoing, I decided it was time to tell our son what had happened.

When I opened the door to Justin's room, he was playing with his
toy trucks, driving them back and forth across the carpet. He looked
so content in his innocence. I felt physically ill knowing that I was
about to wrench that away from him. Hesitating in the doorway, I
thought about how the social worker at the hospital had warned me
that most three-year-olds don't understand what *dead* is. They can't
grasp the concept that there's nothing they can do to bring their loved
one back. And, no matter what an adult may think happens after
death, using euphemisms like *He's gone to a better place, He's moved
beyond this life,* or *He's sleeping peacefully now* only confuses kids more.

But when I sat down on the floor beside him, I knew that Justin
would believe me. I picked up a plastic bulldozer and waited for him
to look up. When he did, I told him that the reason all these friends
had come to our house to help us was that his daddy had died yesterday. I told him that his daddy was never coming home. His eyebrows
quivered, then he started crying quietly, almost calmly, as his gaze
held mine. He didn't move. He didn't speak. He looked sad, but un-
questioning. He understood that Kevin was gone.

What he didn't understand was *why*. And I had no explanations
to offer.

On Thursday, instead of going to his first day of preschool as
planned, Justin got on a plane with me to fly to Wisconsin for Kevin's
funeral. Outside the airplane window, baggage carts shuttled suitcases
and oversized duffels across the tarmac. Justin clung to my arm and
fiddled with his stuffed baby bear as I thought about Kevin—or, more
accurately, as I thought about Kevin's body.

Justin and I weren't the only ones traveling for the funeral. Kevin had to get there too. He was going to be shipped, in his casket, on some plane somewhere, like so much luggage. Was he on our flight? Waiting in a warehouse? Already back in his hometown? I watched the slow parade of bags crawling up the motorized ramp beside us and wondered where Kevin might be as the pieces tumbled, one by one, over the sill of the cargo compartment and out of my sight.

Arriving in Madison was disorienting. Kevin's parents and three brothers were so mired in their own grief that my presence barely registered. To their suffering I was an outsider, distracting and unwelcome, as they circled their wagons in pain. As I drifted along the periphery, I wished we could band together in our shared experience. But I sensed that my very existence was an excruciating reminder: I was still alive, while Kevin was gone. Kevin's mother had already buried an infant daughter thirty-five years ago. To lose a second child was too much for her to bear.

To compound the stress, I was swamped with choices from the moment we arrived. Kevin's family thought they were giving me grace by letting me make every decision, but the burden was unimaginable. By Friday, even simple tasks felt daunting. I ordered arrangements of wildflowers to decorate the church for the service, then cried when I remembered Kevin running up the campus steps to offer me the bouquet he'd picked the day after we'd met. I agonized over coming up with a song he'd loved that would be appropriate to include in a funeral, then scrambled to hire a musician to transcribe it to sheet music for the piano. So many people would be coming to support us, and I was supposed to choose just a few to give the readings. It felt like I was planning the worst wedding ever and had only twenty-four hours to do it.

Saturday was beautiful and awful, healing and traumatic. Most of all, it was one incredibly long blur. The morning began with a visitation, during which Kevin's parents and brothers and I stood by the open casket as other mourners came by to pay their respects. There were so many people I recognized and so many I didn't—probably three hundred in all, over the course of several hours—flooding by in a steady, overwhelming stream. Some moved through quickly, averting their eyes, offering simple condolences. Some lingered, sharing memories of happier times as I awkwardly tried to console them. Many held the rosary close as they paused over Kevin, praying for his soul to pass peacefully from Purgatory into Heaven. As Kevin's older brother handed each guest a remembrance card with a handsome black-and-white photo of Kevin on one side and a picture of his favorite jagged Colorado mountain range on the other, I felt compelled to manage the reactions of others and absorb their grief, just when I most needed emotional support myself.

By the time the service began in the late morning, I was already spent. Kevin's younger brother played the piano. His older brother gave a moving speech about something I formed no memory of but found incredibly thoughtful at the time. A lifelong friend of mine sang a hauntingly beautiful song by one of Kevin's favorite musicians. The priest stood to deliver the sermon—the priest who led Kevin's family parish, who'd known Kevin since he was a toddler, who'd nearly convinced Kevin to enter the priesthood before he'd met me—then offered Communion as congregants stepped forward. My sister-in-law showed a movie of photographs she'd compiled documenting Kevin's life, from babyhood to our travels in Europe just ten days ago. Justin shouted, "Daddy!" and pointed excitedly each time a picture of grown-up Kevin flashed across the screen. I sat on the hard wooden bench, trying to take everything in but acutely aware of how little I was processing in the moment, and said nothing.

It wasn't because I had nothing to say. There was so much I wanted to say—to honor Kevin, to express what a wonderful father and partner he had been, to do him proud. But I just couldn't. And I knew if I tried, I'd fall apart.

After the service had concluded and the guests had begun to wander outside, I looked around the church. The red carpets along the altar and transepts were flooded with flowers and plants that friends had brought as offerings. Their abundance rendered the scene both magnificent and absurd. I had no idea what I was going to do with dozens of potted arrangements, a thousand miles from home. I imagined myself walking down the long center aisle of the airplane the next day, trying to balance them all as Justin trailed behind me, dragging his baby-bear stuffie.

Instead, I found myself walking down the long center aisle of the church, toward the narthex at the back. By the time I stepped out of the tall double doors, Kevin was already being transported—again—from one place to another in a process that I didn't control and couldn't accompany him on, now borne by pallbearers who would set the casket down beside the open grave. Once the parish elders signaled that they were ready, all of us began our collective march across the grassy fields to join them.

We walked. I walked. I pictured Kevin the last time I'd seen him, seen his body, lying still and waxy during the visitation, not looking much like the very alive Kevin I remembered. A few days earlier, the funeral director had asked me what Kevin would want to be buried in. The logical choice was his favorite olive green button-down shirt and tailored pants, along with the handcrafted dress shoes he'd splurged on—the same ones he'd worn on our trip to Europe, up and down those stairs as his legs cramped incessantly. After we'd made a plan, she followed up by asking if there was anything Kevin would be wearing that I wanted to keep.

I was jarred by the thought of anyone undressing him after the funeral. Then I realized that, because he was an organ donor, his doctors would have already removed the skin from his legs to donate for grafting. The ordinariness of clothes, of pants, of shoes seemed bizarre in that circumstance, a patchwork of cotton and leather to cover what was left of a body. But they were his, and they were the pieces he'd chosen when he'd wanted to look his best in life. Why should I remove the shirt that had made Kevin's beautiful green eyes shine?

What good would his worn brown lace-ups do anyone else? Was I expected to save these things for sentimental value, or for our son to wear at some event twenty years in the future? I didn't really care what happened to his things, but every option felt wrong. Who was I to dismantle any part of this man? When the director asked me if I wanted a lock of Kevin's hair, in case Justin ever needed it for genetic testing for medical conditions, I was even more unnerved. I had never considered that death would present so many strange decisions.

But perhaps the most surreal moment had been selecting my own burial plot. Almost as soon as Kevin died, I'd decided that his final resting place should be near his childhood home. Tending to a loved one's grave is very important in Catholic tradition, and I couldn't be sure I'd stay in Fort Collins as my career progressed. I knew his family would want to visit this consecrated site over the years no matter where Justin and I were living. His parents already had plots reserved for themselves in the cemetery beside the church they'd attended since Kevin was barely older than Justin, this church where we'd honor his passing. So I bought one for Kevin beside his mother's. Then I bought another for myself adjacent to his.

Now I was standing in front of those plots, at the edge of a gaping hole in the earth. The day was unseasonably hot, the sun unflinchingly harsh. My dark blouse clung to my back as silver poles suspended Kevin's casket on a platform beside the void. Justin reached his tiny, damp hand up to hold mine. We had been here for ten minutes, or two hours, or four days. I no longer trusted myself to gauge the passage of time.

Blessings were offered.

Grant that our brother may sleep here in peace until You awaken him to glory, for You are the resurrection and the life.

Prayers were recited.

Lord God, whose days are without end and whose mercies are beyond counting, keep us mindful that life is short and the hour of death is unknown. Let Your Spirit guide our days on earth in the ways of holiness and justice, that we may serve You, sure in faith, strong in hope, perfected in love.

Tears were shed.

Remember, Lord, that we are dust: like grass, like a flower of the field.

The cemetery attendants lowered the casket into the ground, and the priest tossed a ceremonial white carnation onto it. And then it was done. It was done.

We all walked back to the church together, our slow progression of mourners trudging along under a cloudless autumn sky. The main emotion I felt was not really an emotion at all, but just complete and utter exhaustion.

Back at home in Colorado the next week, everything seemed inconsequential in the shadow of Kevin's death. But I still had to make food for Justin, maintain routines around naps and bedtime and potty training, and work my full-time job. My parents and sister and grandmother and others who'd flown in to help rotated through our guest room, while local friends raked fallen leaves, repaired broken sprinklers, and filled the freezer with quick-cooking meals. I appreciated anything that made our lives easier, especially since my company allowed only two days of bereavement leave. Cards and packages flowed into our home every day. One faraway friend sent a copy of her favorite acoustic guitar music, which I played for Justin to help him fall asleep at bedtime and to soothe him when he woke crying and shouting, confused. He was acting how I felt but couldn't let myself *be.* There was no space for me to be sad.

But the truth is that I was devastated. I was just better at suppressing my grief. Kevin had always been the one who was good at putting emotions into words, the parent who was in touch with his feelings, the perfect foil to my rational thinking. Now I would have to become this part of him for Justin.

What would Kevin have said if he were the one left behind? I tried to be honest with our son, telling him that it was okay to be sad, that I missed Daddy as much as he did. It was a real effort not to collapse into bed and stay there all day. But while Justin saw me cry many times, he also heard a consistent message that we would get through this together. At least I hope he did. I tried to be extra patient when he had hour-long screaming meltdowns or came to me trembling with nightmares. I knew that I couldn't begin to imagine what this experience would mean for him as he grew up—just that it would define his life even more than it would mine.

As I struggled to adjust to our new reality, my thoughts fogged and floated. I drifted through the days feeling completely detached. Sometimes I found myself reaching down to my left pointer finger to spin Kevin's three-toned gold wedding band, the only thing he'd been wearing that I'd decided to keep. Like when planning the details of the funeral, every decision I was faced with now seemed both daunting and meaningless. I was confused by the mundane tasks as much as by the cataclysmic shifts that had manifested in my life. I didn't know anyone who'd been through a loss like this, and no words could convey how it felt to live it.

The autopsy results came back at the end of October. Kevin's death was declared the result of a congenital cardiac defect. One of the main arteries that fed his heart muscle was narrow and irregularly shaped, compromising blood flow to its electrical control area since birth and causing the cumulative damage that finally sent him into a sudden, irreversible arrhythmia. It explained the pain he'd had in his legs in Switzerland—from decreasingly efficient circulation to his extremities—and it wasn't something we could have fixed. It wasn't something Justin would inherit. I found a little reassurance in these facts.

But having an explanation didn't really change anything. When I let myself peek out of the grief and the numbness, I was also extremely angry. For myself, yes—but especially for Justin. He was too young to have stored up enough memories of Kevin to last him a lifetime. He was too young to get much out of working with a counselor, though we tried. He was too young to have his dad taken away. When did we get to go back to the life I'd chosen for us? It wasn't fair.

My anger was a complicated thing, tangled up in regret, fear, loss, confusion, uncertainty, self-doubt, and vulnerability. I felt a heavy sense of freedom when freedom wasn't something I'd wanted. The world had dropped out from under me, taking with it all my security, all my stability, like a surreal and terrible dream.

But anger felt safer than sadness. Sadness didn't solve anything. Sadness felt passive, like an inevitable reaction to loss. Anger felt active, like motion, like passion, like strength. To channel my anger, I turned to exercise. For years, I had enjoyed hiking and biking on trails with Kevin, scanning for rocks and logs and drop-offs while the terrain sped by beneath me. And I'd loved to play volleyball with friends after a long day in the office. But neither of these outlets worked for me anymore, now that my mind was so scattered and Justin had no one else to stay with in the evenings. I needed distraction rather than focus, solitude rather than teamwork.

Grasping for something different, I discovered swimming. Along the pool's smooth aqua lanes, there was nothing to jump over, nothing to duck under, nothing to guard myself against. The water was always the same, offering its quiet sensory deprivation. I dove in and threw my anger against its placid sheen, thrashing with abandon. I wore myself out. I broke through my own surface. I drained my physical body so deeply that I had no reserves left, and, as I caught my breath, a little calm emerged. Too quickly, though, I adapted. Soon I was barely winded after two miles in the pool. I couldn't swim hard enough to force out my rage, or to help my body allow the rest it needed. Practice was making me stronger in ways that didn't serve me.

And so it was with grief. Where at first I had faltered, I became conditioned in my coping. I worked with a therapist to process my experiences, and my anger didn't show as much. I joined a support group, and my sorrow condensed into a shape that those around me could accept. But I resisted the assumption that grief was an equation I needed to solve. Painful as it was, a part of me longed to sit with my sadness, to feel it fully, to stare it down until I was sure that it would keep me connected with Kevin. As the months slipped by, I was getting used to Kevin's absence in a way I didn't want to.

Kevin's death didn't leave me with *loneliness* so much as *missingness*. I still sensed him there, like a phantom limb, as true as the absence of a piece of my physical self. I thought of a disconcerting photograph I'd rediscovered on my computer recently—one of the last pictures taken of Kevin and me together. As he and I stood on the stairs of the guesthouse we had stayed at in Switzerland in September, Kevin was nearly translucent, fading into the background like a hazy double exposure on old-fashioned film. When we had first seen the photo, we had written it off as a malfunction. But this hadn't happened in any other pictures we'd taken, and we'd used a digital camera. As rational as I usually tried to be, I now had to acknowledge how bizarre this was— and admit that this ephemeral image might signify something more.

With Kevin gone, the parts of me that were parts of him were disappearing too. I constantly tried to relive the most important moments of our fourteen-year relationship in my mind, distraught over the notion of letting a single memory fade before I could cement it. I didn't want to forget anything that would help Justin understand who his father had been and what we had all meant to each other.

But grief distorted everything. It crashed into me, upending my world, stealing huge chunks of time from my life, making my desperation to guard these memories feel all the more distressing. From the moment I learned of Kevin's death, I lost details, dropped threads, and blurred facts, even as I remembered how effortless remembering had used to feel. A friend whose husband had sustained a head injury while skiing remarked on how similar our symptoms were. There was instant confusion on impact, then a slow lifting of the fog over months, but the full sharpness of memory never returned. In a casual conversation, most people couldn't tell that we'd been forever altered. To those who knew us well, though, and to ourselves, we were no longer the people we used to be. How strange it was to look the same to the world when so much had changed inside us.

Maybe this was why finding the letters was such a revelation. Many months after Kevin's death, I was clearing out boxes from the back of our bedroom closet one afternoon when I randomly opened a tattered spiral notebook and discovered two handwritten letters. The first one was addressed to me. Reflecting on his past, Kevin wrote about having come to a place where his life was no longer all about him or his personal accomplishments, and where he no longer cared about material possessions. He criticized his younger self for being too egocentric, too aspirational, too concerned with competition and career. None of that really mattered, he wrote. The meaning of life was in relationships, in the time we spend and the experiences we share with family and friends. He described how this new realization had brought him a level of contentment that was hard to put into words.

The second letter was for Justin. *To my boy*, it opened. *I love you so much, and I always will. As you grow up, my hope for you is that you will not feel compelled to chase being the best at things that other people do. Instead, you should strive to find what's unique within yourself, to be and to become the loved and lovable person that you alone can be.* Every word of it affirmed that being the smartest or the fastest or whatever superlative was imposed by others wasn't important. Every word of it encouraged Justin to live a life of honor, to be a person of his word, to believe in himself no matter how the world might judge him. Every word of it conveyed the love Kevin would always have for us and reassured me that the impact of his life on ours would continue, no matter what I remembered or forgot.

Both of the letters were dated just two months before Kevin had died. I thought of the eagerness he'd always felt about having kids, all while trying not to pressure me before I was ready. Of the Over the Hill birthday party I'd thrown him when, at twenty-nine, he declared himself officially old. Of the grainy photo from Switzerland, his image translucent, ghostly, vanishing in plain sight. Of the ways, in retrospect, I'd noticed Kevin's life accelerating over the past few years, as a sense of deliberateness—even urgency—emerged around his time with loved ones.

I suddenly understood, and there was nothing rational about it: Kevin had known. He had known he was going to leave us. He had been preparing to leave us for a long time before he died. He had given us these huge and generous pieces of himself, these memories and values that would be ours to carry forever. He had ensured that, regardless of what came next, I wouldn't be raising Justin alone.

Kevin has now been gone for longer than he and I were together, and one of my greatest sadnesses still is that we didn't have a sibling for Justin. But our family did eventually grow, and it happened in a way I never would have predicted. When he'd first heard about Kevin's death, our old friend Josh had reached out to me from several states away with the most thoughtful gifts—a beautiful woolen shawl for me and a sweet picture book for Justin—along with a heartfelt note saying that he hoped I knew that Kevin and I had friends who would always be there for Justin and me.

Josh and I had known each other in high school, then reconnected through a chance meeting on the streets of San Francisco as adults. Kevin and Josh had bonded over their shared passion for endurance sports, and all of us had kept in touch over the years, meeting up for leisurely lunches on my work trips to California. The history we shared was unusual and fragmented, but still comforting. I wasn't looking for love. And I knew no one could ever take Kevin's place for me or for Justin. But my friendship with Josh was part of Kevin's legacy too, and our connection continued and deepened over many long-distance phone calls and long weekend visits, becoming the foundation for so much more.

When Justin was five, he asked Josh to marry us. The first time he tried, he pocketed a ring in a jewelry store while we wandered the aisles, awaiting our lunch reservation next door. When the ring clanked to the floor during the extended family luncheon that followed and

I discovered his mischief—mercifully, Josh didn't realize Justin's intentions—he told me he wanted to ask Josh to be his dad.

The second time, a few months later, we were on a trip to Guatemala. We found the city streets carpeted with intricate floral mosaics, stunning and impermanent, an Easter ritual meant to be destroyed by the parades that marched through every day. There, in this season of rebirth, Justin handed Josh a small black box. Inside was the ring I'd ordered before Justin had attempted his own misguided proposal. It was an unusual ring that would represent the unusual story of our partnership. It was crafted from steel-gray tungsten, a rare metal integral to the semiconductors I worked with and known for its resilience and its strong bond formation—for holding things together to help keep them whole. And Josh said yes, to both of us.

Justin is now off at college in Montana studying engineering, and Josh and I live in Poland, a day's drive from the staircases in Switzerland where Kevin's steps first faltered. Alone and together, we're forging our history in new places, and we all spend much of our time exploring mountains and bike trails that Kevin would have loved. Kevin always insisted that having kids would make our travels together better. He was absolutely right. Having Justin has immensely increased my enjoyment of the world, and I see more of Kevin in him every day. Kevin helped us build this family, and he is still part of it.

When he's trying to tell me something, Kevin often signals his presence with a rainbow. As a scientist, I feel skeptical even as I consider this. But I've witnessed it in forms I can't explain with my rational mind: An iridescent prism once appearing in a corner of my kitchen, with no discernible source, as I made dinner and grappled with a difficult work decision. A patch of pigment dancing on my office desktop as I sorted through files to deal with health insurance hassles. Huge stripes of color beaming down from the clouds as I finished a long trail ride, contemplating a move that I was coming to realize wouldn't be good for Justin at that time.

Grief runs through my life in much the same way. Sometimes it's a tiny fragment hovering along the edges, and sometimes it streaks across my entire sky, vibrant and shimmering, calling out for my attention, changing hues depending on the angle of my view. Maybe the colors of grief are the hope, the connection, the sign Kevin offers that he's still here with us, asking us to trust the universe without trying to solve for every unknown.

For now, I think back on Kevin's fading image with reverence and with wonder. I am grateful for the time that he had with Justin, and for what we all still have together. I take the boxes out of our closet, open the old, yellowed notebooks, and hold the letters loosely in my hands. And I celebrate the rainbows most of all.

Eileen ~ Doing the Math

I always do the math. The woman in the produce aisle looks about six months pregnant, and her son looks about twenty-two months old, which means he would have been maybe sixteen months old when she got pregnant with his little brother or sister, and he'll be at least two when the baby is born. She looks like she's in her mid-twenties. I compare my story: I was thirty-four during my first pregnancy, and my first two children would have been less than a year and a half apart. I breathe a sigh of relief at the differences.

As I watch the anonymous woman and her son loading apples into their cart one by one, fragments of equations spin through my mind: How old I was for each milestone and each complication. How much time passed between when I felt ready to try for a family and when Paul did. How long it took me to realize that becoming a mother was going to be the biggest challenge of my life. Sometimes I hate this obsession and the habit it's become. Sometimes I feel better when the calculations reassure me that my family did end up like so many others, even after all these years.

One day, I think, when I'm a frail old woman in a nursing home, I'll sit alone in the glow of the setting sun and rock with a baby doll. Paul and I have smiled over this vision for all our seventeen years together. He knows I've dreamed of being a mother since I was a little girl. He understands why my stomach still knots when I admit the sadness and anger that linger after overcoming infertility—and why I can't quite let go of these struggles, grateful though I am for what we have.

One of my last innocent memories is of sharing a crisp October walk in the park with my twin sister right after we turned thirty-one. I was absolutely mesmerized by all the young moms strolling with their cooing babies among the changing leaves. That winter, when Paul and I talked about our hopes for the coming year, I was thrilled when he agreed that next fall might be a good time to start trying to get pregnant. We celebrated a fresh start by not refilling my birth control prescription in January. Although I felt like a self-conscious teenager buying condoms, I was proud of myself for making a plan to give my body a break after more than ten years on synthetic hormones.

But instead of feeling cleansed, I felt less and less healthy as the months went by. My cramps grew more intense, my bleeding stretched out to a week, and the length of my cycles grew shorter, now averaging only twenty-six days. By the time fall came around again, I was fully exasperated with the well-wishers who kept asking when we were going to have kids. Countering all the mindful preparations—and maybe driving them a little, if I was being honest with myself—was my intuition that something was wrong. In addition to heavy periods, I'd developed debilitating nausea, bloody bowel movements, and rectal spasms that started two days before each period. I worried what my symptoms could mean as I sat on the toilet for hours, my nausea escalating to violent heaves as my trembling hands clutched a trash can in my lap.

In February, with no pregnancy after six cycles of trying and no relief to my worsening symptoms after more than a year off the Pill, I mentioned these episodes to my primary care doctor. She said immediately that she thought I had endometriosis. Over the next few weeks, I read intently about this mysterious disorder in which tissue just like the lining of the uterus grows in deposits outside the uterus, often attaching to the ovaries, fallopian tubes, or bowels, and tries to shed each month. The out-of-place tissue can cause scarring and pain, since it can't flow from the body, then the blockages and inflammation can interfere with getting pregnant.

I pored over every story I could find of other women's experiences, feeling alternately somewhat reassured and completely terrified. I scheduled an appointment at a nearby fertility clinic, then endured blood tests, cervical exams, vaginal ultrasounds, and catheters of dye squirted deep inside me. Reviewing my results, the specialist reiterated my doctor's suspicions of endometriosis on my large intestine—hence the bloody bowel movements and rectal spasms—and put me back on hormones for five months to shut my cycle down.

She encouraged me to give my body another break. But it seemed like such a big step backward, a crushing subtraction when I wanted so badly to add a child to our lives. I tried to appreciate the validation of having a diagnosis that matched my symptoms. I began treatment with a naturopath to optimize my nutrition and an acupuncturist to keep my systems balanced. I calculated that I'd be given clearance to stop the hormones again one full year after we'd first started trying.

Meanwhile, my day job as the director of development at a local school had shifted from a welcome distraction to a source of tremendous pressure. When I had taken the position, I'd seen it as an opportunity to contribute within my community and to save for the expenses of raising a child. Now instead of just the typical purchases of diapers and onesies, we needed to consider budgeting for the exorbitant costs of fertility treatments.

The hardest thing about the job was watching my coworkers go through pregnancies while working harder to cover their maternity leaves and hearing nonstop about other people's kids—especially when the stories came with complaining about surprise second pregnancies or teasing about honeymoon babies. Small children from the preschool and kindergarten classes wandered into our office daily to offer handmade drawings or visit our candy jar.

Sometimes I'd just close my door and cry.

In August, our doctor gave us her blessing to try intrauterine insemination. But after three failed IUI cycles in three months, Paul and I were exhausted and overwhelmed. When our clinic recommended in vitro fertilization, I decided it was time to focus on self-care instead. I joined fertility support groups, scheduled more acupuncture appointments, and spent a year working with a therapist to guide me through cognitive behavioral exercises. An exploratory surgery reassured us that my endometriosis was mild, but blood tests suggested that my ovarian function was low.

We tried on our own for another year, and I still wasn't pregnant. I started grief counseling. I wrote letters to our baby, telling him we were here and we were ready. I asked him why he was waiting so long.

Through that listless winter, reminders of what was missing were everywhere. Holiday cards, even from couples who had started trying after we had, showed two or three children wearing their cutest outfits and toothy grins. Paul and I drifted apart from many of these friends, and I intentionally separated myself from others who seemed to take their families for granted. I felt bitter around women who talked casually about timing conception, bitter toward those who planned for a summer birth then got pregnant easily. I got really good at anticipating when couples were going to announce a new pregnancy and at ducking out of gatherings early. I needed to protect myself.

Paul was frustrated that other women's children upset me so much. "Why are you angry?" he would ask. "That's not our baby." But I was getting desperate. I wanted a baby, my baby. Any baby.

When my ovarian function continued to diminish and Paul's sperm lagged in test after test, we were ready to move to IVF, ready to put our hopes into something new after a long season of seclusion and disappointment. There were drugs to suppress my ovaries to initiate the cycle, drugs to stimulate my eggs to mature, drugs to trigger my ovaries to release the eggs, drugs to decrease the risk of releasing the eggs too early, and drugs to counter the side effects of all these drugs. I asked Paul to manage the medications and the payments, and he owned it. He gave me every single shot, and I never saw a bill. I followed the checklists and numbed myself to the process. I was a machine, just going through the motions. I readied my body to fulfill its requirement of releasing eggs while I imagined a team of doctors standing in wait to receive them.

The retrieval, after more than a month of preparations, revealed fourteen mature follicles—but only five contained eggs. This was not great. Not great at all. As I lay on the cold procedure table with silent tears streaming down my cheeks, I listened to the doctor call out, "Follicle, no egg. Egg. No egg. No egg. No egg. Egg. No egg." I heard *No egg* much more than I heard *Egg*.

Amazingly enough, over the next few days, all five did well and made it through fertilization and incubation. Five times, blue-gloved hands loomed over our specimens with a pipette, and five times those hands inserted a single sperm into a single egg under a microscope to increase our odds of conception, using a technique called intracytoplasmic sperm injection. Five tiny hopes were nurtured in a petri dish while Paul and I went about our lives.

During the transfer three days later, the doctor told me the embryos were going to look like little shooting stars. As I lay back and watched the dark video monitor overhead, I saw a streak of brightness once, twice, as our chosen embryos flashed across the dark sky of the screen. It was surreal and breathtaking and ethereal. Then, suddenly, the day became ordinary again as I walked out of the clinic, pressed the elevator button, got into the car with Paul, and drove home looking exactly the same—but now with the tiniest two babies inside me. I thought of my twin sister and smiled.

As we waited to learn our fate, I used mindfulness strategies my therapist had taught me to quiet the chatter of anxiety in my brain. Every time I started to worry, I would send a message back to myself: *I am healthy. My babies are strong. My body is ready for this.* Calming exercises balanced out the endless string of measurements and mathematics that fertility treatment can become: You chart your cycle for months, figure out which day you're ovulating, and count down the moments until you can justify taking a home pregnancy test to squint in search of a faint pink line. Then, before that milestone arrives, you start to bleed again, so you put the test, unopened, back in your bathroom drawer. After too many months of this, you and your partner endure invasive procedures that you're told will gauge hormone levels, ovarian function, and sperm motility but that instead feel like an unflattering assessment of your self-worth as every data point reminds you that you're less than whole. You take increasing doses of oral medications with names you can barely pronounce. You graduate to measuring liquids in syringes and injecting them into your abdomen. You lie motionless while they count follicles with a probe deep inside you, shielded from your suffering by their gloves and gowns. They scowl at their monitors, doing their own calculations. They retrieve the eggs. They fertilize them. They rank and grade the embryos, like a high school science project. You decide how many to put back and discuss the merits of a Cycle Day 3 versus Cycle Day 5 transfer. You wait for fourteen days—the infamous two-week wait—to allow the medications to clear from your system. You go to the clinic to check your blood hCG level, then wait two more days and check it again and hope it multiplies by two, while your anxiety quadruples. If you're lucky, you count down the days to the seven-week ultrasound where you hope to see a glimmer of a heartbeat, then—if you're luckier still—you count the heart rate and hope it's high enough to move forward beyond the stage where more than twenty percent of pregnancies end in miscarriage.

At the end of our two-week wait, I asked Paul to take the call that would tell us if I had pregnancy hormones in my blood high enough to suggest a successful IVF cycle, then I asked him not to call me with the results. For all three of our IUI attempts, I had taken the calls in my office—and those had never brought happy news. When I returned to work Friday morning after getting my blood drawn, the phone stared me down even though I knew it wouldn't ring. I was sure I wasn't pregnant.

Feeling defeated as the afternoon wore on, I went home early and curled up in bed with my beloved black Lab for a nap. When the jangle of Paul's keys in the door woke me from a deep and dreamless sleep, the bedroom was dark. It was after six o'clock—much later than he usually got home from work. I heard the crinkle of plastic wrap. *Flowers?* My heart leapt. *Paul wouldn't bring me flowers with bad news. He would only get flowers to celebrate.* Then my mind backpedaled. *No, he would bring me flowers to cheer me up.* Paul walked into the bedroom with a stunning bouquet of purple tulips. He sat down beside me, still wearing his coat. And smiling. Purple suddenly became my favorite color.

Pregnant. *Pregnant!* I was ecstatic. Through the lens of impending motherhood, the world looked alive again, radiant with springtime sunshine and awash with splashes of color. I relished the joy of being pregnant as I watched gorgeous summer greenery give way to glowing autumn leaves. Students flocked back onto campus. I chatted with the adorable preschoolers who visited our office. I gazed down at my belly and imagined having my own preschooler someday.

Over Thanksgiving break, thirty weeks into my pregnancy, Paul and I spent an idyllic weekend at the coast. We were as giddy and optimistic as newlyweds, and so grateful to be heading into this holiday season dreaming about meeting our first child instead of deflecting awkward questions from relatives. But as we made our way home along winding forest roads, I started having strange twinges on my right side. When the discomfort suddenly intensified into stabbing pains in my lower abdomen, I called the clinic as Paul listened in with concern.

"Is the baby still moving?" the on-call doctor asked me. *Still moving?* It hadn't occurred to me to consider that the baby could be *not* still moving. I had been focused on getting pregnant for so long that I hadn't allowed myself to think about what could go wrong at this stage.

An hour later, as we got to the hospital triage area, the pain had started to subside. I watched my baby's heart rate hold steady on the monitors through the evening. Extensive blood tests gave no clear explanation for my symptoms. My doctor was very worried I might be having a placental abruption, a separation of the placenta from the wall of the uterus, which can be catastrophic for both mother and baby.

The nurses said that I shouldn't be surprised if I had a baby that day, then were quick to reassure me that my baby would probably be one of the biggest ones in the NICU. I was horrified. But the five days I spent being evaluated by various specialists were completely uneventful, and the baby's bounding pulse never faltered. I went home, still in a little bit of pain, still feeling cautious, and still hoping for an ordinary pregnancy.

Six weeks later, Paul and I went to a New Year's Eve party and lasted less than an hour before abandoning the festivities. Bone-tired and heavily pregnant, I was fast asleep before the stroke of midnight. In the middle of the night, I awoke with waves of increasingly severe rectal pain, just like the pain I used to get with my cycle. Sitting up, I reached for my bedside cup of water, but my hand jolted and the water sloshed across my lap. Paul threw a few things into a bag, and we dragged ourselves to the hospital.

By the time we arrived on the labor and delivery ward, I felt like my intestines were trying to leave my body. Still four weeks from my due date, I doubled over in agony as the screen registered a steady tracing of my baby's heart but not a single contraction. The on-call doctor breezed in and told me I wouldn't be having a baby that night and—less than sympathetically—that I should figure out how to deal with the pain, which couldn't be as bad as I was implying. Over the next few hours, the pain mysteriously vanished. My blood work came back perplexingly normal. When I was discharged yet again, my symptoms were attributed to the baby's head putting pressure on an old pocket of endometriosis.

Back home, I made it through eleven more days on a cocktail of oral morphine, muscle relaxers, and stool softeners. I was so heavily medicated that I couldn't drive. I had planned to continue working until I delivered, but now I couldn't even write legibly. I know I went to the doctor's office for follow-up every two days, but I don't remember any of those appointments.

Just past thirty-seven weeks, I returned to the hospital in what could only be described as rectal labor—and beyond the worst pain I could have possibly imagined before experiencing it. Through thirty hours of writhing on the hospital bed, I watched four shifts of nurses and obstetricians ramp up the labor-enhancing drugs, move me into every position I could tolerate, and cheer me on with eager desperation. When my cervix stalled out at eight centimeters dilated, we all agreed it was time for a cesarean.

Feeling feverish and nauseated as I rolled into the operating room didn't diminish my excitement in the least. I was so ready to meet this baby. My doctor made the first incision and froze.

"Oh my God," she gasped. "She's full of pus." Immediately realizing that whatever was going on was beyond her capabilities to manage alone, she called in a team of surgical specialists. They arrived within minutes, as she delivered my son, Sam. His umbilical cord was wrapped twice around his neck, but he was squirming and perfect, enormous conehead and all. As Paul joined Sam at the warming table, I took in the details—Paul looking tentative in his dark blue scrubs, Sam breathing out a little neighing cry, *6 lb 13 oz* glowing red on the digital scale. Seeing Sam and Paul together kept me calm while the team continued working in a flurry of confusion behind the surgical drape. They soon realized that my large intestine had perforated—probably back at thirty weeks—then had walled off the defect, creating a huge abscess.

I spent Sam's earliest days relying on tubes that supplied three different antibiotics, vast quantities of painkillers, and complete artificial nutrition. I wasn't allowed to eat. I had drains coming out of my abdomen from an open wound and a catheter carrying medication directly to my heart. I overheard the surgeons discussing that, if I didn't heal quickly, they might have to take me back to the operating room to remove part of my digestive tract. I was terrified.

I was also exhausted. Monitors that beeped through the night, a baby who needed to eat every few hours, and a surgery team who visited my room each morning before dawn to poke my belly and ask if I'd been passing gas meant that I was rarely sleeping for more than an hour at a time. A lactation consultant kept coming by to try to convince me to work harder at breastfeeding because Sam was developing jaundice and dropping weight. I was pumping and nursing continuously, but I felt like a failure for not having the energy to make enough milk. Slender to begin with, I had barely gained twenty-five pounds during pregnancy—and now I'd lost that and another fifteen in the week since Sam's birth. The muscles were hanging off me. I had nothing left to give.

Slowly, things started to turn around for all of us. When Sam got supplements of donor milk and went under the bili lights, his jaundice cleared. When I started eating again and drinking protein shakes, I regained muscle mass and weaned off the antibiotics and painkillers one by one. When I had a bowel movement, you'd have thought I'd performed a miracle.

Two weeks after Sam's birth, I was finally strong enough to go home. I wore my scars as a badge of honor. But I did feel a loss that, after all my body had endured, I never quite established enough supply to breastfeed Sam without supplementing. When I pulled a bottle of formula out of my bag at the park, the judgment of other mothers stung—even if my own insecurities had conjured their stares. I wished I could wear a sign that read *You have no idea what I went through to get this baby safe in my arms, so back off!*

Most days, Sam was so easy that Paul and I joked that he was like a fake baby. He made no protests whether fed by breast or bottle and slept in twelve-hour stretches, always waking up happy. Two months after his birth, I had a colonoscopy that showed that my body was recovering well. We reassured ourselves that the complications had all been a result of endometriosis combined with a whole lot of bad luck. I cried tears of relief just to watch Sam grow and smile at me. I couldn't believe he was mine.

Paul and I talked about a second child in the abstract, but we had been advised to wait at least a year. Sex had become so utilitarian during our long fertility journey that it wasn't really a priority for either of us. We certainly didn't expect to get pregnant on our own anyway, given our history, and we weren't looking forward to starting IVF again. Then, one afternoon, when I was leaning over nine-month-old Sam to buckle his car seat after a music class, my breasts ached and recollections of early pregnancy flashed through my mind.

I did a quick calculation and realized that my period was three days late. I hadn't had any of the pain that regularly started two days ahead of the bleeding. My symptoms had never been five days late before. I got back in the car and drove to the drugstore to buy the first home pregnancy test I'd ever needed. Ten minutes later, I walked out with my infant son in one arm and my single small purchase in the other. I drove home, fed Sam lunch, and settled him in for a nap, reveling in the unfamiliar pleasure of my speculation. When I peed on the stick, it lit up like a neon sign.

Scared out of our minds but thrilled, Paul and I shared our

news with friends and family much earlier than we had with Sam. We hadn't even been trying—which was a phrase I couldn't believe I could say after having spent years resenting the happy accidents of others. We consulted with a high-risk obstetrician, who reviewed my medical and surgical records and signed off on us, agreeing that the infection during my pregnancy with Sam had been a fluke. Waves of nausea would strike me suddenly while I sat outside, trying to eat bland crackers and sip ginger ale in the cool winter air, and I appreciated the constant queasiness as a reminder of the hormones surging through my blood.

A few weeks into the second trimester, we had undergone genetic testing that would tell us, among many other things, the sex of the baby. Now, at almost sixteen weeks pregnant, we had the results back, still sealed, and were planning to open the envelope together over a dinner date on Saturday night. But in the predawn hours of Tuesday morning, I woke up in severe pain. As I described it to Paul, and as it happened again and again, he started timing the episodes.

"I think you're in labor," he said quietly. No. I couldn't be. Sam's birthday was tomorrow. I needed to be home to spend the day blowing up balloons, making applesauce cake with cream cheese frosting, and having a pizza party with him. I didn't know what labor should feel like—my labor with Sam had been masked by a massive abdominal infection—but I did know I shouldn't be in labor when I was only four months pregnant. My sister came over while Sam slept, and Paul and I headed to the clinic as soon as it opened.

In her office, my doctor slid cold gel over my belly with the ultrasound wand and found a heartbeat right away. "The baby's moving," she said, sounding almost as relieved as I was. To be cautious, she sent us to see her colleagues in the hospital for a more thorough evaluation. An hour later, the baby's strong heartbeat echoed through the triage room. When we asked the on-call doctor if she could tell us the sex of the baby, she directed us toward the grainy ultrasound screen, showing us a brother for Sam. Paul and I beamed at each other.

But the doctor wasn't smiling when I looked back at her. On the monitor, contractions were registering every two to three minutes. I waited to see what she would suggest to stop them. She shook her head. When she checked my cervix, it was already thinned out and several centimeters dilated. He was on his way.

I protested that this couldn't be happening as Paul's eyes registered the same feelings silently. We leaned together, sobbing for what seemed like hours, while staff orbited around us, charting and monitoring and watching and waiting for us to understand. Finally, I accepted an epidural and closed my eyes, numb in every way as my body slowly moved toward delivering our son. As the clock crept closer to midnight, I willed my body to finish the inevitable. My sons couldn't share a birthday. At 10:54 p.m., with two pushes, Max slipped into my hands.

I was shocked by how much of a fully formed baby he was. Though his body had no reserves of fat, he felt weighty in my arms. The doctor assured me he had died on the way out, with no pain, not strong enough to endure the labor. After a few minutes, it hurt more to look at him than to let him go. I asked the nurse to take him away. I stared blankly at the wall while the doctor massaged my uterus.

The next morning, they wheeled Max to my bedside in a bassinet, like he was a healthy full-term baby. He was bathed and swaddled but still cold from the morgue. My doctor had tears in her eyes. The nurses made handprints and footprints and presented us with a birth certificate. Someone offered to take pictures. I could barely separate what I was feeling physically from what I was feeling emotionally. I just felt weak all over. On Thursday morning, we were discharged with a memory box and pamphlets about our options for Max's remains.

We had missed Sam's first birthday entirely.

I went back to hiding from, avoiding, and ignoring pregnant women. I looked pregnant for weeks. I wore heavy sweaters against the chill and stayed in the house so I wouldn't have to talk to anyone. When I mistimed a walk outside and ran into the mailman, he remarked on how big Sam was getting and congratulated me on expecting our next one. I didn't bother to correct him. I took a sleeping pill every night to numb the pain. On Tuesdays, I had to be asleep before 10:54 p.m. so I couldn't see my clock register the time of Max's birth and death. If I was still awake, I would cry myself to sleep. I missed my baby so much.

Day by day, I rallied, just like I had through infertility. I did my best to enjoy Sam so he would never think his mommy was too sad to play with him. Paul and I worried that Sam might be our only living child because the thought of another pregnancy and the implications for my health were utterly intimidating.

Testing after Max's birth suggested an infection with *E. coli* in my amniotic fluid, and an exploratory surgery showed an unusual tumor within my appendix called a mucinous cystadenoma. Inflamed and enlarged, my appendix was fully adhered to my right fallopian tube, forming a direct conduit for digestive-system bacteria to travel to my uterus. The surgeon told me the mass had probably been sending off little shooting stars of infection since I was pregnant with Sam. I recalled the beautiful shooting stars of my IVF transfer and couldn't reconcile the two images.

"This kind of cancer is exceedingly rare," he tried to reassure me. "You do have a fascinating medical history."

Um, thanks, I thought to myself. *Do I get a biscuit?* I nodded at him absently.

The surgery cured the tumor, and we conceived on our own again, one month before we had planned to thaw our remaining IVF embryos to start another cycle. After a remarkably uncomplicated pregnancy, I delivered our third son one year to the day after the surgery that had removed the tumor and my appendix—along with so much of the doubt and mystery about what had been causing our struggles. We named our third son Maxwell and called him Max, to honor our second son—the much-missed baby we now thought of as Spirit Max—for being brave enough to come first and make the way safe for his little brother.

Sometimes I wonder if women who don't know my story look at me the way I used to look at mothers with two young children, and resent my good fortune. I wonder if women who are still struggling think I'm not one of them. These days, I can enjoy baby showers and smile at pregnant women, but my heart still aches when I see my friend's daughter who was born a few weeks before Spirit Max's due date and think about who Spirit Max would have become. Sometimes I catch a glimpse of other women's lonely eyes in crowded markets and on city streets, doing the calculations that I used to do, that I still fall into sometimes. I wonder if they assume that I take what I have now for granted.

Most days, when people ask me how many children I have, I just say two. But some days I answer that I have three boys, two living. I keep Spirit Max's ashes on my nightstand, where I can see his delicate wooden box, hand carved with tiny hearts, as I sit on my bed and nurse Max or read a story to Sam.

The cruelty of missing Sam's first birthday still haunts me almost two years later. I was away from Sam to be with Spirit Max, but I worry that I wasn't truly present for either of my sons that day. I still regret how quickly I asked the nurse to take Spirit Max away. I wish I'd held him longer. I wish I'd kissed him more. I wish I'd let him rest on my chest for hours and hours, just like I'd done with Sam. I wish I could tell him how sorry I am that my body failed him. I want to keep moving forward, but I don't want to forget.

So many good things have come into my life in the last few years, but—as much as they can push the struggles to the side, displace the memories for a time—nothing can erase the anguish, the isolation, and the endless unmet hopes of infertility and the loss of a baby. These worlds of love and sorrow coexist. Not a day goes by that I don't thank the universe for Sam and Max and think of Spirit Max with gratitude. Not a day goes by that I don't appreciate Paul, who never gave up waiting for our children to come.

I still mark numbers and milestones with a twinge of mourning. Last week, we celebrated our first Thanksgiving together as four. In a month, Sam will turn three. A few months after that, Max will turn one. We honored Spirit Max's birth and death almost two years ago. I'm doing better, but I'm not done working through my grief. No matter how I do the math, the result comes out the same: I can't forget all we've been through, and I can't believe the life we have now. I'll always love my three sons.

CHAPTER 11

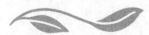

In August, when I was twenty-four weeks pregnant, we set out along the same northbound roads Ian and I had taken to visit Nick and Emily and baby Leo four years earlier. Within a few hours, instead of watching our friends tend to their fragile newborn, Ian and I were sitting with Nick and Emily in a wetlands park and sharing a picnic lunch as our sons tumbled together in the grass.

So much had changed over those years. The passage of time was most visible in Leo's transformation from a four-pound preemie into a lanky preschooler with an infectious giggle—and in Zach's mere existence. But I was also a different person from the one who'd been daunted by the pristine white linens in Nick and Emily's home and by the prospect of holding their baby.

I wasn't angry anymore. I wasn't sad. I had come to understand that I wouldn't be where I was now without what I'd been through. Though I appreciated my struggles for the patience and empathy they'd brought me, I didn't believe that complicated paths had to represent something greater. Sometimes difficulties were just difficult.

In some ways, I—like Tina and Eileen—barely recognized my life when I compared who I was to who I'd used to be. In other ways, nothing essential had changed. Ian and I were still avid adventurers,

and I—like Nancy—was determined not to let pregnancy or parenthood prevent me from doing the things that defined who I was,
especially in the wilderness.

After our visit with Nick and Emily and Leo, we continued our
ten-hour journey north and boarded a ferry that would cross the
watery border between Washington and British Columbia. Our destination was the Sayward Forest along Vancouver Island's northeast
coast, where we'd launch a remote canoeing expedition through a
circuit of lakes and streams and islands. Over the next six days, we
paddled twenty miles and hiked five. We hauled our clothes in dry
bags. We pitched our homemade tent along streams blocked by
beaver dams. We rolled our canoe on a makeshift cart over root-
lined portages and hoisted it to our shoulders when the ground was
too uneven.

While we tried to travel light, stepping off the grid did merit
some additional supplies. Our first aid kit held a copy of my medical records and emergency medications, including one that would
temporarily slow contractions if I had any hint of premature labor.
Our doctor had prescribed it because my placenta was close to my
cervix—nothing near a true placenta previa, and likely to resolve
as the pregnancy progressed, but close enough to warrant caution.
Carrying the jar of small reddish tablets, I knew that I couldn't eliminate all risk. But I wouldn't let fear prevent me from passing down
to my child the love of mountains and rivers that my parents had
inspired in me.

The travel was arduous and our pace was slower than ever before,
especially when we needed to carry Zach on the rougher portages. But
the rewards were immediate. I could see Zach's memories crystallizing
with each new experience: singing and drumming on the bear cans
that stashed our meals, splashing with his fishing net along sandy island beaches, dozing on a camping mat in the shade of a shirt rigged
on a branch. We'd looped a piece of webbing through his favorite orange plastic excavator and clipped it into the boat so he could drag it

along, scooping and dumping contentedly as we navigated the route's intricate passageways.

I loved the wilderness most for its contradictions. Deep in the woods, I felt both a blissful solitude and a deep connection to the wider world. Daily life was at once simpler—with no calendars to be managed or appointments to be scheduled—and more challenging— with maps to be studied, water to be purified, and constantly shifting weather patterns to consider. I missed our home and our friends, yet I never wanted to leave this remote and wondrous place.

The days passed quickly. Within hours of our return to Oregon, I was already reminiscing about floating along those peaceful waterways. Like soon-suppressed memories of labor pain, I'd all but forgotten how heavy our bags had been on the portages and how strong the after-noon winds had felt against our paddles. What I remembered was the palpable satisfaction that this kind of travel brought me.

In the wilderness, as in parenthood, we'd set a course, and we'd mark the route—then, inevitably, we'd have to adjust based on changing conditions. Even as we planned, we acknowledged that most of our experience was beyond our control. But there was such beauty in moving through the landscape consciously and deliberately.

Living with intention echoed through the stories of so many of our friends over the years too: Lydia, whose difficult childhood shaped the caution she felt about relationships of all kinds but led her to peace on her path as an adult. Carolyn, whose children came into her life by luck and choice and circumstances more complicated than any she could have imagined. Mitra, whose longing to be a mother could be fulfilled only when she widened her view of parenthood and chose to follow another calling. In their strength and wisdom, these women discovered new ways to create meaningful relationships for themselves. Genetic ties weren't necessary to forge bonds that en-dured. Sometimes they weren't even enough.

While I felt fortunate to have been born into a supportive bio-logical family, I also had several close friends I thought of as sisters. Zach had known these women as his aunts, and their children as his cousins, for as long as he could remember. As Zach grew old enough to start noticing how physically different we looked from some of these cousins, how far away some of them lived, how much we cherished our rare and too-short visits, he started asking questions about our connections to them.

When he did, so many memories scrolled through my mind. I thought of my phone calls with Tess, our halting and healing conversations stretching late into the night. *Is she really my auntie?* I thought of Zach and Elena bouncing and giggling and tumbling backward together. *Is she really my cousin?* I thought of the relief I'd felt when a close friend had recently had a healthy baby after a devastating miscarriage, and the joy I'd felt in flying across the country to help another when she came home with her son after an early delivery complicated by preeclampsia. *Are we really related?*

My reply was always the same: *Not by blood, but by choice.*

Lydia ~ Given

Later, I found out he had threatened my mother with a knife. But that night, all I heard when my cousin forced his way into our home was a rush of angry voices mixed with slamming doors. My sisters and my brother and I lay terrified in the dark, huddling under a thin blanket on the mattress we all shared on the floor. I was seven years old, the second oldest of our family's five children. I was used to making myself invisible so no one would notice as I listened to the conversations of the adults, and I began to piece together the rest of the story the next morning. My father's sister was furious that my grandparents, who owned the home, were letting us live there. In their family of nine children, my father was eighth in line. As an older sibling, his sister was stung by the injustice of being skipped over in the rightful order of things, so she had sent her son to take the house by force.

Growing up in the Philippines, we moved so many times that I can date my childhood memories with images from each place: A pair of louvered green glass windows. A deep crack in a red concrete floor. A narrow spiral staircase that disappeared into a basement crawl space filled with spiders. At this house, we loved the guava trees that lined the horizon and the fields where my father had planted cabbage and squash. We played hide-and-seek behind the crumbling stone wall that marked the edge of the property. We spent hours catching geckos and stick bugs on the corrugated metal roof. We had already lived in as many different homes as the number of years I'd been alive. After spending the last few months here, I had begun to imagine that, at last, this might be our permanent home. But my cousin's intrusion showed that it was not to be.

My mother must have packed while we slept, because the only thing I remember is hastily collecting a few belongings the next morning. We traveled light. We didn't feel sad about what we'd left behind because we had so little—no toys or games or books. As we walked to town to find a phone and call my father, we were grateful to have shoes, as many of the other children in our neighborhood did not.

When my cousin broke in, my father was living in Saudi Arabia for his job as an engineer. Like so many Filipinos since the early twentieth century, he had to go abroad to find work—sometimes for years at a time—and would send money back home to support us. My siblings and I rarely saw my father, who worked in Japan, the Middle East, and the southern provinces of our island homeland while we stayed with relatives in the north.

Like most families in our village, we had no phone, so we had no way to reach him that night. But it didn't really matter. Even during those rare times when our family was together, my father felt separate from us. With no consistent presence, he held little authority. Each time he tried to help manage his children, my mother would lash out at him for undermining her and silence him with threats of divorce. Each time he left again, she blamed us for coming between them.

My mother, a trained engineer like my father and valedictorian of her high school class, was unable to maintain stable employment in the setting of her chaotic life and our country's corrupt government. Instead of achieving the success her background would have predicted, she took a series of low-paying jobs that left her exhausted and bitter. By day, she taught elementary school, worked as a hospital aid, and opened a street vending cart to sell turon saba, the popular fried plantain treats. By night, she was volatile and violent, unable to express her emotions safely or create the stability her young family needed. The pressures of providing for us robbed her of all energy and patience to be a mother. She didn't understand that I didn't mind not having much. I just wanted to connect with her, even as I watched her grow more and more distant.

In my earliest memories, I see myself sweeping the floor, washing the clothes, helping clear dishes—anything to be near my mother. But my efforts to make her life better were continually misunderstood. She ordered me to keep out of the kitchen, where children were not allowed. She raised new welts on me whenever she came home stressed from work, reinforcing her orders by pinching, slapping, and whipping me with leather belts and slippers. After she told me my crooked teeth made my smile my ugliest feature, I stopped laughing altogether. I didn't know why she was hurting me, but I quickly learned to be in bed, pretending to be asleep, before she got home each night.

To lessen her load, my mother sent me away to stay with relatives for a week or a month or a year at a stretch, consigning me to long, lonely boat trips among the islands even before I began kindergarten. Each time I returned, I bore the brunt of her scorn. While all of us were treated badly, she singled me out as the worst, telling me I had demanded more attention than my siblings ever since I was a colicky baby, and she resented me for it. I felt like an orphan, even in my mother's presence. I don't remember her ever tucking me into bed or hugging me good night. I don't remember her ever saying that she loved me.

While my parents both held college degrees in professional fields, neither had enough money or experience. In the Philippines, a developing country lacking economic opportunities and upward mobility for most of its citizens, this meant severely limited resources and an unstable home for us all. While my parents traveled and pieced together odd jobs, my siblings and I spent our days with a string of hired strangers. I had my first job when I was eight, reselling ice cream in the park. Although I sold it for twice the price I had paid at the market, I couldn't resist eating half my merchandise out of the cooler as I sat alone through the hot summer days. The proceeds were slim.

When I was nine, things finally began to turn around for us financially when my mother rented a storefront at a popular mall. My grandfather, who also ran a shop there, taught her to buy local products—embroidered purses, leather belts, wood carvings of water buffalo—and sell them to tourists. Her business blossomed. Using that income and every other penny they could scrape together, my parents set out to build a house for us on a beautiful hillside overlooking the town. When the house was finished, they were deep in debt and beholden to many friends and relatives who'd contributed funds from their own meager earnings to help, but I finally felt like some security might be coming into our lives.

Then, just a few months after we moved in, we received our legal papers to immigrate to the United States of America. For more than a decade, my parents had hoped and prayed that their application might find its way to someone who saw a need for their skills in the States. They were shocked it had finally happened. So, embracing the dream they had thought would never come true, they sold my mom's thriving business and their newly built house to her younger sister, then borrowed still more money to buy plane tickets for our family of seven.

Early one morning as the sun was rising, we crowded into a dusty red jeepney and started for the airport in Manila. For fourteen hours, we careened over potholed streets and negotiated narrow turns, hoping that none of our four suitcases—containing everything we would bring from our old lives to our new—would get jostled out of the unsecured rooftop cargo bed. We passed our rations around the cab, sharing pieces of fruit, a loaf of stale bread, and a bottle of tepid water. A plastic bag and a sheet of newspaper were our bathroom and our toilet paper.

After a night sleeping on a blanket on the floor at a friend's house in the capital city, we boarded our first airplane and spent the next twenty-three hours traveling through Tokyo and Honolulu to Los Angeles. In our new country, we climbed wide-eyed into a shiny red van. Ahead and behind, the road stretched out into twelve lanes of cars in two directions, going straight forever. We saw no houses or hills or animals wandering the streets. We flew along the smooth highway without a single bump.

When we arrived in the States, I was ten years old and we had less than nothing. Instead of enjoying a network of sixty aunts, uncles, and cousins within a few miles, all our friends and family—save one uncle who'd come before us—were now thousands of miles away. But our parents didn't take commitment lightly. They would never have considered going back. Even if we'd wanted to leave, we couldn't have afforded another set of plane tickets. Every single cent any of us could scrounge went toward paying off debts we still owed in the Philippines and the airfare that had brought us here.

My parents were too proud to apply for public assistance, so we scraped by and did without. Once a week, my mother stocked the pantry with the cheapest foods she could find: tins of salted meat, cans of refried beans, crinkly packages of dessert cakes and instant noodles. After school, we heated the cans directly on the stovetop, then wiped them clean with slices of soft white bread. Our only luxury was a secondhand bike that we shared among all five of us, waiting patiently to be big enough to ride it and finding creative ways to try even when we weren't.

At school, I was an outsider from the moment I stepped into my fourth-grade classroom. Thirty sets of judging eyes stared at my dark skin and my bowl-shaped haircut, given to me by my mom while she reminded me that I'd never be pretty enough to fit in. My threadbare plaid blouses and old brown bell-bottoms—in contrast to everyone else's designer sweatshirts and parachute pants—had been saved from my aunt's school days fifteen years prior. Wearing the same thing several times a week didn't help. Neither did the passing months that made it clear that each outfit was handed down from sister to sister to sister to sister, with none of the fancy new sweaters the other girls had after winter break. Most kids had lunch boxes with pretty patterns or cartoon characters. I carried my food in a grease-stained paper bag that I sheepishly tucked into my pocket to reuse until it fell apart.

The mean girls left messages about me on the bathroom stall doors and whispered giggled insults when they thought I couldn't hear what they were saying. When I complained to my parents, they placed the blame on me, admonishing me to draw less attention to myself. They insisted that words could never hurt us—and that if the other kids hit us, we should hit them back. My sisters and my brother and I coped by seeking each other out at recess where we played with rubber bands and sticks, our broken English giving us the solidarity of shame.

In their workplaces, our parents were struggling to adapt to the culture as much as we were. None of their credentials were recognized in the States, so they would have to redo all their certification exams if they ever hoped to regain their professional titles. For the first few years, my father hauled manure to people's cars at a lumber shop and my mother staffed the cash register at a department store, each earning minimum wage of just over three dollars per hour. They worked for people who were much less educated than they were and served customers who treated them with condescension and mocked their accents.

Beaten down by disappointment, my father began to smoke and drink. He started carrying a gun and firing it sporadically. One day, he pretended to be a boxer, dodging and weaving, hooking right and left as he bounced around me playfully, urging me to fight back. He laughed as I crouched on the ground, my arms shielding my head from his fists, but he had been drinking too much to realize how hard his blows were landing. He hit me so hard above my ear that I slammed into the cabinet and fell to the floor, nearly unconscious. Somewhere behind me, I heard my uncle step in and try to talk him down.

"Tama na, tama na, manóng." *Enough is enough, dear brother.*

My father, usually the one who tried to protect me from my mother, was so drunk that he didn't remember any of it. He stopped drinking after that day, and my parents warned us, again and again, never to talk to anybody about our family affairs. We understood that if the unchecked anger and the verbal, emotional, and physical abuses that were contained behind our closed doors escaped into the public eye, we could be taken away and forced to live with strangers. As terrible as life together was, life apart was unthinkable. So we all kept silent.

Depressed and lonely at ten years old, I was certain that the only way out was to focus on my studies until I was old enough to leave home. The praise of my teachers became a substitute for the love of my family, and I reveled in their positive feedback as I directed all my energy toward academics and art. By middle school, my peers came to see me as creative, smart, and hardworking, and the teasing faded.

By the time I was in high school, I had developed an unwavering faith that there was a purpose to my struggles that would, one day, be revealed to me.

"Every family has problems," my father said when I confronted him about how he treated us. Now that I had friends and spent time in their homes, I knew we weren't normal. As I approached graduation, instead of the liberation I'd envisioned, I felt lost. My grades placed me near the top of my class, but I couldn't afford college. My parents—having finally worked their way through the system and secured professional positions—now had money but were unwilling to help. So I worked three part-time jobs and signed up for a full load of night school classes, scraping together my own tuition just as, a few years earlier, I had paid for my own braces and bus fare to every orthodontist appointment to correct the smile my mother hated so much.

Measuring myself against the expectations of others in this way spurred me on, and my sense of self-worth and success only grew as I transferred to a prestigious university, earned honors in my major, and accepted a demanding job at a high-powered architecture firm. For almost a decade, external validation poured in, along with the thrill of leading multimillion-dollar design projects for world-famous clients. The pace was relentless, the paychecks were grand, and the gratification was heady.

Then, in my early thirties, the life I had worked so hard to create for myself came crashing down. I hid in the bathroom at work, dizzy and lightheaded, trying to breathe through increasingly frequent panic attacks. Trying to review important documents, I couldn't hold one sentence in my mind long enough to tie it to the next line. Depression sapped my creativity. Unable to perform to the exacting standards my colleagues had come to expect from me, I lost my job. Unable to pay the rent, I lost my apartment. All my achievements had done nothing to fix what needed healing deep within me.

Desperate but hopeful, I put aside my ego and asked my parents for their help—or at least their understanding. Though they reluctantly allowed me to stay with them, they made it clear that I was not welcome. I got up early each morning to be gone before they woke up and, after long hours in the library trying to figure out what I should do next, I snuck back into the house quietly each night after they were asleep. I left no wrappers, no food scraps, no evidence of my comings and goings.

On the rare occasions my mother and I crossed paths, she berated me for my weakness. She rolled her eyes as she accused me of exaggerating my plight to make her feel sorry for me. She shamed me for interfering with her life. My father tried to help, but my mother silenced him, just as she had during my childhood. When my parents learned that my brother was between jobs and wanted to move back in, they asked me to leave to make space for him.

Homeless, abandoned, and lost, I could see no way out of the abyss. Thoughts of death pervaded my mind. I willed myself to live when I couldn't find a reason to, rejected by my family when I needed them most. I felt like I was slowly disappearing but that nobody would care—or even notice. My life was coming apart in so many ways that I remember thinking, even in my devastation, that there must be some explanation for my trials. That perhaps I was being broken down to be rebuilt. That perhaps this crisis of meaning would lead to my rebirth. That perhaps there would one day be something more than suffering.

Seeking respite from my solitude, I stumbled upon a retreat house run by the Sisters of Providence. The sisters lived and volunteered within their community in such an unassuming way, dressing like everybody else, pursuing professional lives as nurses and teachers, offering shelter to lost souls like me. Sister Paula poured us cups of chamomile tea and served me a slice of homemade bread while her orange tabby cat kneaded the sofa. As she listened to my story and comforted me, she helped me acknowledge how difficult my life had truly been. She encouraged me to stop blaming myself for all the challenges

I'd encountered. She reflected that our true families are sometimes not the ones we are given but the ones we build ourselves.

Over many weeks, I thought seriously about joining the sisterhood. I pored over their literature, imagining that I could dedicate my life to this. I could find community here. I could count on the sisters to care for me as I would care for others. But I also remembered that Sister Paula, from our very first meeting, had asked me to stay open to all possibilities as I sought my purpose. She had reminded me that there were many ways I could choose to honor the sacred in my life. Devoting myself to service in the name of God would be one. Having a loving marriage would be another.

Her kind words gave me courage, and a much-needed pause. Could there really be some other person out there who could repair the trust my family had left in tatters? On the night of our first conversation, lying in a borrowed bed at the retreat, I sensed God's arms cradling me like a baby. Hope floated over me like a revelation: I was here in this life not to be alone but to give and receive love—the kind of pure, authentic love I was feeling now for the very first time.

Shortly after that extraordinary day, my phone rang and I was surprised to hear the voice of a friend I hadn't spoken to, or even thought of, in years. He had gotten married recently and, eager to help his single friends find the same joy he was feeling, he had met someone he wanted to introduce me to.

When he went on to tell me about Nathaniel, the Filipino American materials scientist who worked such long hours that he didn't have time to find a girlfriend, I cringed. Nothing sounded worse to me than an emotionally unavailable engineer, just like my parents. Still, something about the curious unfolding of recent events hinted that a force greater than my own will might be at play in the timing of this call. Nathaniel's name did mean *given by God*. No matter—I wasn't ready for romance. He would have to wait a couple of months.

As it turned out, Nathaniel was so busy with his work that it was easy for him to be patient. When we finally met for the first time, at our mutual friend's house for dinner, I was not impressed. Though Nathaniel seemed pleasant enough, he had been an hour late to the gathering with no ready excuse. After he left, our friend kept begging me to give him another chance and saying what a great guy he was. At our second meeting a week later, he was late again, this time by half an hour. But he seemed just delighted to be there taking a stroll through the park on a warm spring day.

As we walked, he whistled and chatted and listened to me, asking lots of thoughtful questions. He was modest and funny, quirky and interesting. He occasionally broke into song, which I found both odd and charming. He had a beautiful voice. He kept absentmindedly walking closer and closer to me, not even realizing he was steering me off the path. When I finally ended up slogging through the mud, I asked him to give me more space, and he laughed and moved over, a little oblivious but completely accommodating.

As we spent more time together, Nathaniel's presence grew to feel surprisingly familiar, in a good way. Our natures struck me as perfectly matched yet opposite, like finding the missing partner for a long-forgotten single shoe. Our parents had come from the same province in the Philippines, so we shared a deep bicultural history and spoke the same dialect of Tagalog. We had been raised with common values of commitment, frugality, respect, and self-discipline. But his family had been in the United States for two generations, and they had moved only once, when he was five, while I had never been in any place long enough to establish a sense of belonging. His mother had been a stay-at-home parent with him and his one brother until Nathaniel started kindergarten, while mine had rarely even been around for dinner with the five of us.

Nathaniel made his entrance during the darkest period of my life, offering the light of possibility and renewal. He held my gaze like a dear friend might embrace my hand while listening and speaking with love. His irreverent sense of humor and childlike imagination

helped me learn to laugh again. He was predictable, humble, generous, and sincere, and, around him, I felt safer than I'd ever felt before.

From the beginning, I made it clear to Nathaniel that I did not
want to be a mother. The thought of being tangled in another mess
of parents and children, even as the parent, was more than I could
fathom. To me, family meant not only sacrifice and obligation but
also neglect, instability, violence, abandonment, and fear. Though
he had always imagined being a father, he promised me he understood. I gave him every chance to change his mind about being
with me. He insisted that, as long as we were together, he would be
content.

Nearly two years after we met, and now approaching our mid-
thirties, Nathaniel and I took our oath to become family. As we settled
into married life together, I was happier than ever. What an incredible
feeling to give my love to someone who returned it. Knowing that
I could express my emotions without criticism or judgment, that I
could accept and process my feelings without suppressing or apologizing for them, was freeing. I had never felt so comfortable with and
connected to someone else—or myself.

Still, I was haunted by the conviction that I had done nothing to
deserve this gift. In the dark of night, I would wake with an ache in
my heart as Nathaniel slept peacefully beside me. A voice of doubt
from my childhood rose up. *You're ugly. Stupid. Worse than useless*, it
insisted. *You are the reason for her misery. You should never have been
born, and if she could, she would have given you away. You're nothing
but a burden.*

The pain that this voice inflicted made me want to die. It made
me question all that I was, all that I had been, and all that I could
be. It made me doubt that I could give this amazing man the love he
deserved when I had never learned how to love myself.

But one night, mercifully, a second voice replied. *No*, it assured
me. *She's not your real mother.* At first, I didn't understand. *You came*

from God, the voice replied. *God is your true home, now and always. Though you may struggle, you will never be abandoned. God knows everything about you and everything you've been through. God is always with you, especially in your darkest moments.* Cautiously, I followed the voice. There, I found the secret that had been hiding all these years: I was still just a scared little girl, locked up and lonely, who desperately wanted to be loved by her mother.

Visions of myself holding a tiny infant swaddled in white crept into my dreams. Watching myself hold this beautiful creature, I realized that I had never been unlovable. My given family was just unable to offer me the love I deserved. I didn't have to inherit the misery of the mother I was born to. I could break the cycle of dysfunction by giving a child the love I was never given and allowing my own child to help me grow into the adult I was meant to become.

In understanding myself more deeply, I found sympathy for my mother. Because of the expectations of the culture she had lived in, she had five children under the age of eight by the time she was twenty-six. Her children were born before she'd had time to grow up herself. I admitted that if I had become a mother when I was twenty years younger, I might have been impatient, broken, and bitter too. I accepted the reality that she had done the best she could with what she had been given. I embraced the knowledge that my actions and my attitude were my choice. I began to forgive her.

After two years of believing that sharing his life with me would mean forgoing his desire to have children, Nathaniel was thrilled to hear about my visions of having a baby. We began to daydream together about what kind of parents we wanted to be. After two more years—years of wishing for a child, of medications and surgeries and a heartbreaking miscarriage, of the basic functions of our bodies failing us—I resolved that, although I had been denied connection to my own mother, I would not be denied connection to my child.

Six weeks into our second in vitro fertilization cycle, our doctor beamed her congratulations as she rotated the ultrasound monitor toward me. Our baby was a comma of light, a glowing pause, a silent prayer of perfection given to me in the blessing of this ordinary day. Tears welled up in my eyes as I listened to the beating of this heart for the very first time.

Carolyn ~ Anyone Else's Family

As I stood in the hallway, I heard the phone ring behind the closed door of my home office. The kids were running around giggling while my husband chased after them, trying to get them to brush their teeth and put on something passing for pajamas in the summer heat. They had no idea what the call was about. But I did.

Forty years earlier, when I was growing up in the 1960s, my family hadn't had any of this playful energy. My mother was somber and serious, and my older sister, reserved and wary of new experiences, provided a stark contrast to my outgoing spunk and tendency to trust people implicitly. Our father had left when I was two. We'd never quite been able to make ends meet on the child support payment he sent begrudgingly each month, so my mother's sister moved in to share rent and help take care of us. Our home overflowed with female energy, along with the bickering and fighting that came from trying to contain it in such close quarters.

Even working two full-time office jobs, my mother and my aunt together were barely able to earn one typical man's salary. While they ensured that food, clothing, and shelter were reliably available, emotional nurturing was not. At dinnertime, no one asked what I was thinking. No one wanted to know about my day. There was just the clinking of the cutlery as we stared down at meticulously plated meals in our sparsely furnished Portland apartment. I quickly learned to guard my emotions from my family and to rely instead on my friends for support.

When I was a freshman in high school, I fell for Will. A three-sport varsity athlete, vice president of the sophomore class, and a hardworking student with an after-school job, he was a sweetheart all around. His family was even poorer than mine. His mom struggled to put food on the table for her five children, especially when Will's father was drinking, which was most of the time. Still, their home always seemed so welcoming, so full of messy love and easy laughter. I longed to be part of something like that.

Will and I had a tumultuous relationship, but I was the cause of most of the drama. "Why don't you want to spend Friday night *and* Saturday with me?" I would shout across the school parking lot as I stormed away. Every time I came back to him with my needy and demanding immaturity, he was stable and comforting. Our chemistry was intense. It was the closest thing I had ever known to love.

In March of my junior year, my period didn't come. I had been dreading this day for such a long time, but I was also kind of amazed it hadn't happened sooner since Will and I had been having sex for well over a year using only a hazy sense of the rhythm method. No one had taught me about sex—not my mother, not my sister, not my aunt, not even health class at school—but I knew just enough to understand that I was playing with fire. My period had been regular since it had started in sixth grade. I'd never once been late before. Home pregnancy tests wouldn't be invented for ten more years but, at sixteen, I knew my body well enough to know that there was no better explanation.

I couldn't tell my mother. She was emotionally shut down to all the world and especially unapproachable to me. If I told my aunt or my sister, my mother would end up involved too, and our relationship didn't have the foundation to support something this big. I was devastated when I thought about what my friends would think. Accidental pregnancies were for rebellious sluts who didn't take care of themselves. This wasn't supposed to happen to well-behaved young ladies with good grades and steady boyfriends. Nice girls like me didn't get knocked up.

Will called during his break from work one day. He wondered why he hadn't heard from me in a couple of weeks after an argument we'd had. I stammered as I searched for an excuse for my silence.

Slowly, the possibility dawned on him. "Are . . . you . . . pregnant?"

"I think I might be," I whispered, and told him my period was now three weeks late.

Will was completely unnerved. The next day, when I passed him in the school hallway, he wouldn't look at me. Instead, shockingly out of character, he mumbled degrading comments under his breath and snickered to his friends, leaving me feeling even more worthless than I already did.

Terrified to risk seeing anyone my family knew, I made an appointment at a clinic across town. When the nurse handed me a cup, I skulked into the bathroom and gave a urine sample. Five days later, I called the clinic to get the results that confirmed what I already knew.

After school, my girlfriends and I still giggled and gossiped. We rode the bus downtown to people-watch along the waterfront. We wandered through the ornate shops of Chinatown. We shared corned beef sandwiches from the neighborhood deli. But I could feel myself pulling away from them, nostalgic for the lighthearted fun and innocence I had taken for granted. My secret was transforming me into a different person.

One day as we watched a soap opera together, I was startled to hear one of my friends exclaim, "Hey, Carolyn! There's this crazy rumor going around that you're pregnant!" Two others leaned into me, howling at the sheer ridiculousness of her suggestion, as a jingle advertising laundry detergent echoed on the black-and-white screen in front of us. I looked down at my hands and burst into tears. Immediately all three of them stopped laughing and just hugged me without saying a word.

Desperate to end the pregnancy, I tried everything I'd heard of that might cause a miscarriage. I took scorchingly hot baths. I threw myself down the stairs headfirst. I asked Will to punch me in the belly, then got mad at him when he actually did. In my apartment's shared basement, among the olive green lockers and dank smell of old blankets, I drank a bottle of castor oil and slumped down, waiting for a miracle. I don't know what I expected.

Abortion was illegal, but I had heard about a shady clinic in a nearby town. My weeks of effort trying to find out how to get an appointment there turned up nothing but dead ends. Instead, every month, I took the bus to the obstetrician's office after school. In June, after his nurse had weighed me and measured my belly, my doctor took me into his office and sat me down.

"Carolyn, you have a decision to make," he said to me quietly. "Do you want to keep this child and marry the father? If not, I can arrange for a private adoption." His tone was gentle but patronizing. "Don't you think this baby deserves a name?"

I thought about Will. He had been such a stellar kid when I'd met him. Now, any ambitions he used to have were fading into a haze of drugs and alcohol. He had just enlisted in the Army at the peak of the Vietnam War, and the prospect of his being sent overseas loomed large. As much as I loved him, I understood that becoming his wife would lead to disaster for all three of us. Determined to continue my education and break the cycle of economic oppression that the women in my family had toiled under for generations, I also knew that networks of social services for young parents didn't exist and that no universities would welcome me with a one-year-old.

I thought about my family. I couldn't live at home and subject my child to the same dysfunctional upbringing I'd endured. I—we—had to escape that. I didn't want my child to grow up in anyone else's family, but I didn't think it was fair to bring a child into the family I was in right now either. Dreaming of something better for my child, I didn't feel like I had a choice at all. I told my doctor we should plan for an adoption.

Now in this final month of the school year, I was almost halfway to my due date. My family was so checked out that they hadn't even noticed my changing shape as the weather got warmer and the clothes got smaller. Midriff crop tops, fitted bell-bottoms, geometric minidresses, short shorts: my friends admired the latest fashions in window displays while I took the twice-a-year clothing allowance my mother had given me and snuck off to the maternity department. I eyed myself in the dressing room mirror. Turning from side to side, I tried to decide whether each outfit made my pregnancy less obvious or highlighted it. After nearly an hour, I walked to the register, clutching a navy-and-green chiffon wrap top, three pairs of elastic-waist pants, and several loosely flowing tunics with distracting multicolor patterns. Leaving the store with my purchases, I knew I had run out of ways to put off what had to come next.

I felt constantly sick to my stomach. But it wasn't the queasiness of morning sickness. It was a sinking dread about telling my mother. Each day I would wake up and resolve, again, to muster the courage to do it. But shame and fear always stopped me. We went through that whole summer barely saying a word to each other.

In September, I moved in with one of my best friend's sisters. Pam was a recently divorced single mother raising two young sons on her own. I would take care of the kids while she worked, and in exchange I could live there. Knowing that girls who looked like me were not welcome in mainstream education—nearly seven months in, I could no longer hide my pregnancy—I was also sure someone from school would call my mom as soon as they noticed I hadn't shown up. A few days after classes had started without me, I knew I had to tell her.

So I wrote her a letter. It took me three days and as many pages to get the words just right. I told her everything. I said I was sorry but that I had a plan all figured out. *Please don't call until you have collected yourself*, I wrote, *because I can't bear to hear you cry.* I set the letter on the kitchen counter on a Friday afternoon and left with my small red suitcase.

My mother discovered the letter when she got home from work that night and called me immediately, distraught. My voice, in contrast, was stoic as I recited directions to Pam's house. When she and my aunt arrived, my mother and I both dissolved into tears. My aunt drove us all back to our apartment, where we could talk privately—and where she asked most of the questions while my mother continued to weep. Finally, regaining my composure, I reassured them that I was taking responsibility. I was being monitored by an experienced obstetrician. I exercised regularly, took vitamins, and cooked healthy meals. Will and I were still together, and he treated me well, even though we both knew we might not last. I had quit smoking as soon as Pam had told me she'd heard cigarettes could prevent the baby from gaining enough weight. I was trying to be the best mother I could be.

My academic ambitions never faltered either. Each weeknight through the fall, I hustled out the door to the bus stop as soon as Pam got home from work. It was an hour's ride from the sleepy west-side farm community where I was living to the urban campus where I studied civics, writing, and biology in a dimly lit college basement. I spent each evening in a room full of young men and women who were trying to pull their lives together after various detours—unintended pregnancies, school expulsions, minor troubles with the law. A room full of misfits, just like me.

By early November, the weather had turned cold and blustery. I was on the phone with a friend late one weekend night, tiptoeing around while the boys slept and Pam attended a party two towns over. The third time I excused myself to use the bathroom, complaining about increasing discomfort and gas pain, my friend said that it sounded like labor.

I doubted it. My doctor had told me I was due at the end of the month, not the beginning. Then again, I wasn't sure exactly when I had gotten pregnant. And I had spent the whole day cleaning the apartment in a burst of energy, which I'd heard could happen right before birth. I got off the phone with her and called my mom. I knew she would be home. For once, I was grateful that her world was so predictable.

By the time she and my aunt got across town to pick me up an hour later, I was in full-blown labor. We didn't have any way to reach Pam while she was out, so my aunt stayed with the kids while my mom guided me into the passenger seat of her old blue station wagon. As we drove, she gripped the steering wheel and stared straight ahead without saying a word.

Everything hurt so much. I curled into myself on the car's cracked vinyl bench and felt more alone than I ever had before. I didn't know what was going on inside my body, and I had no idea what to expect. I was riding waves of hormones and impulses beyond my control or comprehension, withdrawing deeper into the pain with each contraction. When I opened my eyes and looked up at the sky out the car window, tall shadows of trees swayed in cold, damp gusts along the road. Finally, the car stopped, and I saw that we had arrived at the hospital at the edge of town, a squat beige building surrounded by fields and foothills. I closed my eyes again.

Somehow, we ended up inside. In the shadowy labor room, people scurried in and out but I barely noticed. I can't remember if my mother stayed. I do remember one kind young nurse who held my hand and wiped my brow. The doctor must have put me under because I didn't see my baby being born a few hours later.

As I came out of my fog the next morning, another nurse told me I'd had a girl. A daughter. She wasn't too early. She was healthy. She weighed more than six pounds. I knew immediately that I couldn't meet her. That if I saw her I wouldn't be able to look away. That if I held her I wouldn't be able to put her down.

The obstetrician kept me in the hospital for five agonizing days while he helped finalize her adoption. When the lawyer brought me forms to sign to relinquish her, he asked me if I knew the birth father. *Of course I do*, I thought, offended. I held myself on a moral high ground apart from those other girls who slept around. In a situation the whole world kept telling me was disgraceful, I clung proudly to this single badge of honor. Will and I had been together for more than three years. We had a deep and intimate relationship, even if it wasn't perfect. Will had even come by to visit me several times—and had gone to hold our baby when I couldn't bear to.

In a small act of kindness, they didn't put me in the maternity ward after she was born. I didn't have to share a room with three other women tending lovingly to their newborns. But I was still close enough to the nursery, where the babies were lined up in rolling cots, that I could hear them crying all the time. It was heartbreaking. A chorus of voices, and I didn't know which one was my daughter. I couldn't respond to her needs. I couldn't be with her because I had to protect myself.

So every time I came out of my room, I turned the other way. I turned away from the nursery, away from the pull of relying on my family, away from the heaviness of having to go back to my mom's house with a newborn. I wouldn't walk by the babies when I left. I never looked for her in the line of helpless, swaddled creatures. I never saw my daughter.

When I was discharged from the hospital, my mother came to get me. Again, I climbed into the passenger seat feeling overwhelmingly alone and confused about what was happening to me. Again, she gripped the steering wheel and stared straight ahead. We drove in silence, backtracking along the same route we had taken to the hospital five days earlier.

At home without my baby, I bound my breasts to stanch the flow of milk and sat delicately at the dinner table while the stitches from my tearing healed. I lay around on my bed listening to music while I stared at the tiled ceiling. I went back to evening classes four days later and somehow finished the first semester of my senior year. Looking back, I don't know if I had postpartum depression or if I was having a normal reaction to the trauma I'd just been through. I felt a profound emptiness, far beyond sadness. I knew I had done the right thing for both of us. But that didn't lessen my sense of loss.

At the beginning of January, as all my friends were settling into their routines at school after winter break, my mother and I met with the dean of women to petition that I be readmitted to my public high school.

"You must never speak about this," she said, looking back and forth between us with a stern glare, not even naming what *this* might be. "You are not allowed to run for student body office, and you may not try out for Rose Festival Princess."

I nodded and tried to look grateful as she treated me like I had just been convicted of a felony. But any limitations she could impose were irrelevant. I felt so different from most of my peers that competing for these coveted high school honors was the furthest thing from my mind.

My classmates embraced me on my return. Though they couldn't understand what I'd been through, everyone knew I'd had a baby. My close friends listened and hugged me on those rare occasions when I opened up a little about feeling sad, missing her, and wondering where she was. As I drifted through my last few months of high school, everyone seemed so young. I'd had such a pivotal adult experience, so life altering and yet so separate from the place I was in now, that I was still trying to reconcile the two halves of my world.

For years, I kept walking straight ahead, just as I had forced myself to pass by my daughter's hospital nursery, without a backward glance. In college, I signed up for more credits than all my friends and made the dean's list every semester. I had sacrificed my child so I could pursue my education, so she and I could both escape the fate of recreating the childhood I had experienced. I needed my accomplishments to justify allowing someone else to raise my daughter, to prove that giving her up hadn't been for nothing. In every challenge lay the possibility of redemption.

After college, I dabbled and wandered, working in a brokerage firm, tutoring children with disabilities, selling photocopiers, and waiting tables. Will and I drifted apart and never found our way back to each other. By the time I was twenty-six, I'd had two more pregnancies with two different partners in spite of using birth control faithfully. The first time, we'd already split up before I found out. The second time, pregnant with twins, I was in a dissolving marriage.

I felt overwhelmingly grateful that abortion had become legal five years after my first pregnancy. I was so relieved to realize that I wouldn't have to go through adoption again, or feel like I had to choose to parent when I wasn't ready. I finally had control over my own body. Even so, the humiliation I felt over having to deal with unplanned pregnancies consumed me and brought me back to my daughter's birth each time.

Then I met Landon. Like with Will, one of the first things that drew me to him was his large and vibrant family, a pleasantly screwed-up clan who could always be counted on for lively conversations around the dinner table. They were old money and high status, with a prominent name around town. Under this unspoken pressure, Landon struggled with self-doubt and depression. I thought if we were together, I could help him reconnect to his family and take better care of himself.

Though we cared deeply for each other, our relationship was never very physical. We had sex on Sunday mornings. Only. "Hey, do you think we could do it on a Tuesday sometime?" I would tease. "Let's go for it in the back of the car." By the time we felt ready to start a family, a few years into our marriage and a few years into my thirties, we were having sex even less often. We stopped using birth control, and I got pregnant twice in eleven months—the only two times we had had sex that year—but miscarried both pregnancies.

The second time, I had been feeling so hopeful. But as soon as the spotting started, in the bathroom at the upscale department store where I was working, I knew what was happening. I forced a smile and went back out to the sales floor, walking in a daze among the businesswomen browsing high heels and tailored blazers on their lunch breaks. Soon I was bleeding heavily. I retreated to the break room. I called Landon and asked him to meet me at home to take me to the hospital.

At home, I began to feel like I was going to pass out, so I lay down on some towels in the bathroom. When Landon finally arrived an hour later, he stood over me with a stack of five shirts on thin metal hangers slung over his shoulder and a blank expression on his face.

He had stopped to pick up his dry cleaning. He was doing errands while I was bleeding on the floor. He had become yet another person in my life who was not emotionally present for me when I needed him.

But my disappointment with Landon's behavior couldn't outweigh my desperation to have a family. I'd been pregnant five times with six babies over twenty years, and I didn't have a child of my own to raise. Trying again with Landon still seemed like my best option. The first doctor I met with told me my progesterone hormone level was low, so I started taking fertility drugs, and Landon did his part into a plastic cup.

While we were going through rounds of artificial insemination, I also started to wonder if we'd be up for considering adoption. As I took the first tentative steps into learning about the process, I marveled that agencies now connected birth mothers with people who were seeking children. Rather than the secretive middleman handoff coordinated by my doctor, which had done nothing to lessen my sense of shame and failure, birth mothers could actively select the families their children would grow up in—and even maintain ongoing relationships with these families. I was intrigued.

Meanwhile, none of the medical efforts that Landon and I had tried were working. Landon's heavy drinking and constant smoking, which had only escalated over our six years together, probably weren't helping. I didn't want to do extensive testing to figure out the cause of the miscarriages. I wasn't interested in in vitro fertilization. Adoption, on the other hand, was starting to make more and more sense to me. I had openly shared the story of my daughter's birth with Landon, and he was always compassionate when we talked about that part of my history. Soon, I realized that I was genuinely excited about the possibility of building our family through adoption.

We drafted a profile and submitted a picture. I wrote an eager letter to the women who would be considering us. I was keenly aware that what I shared was all they'd have to draw on as they fantasized about the life they were choosing for their unborn child—and it was quite surreal to realize that they were now in the same situation I'd faced so long ago. But they could see into my life, while I had been asked to blindly trust my doctor to give my baby to a family that he saw fit. I imagined these birth mothers flipping through binders of hopeful would-be parents, scanning our glossy photos, scrutinizing our lives reduced to summaries. I thought of my own daughter out in the world being raised by someone else while I waited to see if I would be anyone's mother.

Then Grace chose us. As we arranged to meet her, we didn't know that our names had only recently been added to the listings, didn't realize that she had pored over the pages dozens of times before without finding anyone she could imagine raising her child, didn't know that we were suddenly at the top of her list. We didn't know she'd found us only because she was having second thoughts about the family she'd originally chosen. We just knew we'd been summoned to audition.

We drove south and she drove north, and we met at the adoption agency in Eugene, a neutral location between our two homes. When we sat down together over tea in a homey conference room, Grace was sweet and soft-spoken. We learned that her boyfriend had denied paternity. She was older than I had been, in her early twenties, but she was every bit as alone.

My letter to birth mothers, a central part of our adoption profile, had been absolutely heartfelt, but it hadn't told my whole story. We had been encouraged to keep upbeat in our communications, focusing on why we wanted to be parents and avoiding mention of losses, regrets, or infertility. When we met Grace, everything poured out. She didn't ask many questions. She seemed grateful to know more about us, but she didn't really need to. My life resonated with hers. She was ready to trust her sense that we should raise this child.

We arranged an open adoption. Adoption laws in the United States had changed quickly and drastically since my daughter had been born. In the 1960s, adoption was shrouded in secrecy. Adoptive parents were assured that if they were good parents, their children would have no questions about their backgrounds or origins. In the 1970s, a few states began facilitating the anonymous sharing of information between adoptive and birth families, acknowledging the potential significance of adoption to a person's identity. In the 1980s, as scientific advances made family medical history both more relevant and more useful, birth parents started to volunteer genetic and medical information to be passed on to adoptive families. Many birth mothers were offered the opportunity to select their child's adoptive family from portfolios, just like the one we'd designed, and to be involved in designing an adoption plan. By the 1990s, most adoption experiences looked much more like the one we were arranging with Grace than the one I'd been through with my daughter.

When we got the phone call that we had a son—a son!—one sweltering August morning six weeks later, Landon and I were packed and flying down the highway within an hour. The caseworker met us in the maternity ward. We all knew that Grace could still change her mind, since the law allowed the birth family several months to rescind their waiver of parental rights. But I sensed that she was firm in her convictions, just as I had been when I'd relinquished my daughter. I couldn't imagine the heartbreak of losing this baby now.

I walked to the nursery window and saw Cole. With his long, dark lashes and bright red hair, he stood out from all the other babies around him as my beautiful new son, my little bun-bun boy. As I watched him sleep, a reflection glinted off the glass and my gaze shifted to a girl in baggy clothes shuffling down the hall. It was Grace, with her mother's arm around her. They leaned together, backs toward me. The incongruously cheerful sun shone through a huge picture window as they began to walk slowly, somberly, away.

I remembered exactly how it had felt to take those first big steps away from my baby. Grace and I had so much in common, but at that moment, the same circumstances that were bringing me immeasurable joy were inflicting complicated pain on her. I began to cry as a part of me tore away to follow her. Then I realized why Grace had picked us. She knew I would carry not just her son away from the hospital but also the gratitude of finally being the one on the other side of the adoption.

Suddenly, it was just the three of us. Landon and I were so excited, so overwhelmed, and so, so scared. We had become instant parents. Our days and nights were a blur of diapers and bottles and lullabies in a narrow rocking chair. We passed the hottest summer hours at our good friends' pool, bringing Cole into the water when he was just a few weeks old. I spread a beach towel over a chaise lounge in the shade and set Cole on his back, then spent the afternoon bicycling his legs and blowing raspberries on his tummy. I marveled at his chubby little arms as I bobbed with him in the shallow end, both of us laughing each time the water splashed onto his cheeks and dripped off his beautiful eyelashes. When I passed him around our crowd of admirers, he smiled at every new face he saw. People were constantly dropping by our home to bring gifts and cards and food, welcoming us back to the community. Our friends and family threw us two baby showers. It was as if this precious little boy had always been part of our lives.

But as our circles expanded, our marriage faltered. Landon began to drink even more heavily, slumping in his burgundy recliner after each failed business deal, staring at the television while Cole chattered and played on the floor beside him. The outspoken and passionate parts of Landon's personality, which I had found so charming and engaging before we were parents, turned volatile and unpredictable. The sarcasm that used to seem like witty banter turned mean and edgy, then escalated to verbal abuse. When Cole was four, I realized I would be better off parenting on my own than with Landon.

Just a few months later, I met a warm, handsome banker named

Bryan at a dinner with mutual friends. I was in absolutely no position to get involved in a new relationship, and he, too, was in the midst of untangling himself from a loveless marriage. I kept him at arm's length as I tried to heal myself and sort out my life and Cole's. But his kindness and his patience were boundless. We couldn't deny what a wonderful match we were, in spite of the terrible timing. We fell hard for each other. Within a year, Bryan and I had created a blended family with Cole and with Bryan's daughter, Lara, both precocious four-year-olds.

As our kids grew up, I loved being a mother and I continued to wonder about my daughter. I couldn't ignore my intuition that she wanted me to find her. In 1998, an Oregon ballot measure allowed adult adoptees access to original birth certificates for the first time in the state's history. This legal blow to confidentiality and sealed records was stalled by challenges to the measure's constitutionality—and by some birth mothers, now older and middle-aged women who were horrified by the threat of having their pasts come back to find them. I submitted a request to be connected with my daughter, which would authorize state offices to give her my contact information if she sought it. I volunteered to pay for any costs associated with the search.

Two years passed, and I hadn't heard back. Still, I was convinced that our paths were converging as I fantasized about her out there looking for me. In June 2000, I heard that the measure's constitutionality had been upheld and that it had finally gone fully into effect.

One steamy summer afternoon just a few weeks later—on a day that reminded me of the day we'd received the call announcing Cole's birth—I was at my mom's place watering her plants while she was on vacation. More than thirty years after I had moved out, she and my aunt still lived together in that same small apartment, in their same small world. Their elderly neighbor, sweetly nosy, always with half an eye out the apartment window watching the neighborhood goings-on, stepped outside.

"Carolyn, I just wanted to tell you . . ." The hair on the back of my neck stood up. I suddenly knew what she was going to say as if I had been waiting for this message all my life. "This pretty young gal came by here the other day asking about you. She gave me this card." I reached for it before she even held it out.

I thanked her calmly and turned to pluck a few brown leaves from the hanging plants as if nothing remarkable had just happened. As soon as their neighbor stepped back inside, I called Bryan, my fingers shaking as I dialed. "Honey, this is it," I whispered, barely able to contain my growing excitement. He warned me not to get my hopes up. But what else could it be?

I carried the card in my pocket all day, taking it out from time to time to look at it. Her name was Tracy. She lived in California. She was all I could think about as I caught up on paying bills, then collected Cole and Lara, now ten years old, from camp.

When we got back that afternoon, I snuck away to my home office. I was thrilled and confused and elated and terrified. I was determined to call her. I looked down at the card again. Its delicate script was accented by the commanding green-and-white university crest positioned to its left. Until now, I had been so taken with finally knowing her name that I hadn't noticed the rest. She had a doctorate and was an associate professor. Her credentials took my breath away a little bit. Then I got goose bumps. Whatever else my fears had been for her all those years, I now held clear evidence that, at least by some objective measure, she was okay. That she was living a good life. That she had found success.

Finally, I picked up the phone and dialed. It rang and rang. I was relieved to get the recording. I marveled at the sound of her voice saying her name. After the beep, I hesitated, then introduced myself. I was trembling as I continued, "You left a card at my mother's house this morning, and I'm just reaching out to you."

A few hours passed. Soon, the kids were buzzing around with a level of almost-bedtime stalling that only summer weeknights with nine o'clock sunsets can inspire. I registered the ringing of the phone, two doors down in the office, a beat after it had started. Why hadn't I given her my home number on the message? I must have wanted to preserve that little bit of separation, that sliver of privacy, while I waited to discover if she was who I thought she was.

I opened the door and picked up the phone on its fifth ring. "This is Carolyn," I said, my voice unnaturally steady and business-line dignified.

"Oh!" Her voice caught. "Yes." She tried to regain her composure. "My name is Tracy and I have reason to believe you're my birth mother."

"Really?" I breathed out slowly. "Oh, I was hoping. I've been waiting for this call for so many years."

"Really?"

"Yeah."

Silence.

"You know," I ventured. "I am dying to talk to you. You have no idea. But I've got the kids here and I need a quiet place and that's just not available to me right now. Can I call you back?"

"Yeah."

I hung up and stepped into the hallway. I beamed at Bryan.

"Gather round," I said to Cole and Lara. "I've got a story to tell."

It was an intense few weeks of history unfolding. Cole and Lara were in awe to learn that they had another sibling. I tried to answer all their questions honestly, and I explained that I had never told them before because I hadn't thought they were quite ready to hear about her. To them, Tracy was an exotic and mysterious new person who had suddenly entered their lives. To me, Tracy was a familiar and beloved young woman I had carried with me for decades and would finally get to meet. For all of us, it was a miraculous time.

In the twenty-three years since that night, Tracy and I have become very close. I've learned a lot about her childhood. She was raised not far from the hospital where she was born, by a caring couple in a stable home, with a younger brother who was also adopted. She always felt loved and cherished. But she also always felt different. She struggled with her parents' guarded, insular views—views much like those of my own mother. She longed to break free from the constraints of their shelter, to seek her people, to live generously, to tell her story. Every impulse within her insisted that the world was large.

When Tracy and I talk now, we connect so easily that it's hard to imagine we were apart for the first thirty-one years of her life. She tells me I'm exactly the kind of person that she grew up fantasizing might be her mother. This thought makes me smile, but the assumptions behind it also make me uncomfortable. She sees my passion for interior design, my long career as a businesswoman, and my attention to style and fashion, and she imagines the mother that the person I am now might have been. But I haven't always been this person. I might never have become this person if I hadn't chosen adoption for us.

While Tracy was growing up, I was growing up too.

Tracy is now in her mid-fifties and I just turned seventy, and we have a real relationship. But the love I feel for her is not based on maternal instincts. It's a love we've had to learn. It's a love we don't take for granted. It's a love that needed mending after I forced myself to shut off something deep inside when I walked through those hospital doors.

My family doesn't look like anyone else's family. It's far different from what I ever would have envisioned, and it's full of the kind of gratitude that can be born only of imperfection, of seeking trust and acceptance and forgiveness. All my life I've been cobbling my family together out of luck and risk and longing, out of choices that I wished I could have taken back at the time but that have given me all that I have. Tracy and I share an understanding that the forces that kept us apart—and that ultimately brought us back together—are far beyond the scope of our individual stories. Our bond comes from filling a role in each other's lives that no one else could fill. It's not about childhood, or even parenthood. It's about adulthood. Personhood. It's about building connections beyond what we're born into.

The first time Tracy and I met, about a month after we first spoke on the phone, I sat before her in amazement. I couldn't believe I was looking at my daughter. Here was the considerate and thoughtful woman who had insisted on booking and paying for a room at the nicest hotel in town, then filled it with baskets of fruit and wine and cheese to celebrate my arrival. Here was the accomplished professional who now taught on the same university campus where I had spent countless evenings in a dark basement as a scared teenager, desperately trying to make our futures better than circumstances predicted they would be. Here was the mother-to-be who was twenty-two weeks pregnant with my first grandchild.

After more than three decades apart, we were finally together, face-to-face in her living room. We were family, forever, with a love that was timeless and tangled and knotty and pure. I was her mother and not her mother, and she had been my daughter through it all. As we kicked off our sandals to rest our legs on her couch, I felt awkward and overjoyed and so very grateful to be back in each other's lives at last. I picked up her feet and cradled them in my hands like a newborn's. We laughed together as, one by one, I counted all ten of her delicate, perfect toes.

Mitra ~ Other Women's Children

Fajr. First light appears on the eastern horizon. Allahu Akbar. Allahu Akbar. Allahu Akbar. Allahu Akbar. *God is the greatest.* Assalatu khayrum minan naum. Assalatu khayrum minan naum. *Prayer is better than sleep.*

Maybe I became a woman in middle school, when I first got my period. My awareness dawned with my changing body. The popular girls were blonde and petite and perfectly styled, with delicate names that ended in *y* or *ie*. I was none of those things. Big-boned and stocky, I had thick eyebrows, a shadowy mustache, and a name that marked me as Persian. I felt very unfeminine as I tomboyed around in my favorite cutoffs and high-top sneakers. I understood the ideal that women were expected to uphold, but I knew that I couldn't pull it off. I didn't bother trying to fake it.

In most of the visible ways, my childhood was a happy one. We spent summer vacations at a lakeside park in central Oregon, splashing in the turquoise water and hiking among the junipers and pines. I yawned over the stories my dad told, then told again, as we huddled beside the campfire. I lived in the same pretty-nice house for my entire childhood and attended the same pretty-good school from kindergarten through eighth grade. I never went to bed hungry. I felt this stability, and I understood it as love.

But as I got older, I began to see the flaws in our narrative. On the surface, we were living the American Dream. My father had emigrated from Iran in his twenties, established himself professionally as a television cameraman, and built a respectable life for us all. What we didn't talk about was the fact that my mother had been forced out of high school for getting pregnant with me when she was seventeen, and my father, eleven years her senior, had married and then divorced her right after I was born, marrying my stepmother, taking in her two daughters, and obtaining full custody of me by the time I was fourteen months old. I called my stepmother Mom, but I was another woman's child.

My father upheld his promise not to speak ill of my mother around me. The result was that we barely spoke of her at all. I felt no special connection to her, and the erratically scheduled weekends we spent together felt strained, like visiting a cousin I had met at a holiday gathering. Our focus was on the family who lived in our home. My mother was always an outsider to that.

By the beginning of high school, I felt restless under the weight of my father's uneven imposition of old-world cultural expectations. While he wouldn't let me engage with Islamic religious traditions or learn Farsi for fear of drawing more attention to our foreign heritage, he insisted that spending time with family should be central to my life. But I needed time alone. My bedroom was my haven, where I could retreat to write poetry and turn up the stereo to drown out the arguing, to mute my father's anger when my stepmother resisted his will as the head of the family. And I needed time with friends. I was starting to find my people, and I saw other kids my age becoming more and more independent. I just wanted to be a normal American teenager at the mall, making my own choices too.

Since I knew I couldn't get away with sneaking out after hours, I started using the school day to escape. After lunch break, my friends and I would go to whoever's house was empty while their parents were gone for work. All afternoon, we'd lie around listening to hip-hop music and drinking horrible wine, the worst of the worst, bottom-shelf blends made with cheap fruit and extra sugar and artificial flavors that tasted like cough syrup. We learned to time things so we got home right about when our families expected us to be done with classes. I'm not sure my parents would have even noticed my truancy if I hadn't gotten pregnant.

Zuhr. The sun has reached its highest point in the sky, and it will soon descend. Ashhadu anna la ila illAllah. Ashhadu anna la ila illAllah. *I testify that there is no God but Allah.* Ashhadu anna Muhammadan rasul Allah. Ashhadu anna Muhammadan rasul Allah. *I testify that Muhammad is God's Prophet.*

Maybe I became a woman at sixteen, when my stepmother brought me to the clinic to get an abortion. In our just-barely-middle-class family, I trusted her unwavering resolve that abortion was the only way forward. I went along with the assumption that I would not take the path my mother had taken in having me. It was a complicated, grown-up experience, so I turned inward and protected myself by staying on the surface of my thoughts: *Okay. Well. That's done. I was pregnant and now I'm not, and I don't have to worry about that anymore.* Stuck between expectation and desire, between wishing for something different and knowing that this was the way it would be, I understood even then that every choice available to me was both right and wrong.

I drifted through the last few years of high school with little direction and no one in my life to model making a deliberate plan for the future. Taking on odd jobs to earn spending money, I discovered another unfortunate side of womanhood. The manager at the burger drive-through where I worked many evenings and weekends was an older man. Running his fingers through his greasy hair as he watched his crew of young women chop tomatoes and fry french fries in our tight striped uniforms, he lorded his authority over us with a lecherous self-importance. As I stood at the prep counter, he would walk by me, his breath hot on my neck, his rail-thin frame pressed a little too close, and his hand would graze my backside. It never occurred to me that I could report his behavior or ask for help. Although I was still a child, I understood that this was something women learned to tolerate. Life was a thing that was happening to me, and I chose my next steps as they came, from whatever options presented themselves.

That was the same way I joined the Navy during spring of my senior year. I was wandering around downtown with a friend after school one day when she asked if we could stop by the local office to sign her enlistment paperwork. When we walked in, she introduced me, and the man behind the counter asked if I wanted to join the Navy too. I barely paused before replying, "Sure." I didn't have a different plan. I just wanted to get away from home, and this felt like a responsible way to delay thinking about what I was going to do with my life. Within seven minutes of walking in the door, I had enlisted.

Twelve days after graduation, I reported to the Long Beach Naval Station with a duffel and an emerging sense of determination. My father had been shocked, outraged even, that I'd agreed to this. I'd never visited California or been on a boat larger than the fifteen-foot skiff we sometimes took out fishing along the dam on our summer lake trips. He had expected I'd live in his house under his watch, under his jurisdiction, until I got married. But he couldn't stop me. At eighteen, I was a legal adult, and I'd signed a binding contract. I hadn't even known I had that kind of power.

Over the next four years, I worked all over the world, including on two six-month deployments in the Western Pacific that brought me from Hawaii to Guam, then through Japan, the Philippines, Thailand, and Sri Lanka, and as far afield as the port city of Dubai while the Gulf War raged in the Middle East. Day by day, I served on the team that made our boat go. For six-hour stretches, I watched the water level on two boilers for the steam-powered craft, tipping a giant wheel a little this way or a little that way to make sure all the measurements stayed perfectly calibrated. I spent the six hours of downtime between my shifts trying to recover from the debilitating motion sickness that had come as a total surprise my first day on board. And then I did it all again, in alternating blocks of six hours, for weeks and weeks with no respite.

In the middle of the night, to break up the monotony, I would often find myself in the bowels of the ship with men I barely knew, consenting to things I didn't question at the time. Sleeping around was my way out of heartbreak. The boyfriend who had gotten me pregnant never talked to me again after I'd told him I was having an abortion. The next guy I'd dated had cheated on me with my best friend. These betrayals made me feel expendable, replaceable, alone. Well, I could detach myself too. I could devalue relationships before others devalued me. I didn't have to care.

Military service was more rewarding than I'd expected. Its routines played into my need for order, and I appreciated knowing the standards I would be held to. But some days, I felt removed from my truest self, like I was observing my experiences from the vantage point of someone else. Because my need for order came from insecurities that had been laid down in childhood, I had to push aside any traces of self-examination in order to function at the level my position demanded. When I completed my last tour of duty at twenty-two and accepted an honorable discharge, I was ready to go home.

Except I had no home to go to. My father and stepmother had divorced while I was overseas and now lived separately, in their own small apartments. They had sold the house I'd grown up in before I'd had a chance to go through my belongings or choose family keep-sakes. Everything was gone.

With nothing to ground me, I floated around Southern California for a few months, then moved to Virginia to try to make a go of things with a guy I'd been dating in the Navy, then went back to Portland to crash with one friend, then another, then an old boyfriend. I even tried living with my mom for a few months, but I quickly realized that I needed my own space. When I learned about friends from my high school crowd who'd gotten deeper into hard drugs while I was gone, I realized that joining the military may have been the smartest thing I'd ever done. I couldn't have known my time away would end up coincid-ing with a huge rise in crack cocaine use in my neighborhood. Seven of my classmates hadn't survived.

I was grateful for the structure and direction the Navy had pro-vided. But now I was drifting again, with no real plan. By the time a year had passed, I had landed in a small studio across the street from a convenience store. So, naturally, I got a job at the store, and walked the two hundred steps to work each morning. But what had started as a job of convenience—in all senses of the word—would soon lead me to an essential discovery about myself.

One day, a young woman walked in with a child of maybe nine or ten years old. He picked up a bag of chips and threw it at her. He took a soda from the refrigerator and stomped it on the ground. She quietly, patiently, redirected him, then walked him to the counter and paid for the things he had destroyed, along with her small basket of tissues, gum, and pencils.

After they left, I couldn't stop wondering about their story. He looked way too old for this behavior, but she seemed unfazed by it.

And I hadn't felt irritated or upset while they were in the store either. I had felt curious. When they came in again a few weeks later, along with two other kids, I learned they were from a group home, four blocks away, for developmentally disabled children. And when I asked if they were hiring, I was thrilled that her response was "Always."

As soon as I started working there, I learned how demanding the work really was. The kids could be a handful, with unpredictable behavior and violent outbursts. But my days were so rewarding. Even a project as minor as installing shampoo and bodywash dispensers above the bathtub and coaching a teen to take a shower independently for the first time in his life felt important and empowering. I found so much joy in living in the present with children and using my creativity to make their lives better, knowing the love I spread in this way would reverberate beyond my small actions.

Over my three years there, I watched these amazing kids grow and accomplish more than they had been told they were capable of. But I kept feeling like we should be cultivating a better life for them. The real challenge was the lack of resources. Any financial support the organization could piece together from families and from governmental sources was meager. The food was terrible. There were no plants or books or colorful posters to brighten the space. Instead, every room felt burdened by an absence I couldn't quite name. I knew that these kids, all kids, deserved more.

Asr. The sun has reached the midpoint of descent, the balance between its peak and its disappearance. Hayya alas salah. Hayya alas salah. *Come to prayer.* Hayya alal falah. Hayya alal falah. *Come to security. Come to salvation.*

Did I become a woman when I discovered my life's true work and followed my calling to be with children? When I found my way to Islam? When I met the man that I would marry?

At the party on that warm, sunlit beach, I was captivated by Elijah. Ten years and a lifetime had passed since we had crossed paths once before, briefly, introduced by a friend when I was fifteen. He was still super cute, to be sure, with his strong chest, full lips, sharp style, and confident stance, holding a camera instead of a drink or a joint—a stark and appealing contrast to most of the guys I was used to hanging out with. But my attraction to him was a force beyond the physical. I was overpowered by a conviction that we were supposed to be together. As the event wound down, I realized I had talked to everyone else there, but all I wanted was to be standing right beside Elijah.

So I walked up to him and asked, "Do you remember me?" At first he didn't, but when I told him my name, he flashed a huge smile. "Well," I blurted out, "I'm about to leave but I'm not married and I don't have a boyfriend." He raised an eyebrow at me and gave a skeptical laugh. This boldness was so out of character that I was a bit taken aback by myself too. Then, when he spoke, his deep, sonorous voice stirred something within me I'd never felt before. He was so straightforward, so genuine, that he made me feel instantly safe. There was no sense that he wanted something from me, as I had become used to from other men. There was no pretense, just a pleasure in the reconnection. Within five minutes, I knew this moment would draw a line between what had come before and what would be. I knew Elijah was the person I would spend the rest of my life with.

By the end of the week, we were sharing the worst meal I'd ever made, a concoction of leathery chicken drowned in alfredo sauce and cooked on a plug-in single burner in my tiny apartment. But we were also playing dominoes and sipping wine and thoroughly enjoying each other's company. Within six months, he was introducing me to his three children from two prior relationships, and I soon became like a second mother to the youngest one.

Jahan was three years old when Elijah and I got together. What I remember most about our time with Jahan was the laughter. I hadn't given birth to this amazing creature, but she was my baby. Even as a preschooler, she had a big personality and a spunky sense of humor that meshed perfectly with mine. Her clever, irreverent observations—like when she asked Elijah why he was wearing high heels as his oversized slipper socks poked out from the back of his foot at a silly angle—filled our home with light.

We took to each other so naturally, even as we navigated the challenges and boundary testing that are an inevitable part of coparenting. When Jahan was with us, we adapted our routines to welcome her. We ate dinner early, maintained a consistent bedtime, and read together every night. We moved to a larger apartment that had a spare room. As Jahan split her time between two homes, her mother and I became so close, our relationship so loving and collaborative, that it continually surprised me. The partnerships we built and nurtured were so different from what I'd experienced as a stepchild growing up. Together, Elijah and her mom and I made a choice to create this family for Jahan, to put the love of a child above the grievances of adults.

Even as we moved forward together, Elijah and I didn't have a plan. We were just happy to have found each other. Over the next few years, I went to college, got my degree, and followed my passion for working with children. I juggled nannying, teaching at a nearby preschool, and looking after Jahan. Pieced together as my days sometimes felt, I was finally seeing some defining themes about who I was and where I fit in the world. I was starting to understand that my life could have a bigger purpose than living day-to-day and accepting what came along.

This was also when—and probably why—Elijah's Muslim faith became even more intriguing to me. As he prayed or read the Qur'an, he seemed so at peace. His humble, unassuming grace seemed to come from deep within these traditions, and I had so many questions. Soon, we were talking for hours about the history of the religion, the teachings of its culture, the guiding principles at work. For my birthday that winter, he presented me with my own copy of the sacred text, a beautiful dark green volume binding parchment-like pages. He wrote out the five daily prayers for me in delicate lettering. And he gave me a gorgeous deep red prayer rug adorned with intricately woven flowers and the softest fringe.

As much as Islam appealed to me, I had trouble reconciling its problematic history of discrimination with the purity I saw in its teachings. The Prophet Muhammad in the seventh century had declared that all people are created equal. His teachings hold that diversity in human appearance reflects the vast and varied beauty of the Creator Himself and that only personal piety and righteousness, not physical characteristics, can determine superiority of any one individual over another. The Qur'an affirms gender equality just as explicitly. But in some modern Muslim communities, racial tensions run high and women and girls are treated as second-class citizens.

I pushed Elijah to question these discrepancies too. How, as a liberated man, could he justify the harms perpetuated in the name of Islam on women in Iran? How, as a Black man, could he follow any tradition whose proponents deliberately othered a vulnerable group, then oppressed them based on that otherness in order to elevate another group to power? Through our conversations and explorations, we committed to our beliefs that the misguided cruelties some humans chose to inflict were never true Islam. These faults emerged where the complexities of politics and history overshadowed the deeper intents of the faith. If I chose to become a follower, I would know Allah in my own way.

Growing up Persian, I had been discouraged from exploring Islam for other reasons. Although we didn't eat pork because it wasn't halal, and I noticed my grandmother, the only member of my family who wore hijab, praying when we visited, my dad never prayed. He had gone out of his way to assimilate and encouraged me to do the same, to prevent me from feeling any more different than I already did.

I understood my father's concerns. When I was nine, at the height of the Iranian hostage crisis, I'd overheard a boy in my class say that he thought they should chop me up and send me back where I came from. But I'd been born just two miles away from the elementary school where we stood. My stepsisters—my very pale, very blonde stepsisters—looked like the trendy models in teen-magazine fashion spreads, while my skin got distressingly darker every summer as I grew up. Even many years later, as a teacher setting up my preschool classroom to welcome the children one September morning, I heard parents at drop-off talking about a terrorist attack in New York City and felt conspicuous. Did I imagine that their voices grew hushed when I looked their way? By the time I got home and turned on the television, every station was playing an endless loop of airplanes crashing into buildings, as the Twin Towers crumbled and crumbled, again and again.

My stepmom told me to cover the tattoo on my leg, looking down at the intricate script. "There's going to be backlash," she warned, "and that's going to mark you." She was right. Sometimes people would tell me that my name was beautiful and ask me its origins. When I replied that it was Persian, or when they learned that my tattoo spelled out my name in Farsi, they seemed taken aback. The awkward, uncomfortable silence that followed said more than any words they could have spoken.

But the first time I read the Qur'an, I felt like it was speaking directly to me. It was so beautiful in its calling to be more, in its imploring to seek meaning beyond the ordinary. It explained on such a simple level how to be: How to interact with nature. How to spread kindness to others. How to hold yourself accountable. How to consider the ways in which your actions, words, and presence affect the world around you. It found me in the process of changes I was already seeking. I was striving to be a better human. Islam presented itself, and I set out on its path.

Other paths were less clear. Growing up, I had never expected marriage and children and a house in the suburbs, especially after watching my father's American Dream go sideways. Then, over time, my love for Jahan and my continued work with children made me think I might want a baby of my own. But even after Elijah and I had been together for more than five years without using contraception, I'd never missed a period. Being the not-planners that we were, we had just thought it would happen eventually.

Now well into my thirties, I started to feel a longing. I wanted to be sitting in a circle with other women and their kids, hanging out at barbecues with my friends and my baby, Elijah's baby, our baby. I wanted to be part of mom culture. I wondered if there might be some easily fixable explanation for why I hadn't gotten pregnant. I was deficient in some essential vitamin, maybe, or they just needed to scrape something away to make my uterus more ready. My doctor ran a panel of blood tests, and everything looked fine. But we didn't have the money to go deeper into exploring fertility treatments, adoption, or surrogacy. Elijah was an aspiring filmmaker and I taught preschool. We lived in our two-bedroom apartment and pieced together a decent living, but there was no cushion for extras. We kept waiting, hoping, and trying without trying. We left it to a power greater than ourselves.

While Elijah struggled with his own direction as an artist, quitting a soul-crushing shipping job and teaching himself to code to keep a paycheck coming in, I had become disenchanted with my job lately too. I still loved working with the kids and families at my preschool. But something was missing. The banality of it all—the fluorescent lights and plastic toys and splatter of caked-on applesauce along a row of high chairs—was wearing on me. I thought about it. I prayed about it. I wondered what was next. I threw it out into the universe and asked for guidance.

Within a week, I bumped into an old friend at a coffee shop. I remembered that she ran a small Montessori-inspired preschool. Montessori education had intrigued me for years for its emphasis on following the lead of the children themselves, on fostering love of learning by tapping into students' natural desire for knowledge and self-actualization even from the youngest age.

"Do you have a job for me?" I asked, half joking. But she did. She actually did. I gave my two weeks' notice at work the next day.

The first time I stepped into her classroom, I felt like I was coming home. Cups full of wildflowers adorned tiny bookshelves. Low wooden chairs paired with low wooden tables, just the right size for toddlers to sit at while sewing buttons and sorting beads. From the kitchen, where all the meals were cooked from scratch, came the smell of savory herbs and fresh-baked bread. Every nerve in my body felt soothed, every fiber at peace. This was my place. These were my people. This was where all the other long, wandering paths had led me.

In the infant room, so sweetly nicknamed the nest, the joys of teaching the youngest children quickly became my world. In the springtime, we danced among the daffodils. In the summer, we ate fresh plums off the trees. In the fall, we listened to the music of our wind chimes. As winter approached, a few parents told me that the little ones who could walk had taken to tucking them in, drawing a cozy blanket up to their parents' chests and patting their backs, comforting their families at home just as we comforted the babies themselves at nap time. Through all the seasons of their lives, I surrounded these children with care and compassion to teach them they were worthy of laughter, respect, and joy. It meant so much to me to be one of the first points of contact beyond their families, one of the first outsiders to show them that people can be kind and the world can be good. Every day, I was planting the seeds of love.

My work gave me the privilege of creating a nurturing environment for other women's children. But I immediately understood that I was mothering the mothers of these children too, helping them navigate the challenges of new parenthood and the impossible tensions inherent in being a woman who is called to do many things at once. Every day, I hoped the mothers felt like they were just bringing their babies to another part of the village while they went to their own jobs, so we could all take care of each other. Their trust was such a blessing.

Sometimes a mother would ask me my opinion on baby-led weaning, or safe cosleeping, or the best first foods for an infant. I had thoughts. I had read articles. I had made decisions for Jahan and designed parts of our preschool programs. But only the woman standing before me was this child's mother. So I would just turn the question back to her: "What feels right to you?" Whatever her answer, my reply was the same: "Well. There you go." I wanted to affirm to her that, as protector of this baby, she knew in her heart what was right. I was determined to help other women remember that, in the noise of the world, we must not lose sight of our instincts. We must not doubt our own truths.

Maghrib. Sunset. The beginning of the Islamic day, the true first prayer. Allahu Akbar. Allahu Akbar. *God is the greatest.*

I'm fifty-two now, and the idea of having babies is long gone for me. Like the Islamic day that starts when the sun descends, maybe my fullest life of womanhood is just beginning, as I move into a deeper understanding of who I am and who I was never meant to be.

For a long time, I lived in an in-between space. Some women choose to parent, and some women choose not to parent, but I never quite made a choice. Like in so many things, I followed what came. I relinquished control. I questioned and wondered and waited, never knowing if my life was about to change. There wasn't a moment when Elijah and I decided to start trying to have a baby, and there wasn't a point when we stopped. Although never getting pregnant again brought me a lot of heartache, holding the idea loosely also made my grief a little less. I think the continual cycles of hope and expectation and disappointment and loss that might have come from deliberate intention would have torn me down. Instead, as the years passed, the light of possibility dimmed so gradually that I recognized its absence only when it had fully disappeared below the horizon.

Elijah reminds me, in his kind and calming way, that if I had had a child, I might not be able to do the work I do. He says maybe my purpose on this earth was never just to raise one child but to mother the many children in my care—to be a mother for a whole community. He reminds me of the special connection I have with babies, how I get a smile, a look, an exchange of excitement and hope from almost every single one I meet, as we both glimpse the possibilities in each other.

My days overflow with work and family and creativity and faith.

I've taught at the same preschool for fifteen years now, that same preschool with the wooden chairs and fresh-baked bread and daffodils, pouring love into other women's children. It's hard to imagine giving my energy to these tiny, wonderful people all day and then going home to be the mother I would want to be to my own child. Instead, I spend quiet evenings reading, cooking, and talking with my husband and our friends. I immerse myself in creative projects, sketching flowers and mushrooms from our yard, weaving bright threads into whole cloth, scribbling to capture the movement of a tree in the breeze with a swing hanging down. I center myself in who I aspire to be, building a home that is authentic and kind and welcoming to others. I connect and create. I rest and I pray. I let go of the idea of things being perfect, knowing that the only perfect creation comes from Allah.

I have so many blessings. Not having one specific blessing I thought I would have doesn't negate all the others. Our society too often treats women who can no longer bear children, or who have never borne children, as expendable, but my life is richer and more productive than ever before. Does the fact that there wouldn't really be room for a child amid all this other abundance in my life mean that I'm at peace with not having had a baby of my own? I don't know. Not necessarily. But my story doesn't feel as heavy as it used to. I can step back and look at how I've constructed meaning for myself, and be content.

Being content is not about being worthy. Worth is not determined in this life, and virtue is not for humans to judge. Sometimes I feel like I'm not a very good Muslim. Physically, I'm not able to fast anymore, and I hardly ever get in all five of my prayers. Still, I can remind myself that, even when I fall short of expectations, I am a child of the divine. I can aspire to grow in compassion and in service every day. I can love the ritual of kneeling down on the same beautiful red prayer rug and reading from the same cherished green holy book my husband gave me nearly thirty years ago. I can be thankful for another chance to strive, to connect, to make a friend laugh, to seek joy for myself and to offer it to others. I can wake up and choose gratitude.

After visiting Iran for the first time a few years ago, I can't see myself as anything other than a Persian woman. In Persepolis, I walked among the pillars of the ceremonial capital where the king had held court at the height of the empire's power more than two thousand years ago. I ran my fingers along intricate carvings of processionals, taking in the figures of herders leading sheep to market, supplicants carrying chests of treasures, and noblemen dressed in military garb, and I felt my touch absorb their long and storied traditions. I climbed along the mountainside, and, looking down into the ruins of this glorious civilization, I marveled at the bounty of wealth and skill and artistry my ancestors had amassed while so many in their era were just trying to survive.

In Nowshahr, at my father's home along the Caspian Sea, meeting my four aunts in person for the first time was magical. I saw myself in each of them, and I finally understood where I came from. They *were* where I came from. The chaos of being together was an embrace, and love was woven into everything—the teasing with kindness, the calling out quirks, the chance to be all up in each other's business like that was where we were always meant to be. These women had loved me long before they had even touched my hand. How differently would my life have unfolded if they had been part of it earlier?

Since that trip, I've started opening doors that have been heavily bolted shut since my childhood by reconnecting with another important woman in my family: my mother. Although we were never estranged, our relationship always seemed fickle, and neither of us came away feeling good on the infrequent occasions that we did see each other. A few years ago, I decided I was done with this narrative. I wanted to try something new, something that wasn't grounded in regret and in memories of loss. I wanted to heal from our past, to seek—and to offer—understanding and forgiveness for all the ways trauma has shaped our lives, both individually and together.

When I first reached out with this mindset, the pain of life was weighing heavily on my mother. So many things felt out of balance in the world. Her own mother had been slowly disappearing for years, the relentless progression of dementia stealing her selfhood and taking with it any hope of resolving the deep rifts in their relationship. To bring some light into our lives, I proposed to my mother that we send each other a message of gratitude every day.

The next morning, we began. My notes were about simple things: Appreciating a cup of steaming hot coffee. Enjoying a smile I'd shared with Elijah. Hearing the song of a bird in the yard. As our connection deepened, we started getting together more often, and with true joy for the first time. Our messages moved into ways we were thankful for each other: Being happy we'd gotten to go on a walk in the park. Celebrating an afternoon when we sat in her kitchen and laughed. Feeling grateful to be reunited in this new moment of our lives.

From the beginning, my mom responded in kind, and day after day after day after day, we continued. We've gone on for more than three years now, never missing a day. This touch point has become more reliable in my life than prayer, reminding me that *love* is a verb. Love is an action I can take every day—in the teachings I pass on to babies, in the relationships I have with my stepkids, in the commitment I offer in marriage, in the devotion I bring to my faith, in the healing I seek with my mother.

That doesn't mean every day is easy. Sometimes I have to search hard to find my gratitude. When I tell my mom that all I can think of to appreciate is that someone invented sunglasses, she knows I'm probably not exactly thriving. But being authentic in this way, even when we're feeling low, is a promise to be a safe place for each other.

Over time, as our relationship has deepened, my mother has told me more about her story too. She's told me what it was like to be seventeen years old, pregnant by a much older man. And she's told me our story. She's told me about how it felt to have her tiny, sweet baby taken away with no one to advocate for her, to listen to her, to offer her the choice to mother her child. I've thought about how, when I got pregnant as a teenager too, no one advocated for me, or asked me what I wanted, or checked in to see how I was doing after the abortion. Our stories are so different but so much the same. She and I both did what was expected without question, trying to find our way through the world on our own. Neither of us had gotten the support we needed, poor lonely children that we were. Neither of us had been offered the chance to be the mothers we might have been.

I feel like I owe my mom an apology for never really seeing her until now. Before these past few years, I saw her only how others had told me to. I hadn't thought to question their assumptions, or my own. I'm not sure if I was even open to thinking something different or listening to her story. She never offered, and I never asked. But she went on believing in me all along, while I didn't even know enough about her to know what to believe about her.

In reaching out to my mother and in sending compassion to my childhood self, I've begun to forgive us all for the past. I'm so thankful that my mother and I are back in each other's lives in a meaningful way and that she is truly, finally, part of my family. Either one of us could have given up long ago. But somehow we stuck it out. It saddens me to think about all the things we've missed, and I wish I could go back and reclaim the time we've lost. I resent the false narrative that my mother and I couldn't have made it on our own just because she was young and alone. I feel like I was cheated out of something I didn't even realize was possible, under the guise of protecting me. But this is where we are now, and now we can move forward together. In spite of our trauma—and, in part, because of our trauma—we are imperfectly, beautifully, exactly who we are meant to be.

Isha. The sun's light has departed the western sky. The night has begun. La ilaha illAllah. *There is no God but Allah.*

Some things we are born into, and some we must become. We humans are so powerful in shaping our own destinies in some ways. In others, we're like dust. We choose, and then we don't. The wind blows, and we float away. We crash, we burn, we dissolve into nothing. But scattered among the ruins of our struggles is evidence of the great beauty we once created, and of what our legacies might become. I will still be a woman long after I leave this life, carried forever in the memories of the children I have cared for, and in the children of their children, and somewhere deeper in the children of those children too.

Womanhood is not the same as motherhood, and motherhood is vast. Motherhood, for me, has been a gradual shift away from possibility, toward an ongoing acceptance of the ways I can nurture those around me with love, and now it means movement into a place where I feel no limits.

The day will end, and I will rest. Then I will begin again.

VI:

DELIVERING

CHAPTER 12

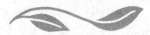

Cora Terese was born on a blustery fall morning, two and a half years after Zach, nine weeks after I finished residency. In choosing her name, we hoped that *Cora* would honor the cycles of life, through its seasons of growth and loss and beginnings and endings, and *Terese* would mark her connection to the healers of the world.

On the day of her birth, we checked into the hospital before sunrise. I watched the monitors trace our heartbeats. I stood up from the bed and walked myself to the operating room. The fog was thick outside the hallway windows as I passed by, and the sky was just beginning to brighten. The trees were the deepest shade of November red I'd ever seen.

In the OR, I hoisted myself onto the surgical table and draped my arms over the shoulders of my physician—the same physician who had saved my life twice, with surgeries for the ectopic and for the molar pregnancy. Devorah and I leaned forehead to forehead, closing our eyes and breathing deeply, as I curled my back for the anesthesiologist to place a spinal anesthetic. Twenty minutes later, Devorah lifted our daughter from my body and held her up as Ian reached a gloved hand across the blue paper drapes to cut her umbilical cord.

Cora's birth was healing. It was empowering. It was everything I had thought a cesarean delivery could never be when I had been devastated by needing one to deliver Zach. No longer bound to the hospital where I'd been a trainee, I had transferred my care to Devorah's clinic in time for delivery. With Cora's arrival, our story had finally come full circle—for me, for Ian, for Devorah, for this child, for our family. At our three-day postpartum clinic checkup, Devorah held my tiny daughter close to her chest and whispered, "You chose well, kiddo. You're going to have a life full of adventure."

Getting to this moment had been an adventure in itself, infinitely more complicated than I could have anticipated. Of the three-year family medicine residency that I had started when Zach was the size of a poppy seed, I had spent all but ten months pregnant or breast-feeding. Learning to be a doctor while learning to be a mother was doubly humbling. Residency had sometimes felt all-consuming and sometimes like the least of my concerns.

For many years, I found it impossible to make sense of everything that had happened, that was happening, to us. Stories are always harder to tell in the present tense. But knowing at least this much about the direction our narrative takes, it's no longer too painful to share the beginning.

In hindsight, so much blurs together, but what does remain are memories of individuals, of the wise and resilient women I've been honored to call my patients, my colleagues, my friends, and my family along the way. We've stood together in the face of ambiguity and complexity. We've grown stronger even when our physical selves have failed us. We've found each other as we've built the families we weren't born into.

At the intersections of these relationships, I've discovered some of my most rewarding connections. Women I first met as patients have later become friends. Friends have become colleagues as we've delved into common interests through our work. Colleagues have come to my clinic for care, and I've shared my own story whenever I could.

Devorah and I don't see each other as often as I wish we did. We live on opposite sides of town, and work and family commitments have a way of letting the days slip away from us. But she's become one of my most treasured friends. When we sat together in that cold and scary emergency room, when I was trying to become a mother and nothing was working out as I'd hoped, she was one of the first people to really listen to me. Listening to each other has always been at the core of our connection.

When Devorah became a mother herself, I was grateful for the chance to offer what I could from the perspective of being a few steps ahead: advice about swaddling her newborn to get a long nap, tips on maintaining a comfortable latch for breastfeeding, the gift of a cozy fleece snowsuit to take her toddler hiking in winter. I wanted to give her something, anything, after all that she had given me.

As our lives unfold and our families grow, I hope I can find other ways to support her. I hope that we'll still be there for each other in whatever comes next for both of us. Because looking back on our history—mine, Devorah's, my other friends' and patients'—I realize that the boundaries are even blurrier than I'd realized. We are all the healers. We are all the healed. We heal ourselves as we heal each other.

When I think of everything Devorah has done for me, I know that mine is a debt that can never be repaid. But as we raise our children together, watching them climb on tree stumps and play board games and share meals in the yard, I know that we're creating something meaningful just by living with intention, just by staying in each other's lives.

And I think, on most days, that maybe that's what matters.

Devorah ~ A Good Story

My mother loved a good story. She dreamed of becoming a writer and telling her own stories, but all that remains of her writing lingers on scraps of paper that I keep in a box of her things. Running around after us, juggling her hours as a social worker, taking care of my elderly grandmother after my grandfather died, and investing in her own marriage, she didn't find much time for reflection. Even I, the eldest of three but just eight years old when my youngest sibling was born, could sense that.

Stacks of the novels she loved to read, all unfinished, covered her bedside table. Short stories fit more naturally into those in-between moments my mother allowed herself to carve out. Her short story books looked thicker than novels to my young eyes, but when she let one fall open and started reading, then looked back at me intently, I understood.

"You can jump in anywhere," she said. "Every story holds together. A new world spun in just a few minutes. Anyone can make time for that."

For years, my mother worked at the same school my brother and my sister and I attended. Each morning, after my father left for his psychology practice, my mother drove us there and walked us to our classrooms before settling into her office just down the hall. Each afternoon, after the dismissal bell rang, the three of us found our way back to her and lined up in a row of chairs with our homework on our laps as she frantically tried to do a few more things before leaving— even though most days she'd already been on phone calls all through lunch and would review reports well into the evening.

Keeping on top of ordinary tasks seemed a constant challenge. Many days, when we got home and realized our fridge was empty, my mother would pile us into the car again and backtrack to the grocery store. Then, exhausted, she'd fall asleep on the couch while we cooked. She gave so much to everyone who depended on her that she had very little left for herself. She always seemed to struggle with balance, and I don't think she ever attained it.

Still, I admired her. She was a devoted mother, a gifted communicator, a champion of women's rights, and a stable support for families in crisis. With her as my role model, I saw who I was and who I might become: When I needed glasses at eight, just as she had. When I still hadn't started my period at fourteen, just as she hadn't at that age. "We're late bloomers," she reassured me. I felt more deeply connected to her with each passing year.

Three years after finishing college, I decided to apply to medical school. I'd been living and working in California, far from my Midwestern family. The first person I called was my mom. I took for granted that she'd be thrilled, envisioning the stereotypic pride I imagined parents feel when their child is planning to become a doctor. For years, I had relied on her as my closest confidante. We'd had countless conversations about this big decision. But when I told her, she just said, "Oh, good, okay," and sounded kind of distracted. "That's great. I'm glad you finally decided." Her response fell flat.

As we talked, she admitted that she was worried my training would delay my chances to get married and start a family. She longed to be a grandmother. I knew I wanted children, but my boyfriend, Alex, and I had been together for only a year. I wasn't sure he was the one. Having kids just wasn't part of my focus then, in my mid-twenties. Her disappointment stung.

Medical training was predictably all-consuming, and I missed my mother more than ever. Toward the end of my third year of medical school, she flew across the country to visit me for a week. Her presence was such a relief after a year of clinical rotations. To feel unconditional acceptance and joy in each other's company was just what I needed, especially in the wake of so many long months of being scrutinized and judged by people who didn't really know me.

I loved it when she came with me everywhere, like my shadow.

She was so eager to understand my life. We wandered around the steamy July campus together and met up with Alex to walk on the beach. We dined at my favorite restaurants, where she would invariably order the salad she thought she should want and then proceed to eat at least half the fries that had come with my sandwich. She read her beloved short story collections alongside me in the library while I studied late into the night.

One evening, she joined me to watch a panel discussion coordinated by a reproductive rights advocacy group. In that basement auditorium, as my fellow students told stories full of vulnerability and truth, she looked unusually pensive. When the event was almost over, one of the leaders of the group invited audience members to share their own experiences. I was stunned when my mother was the first to raise her hand.

She recounted the fears she and her friends had lived with during college in the 1960s, when abortion was illegal and often unsafe and birth control options were limited. Condoms were unreliable, old-style intrauterine devices could jeopardize fertility, contraceptive rings and patches and shots and implants didn't exist yet, and the Pill was such a crude new technology that its high hormone levels left women constantly queasy and with a significantly increased risk of blood clots. Faced with these options, many women relied on hope and faith. But everyone had known classmates who had disappeared, later returning with stories they couldn't tell, from months that had been distinctly carved out of their lives. It was a time I'd never heard her talk about. She'd had a whole life before she'd had me.

Later that night, when I asked her why she hadn't told me these stories before, she shrugged. "Truly, Devorah," she said to me, "I've never had a reason or an opportunity to talk to you about what life was like for us before *Roe v. Wade*. I'm glad I never had to take you to the clinic for an abortion. And I'm so grateful that if you had needed one, it's safe now." My friends were coming up to me for weeks after her visit to tell me how amazing my mom was, and I just smiled, appreciating her even more.

Two months later, as I was beginning my final year of medical school, my phone rang in the middle of the night. I picked it up and heard my dad sobbing on the other end. Bleary with sleep and confused by my father's halting words, I nudged Alex awake beside me. All I could understand was that there had been a fire in my childhood home in Chicago, where my parents both still lived.

Later, the details emerged. In the early evening, my mother had gone up to bed to read, while my father had dozed off in his chair in front of the television. A few hours later, he woke to a blaring fire alarm and a house full of smoke. He raced upstairs to the bedroom and pulled frantically on the door. He managed to get it open against the back pressure of the tremendous heat, only to have it slam shut again immediately. He crawled down the stairs to the kitchen to call 911. That was where the paramedics found him, passed out on the floor, phone cord dangling. My mother didn't survive.

I hung up my own phone, reeling. *This isn't what happens to normal people*, my mind insisted. It was late September, and summer had come to an abrupt end. I couldn't imagine the shelter of my childhood now charred and crumbling—let alone begin to understand what life would look like without my mother. I had always taken for granted that I could talk to her about anything. Now, I was headed into the most difficult stretch of medical school without her comfort or support. In the next few months, I would have to commit to a specialty, complete advanced rotations, and apply to residencies. Alex and I had been discussing if he should come with me wherever I got a job, if our relationship was ready for that level of commitment. With my mother's death, I was in absolutely no position to make life-altering decisions thoughtfully.

Even while I had trouble sorting out the details of the present, I felt compelled to envision the future. A few days after she died, I turned to Alex and asked, "If we ever have a daughter, can we name her Ellen?" Alex agreed without hesitation. I already longed to recapture my mother's spirit by carrying on her name, even though I knew we were nowhere near ready to have children.

In October, I did a rotation in emergency medicine. On my fourth shift there, I picked up the chart outside the pale blue drape of the next patient I had been assigned: *51 y.o. white female, brought in w/ 2nd & 3rd degree burns over legs/abdomen, injuries sustained at job as a line cook.* I turned around and walked up to the senior resident.

"You need to reassign me," I said. "Please."

She looked at me with exasperation. "You don't get to make that choice," she said flatly.

I hesitated. "I'm really sorry to do this to you," I said slowly, "but my mom died in a fire three weeks ago, and I cannot take care of that patient. I don't care if you fail me. But I'm not going in there."

Another long pause. "I'm so sorry. Fair enough."

I could see her wishing she could undo knowing what I had just told her. I hadn't wanted to share this raw, fresh tragedy with her either. We stood there awkwardly. The chaos of the emergency department never slowed.

"You could take a leave of absence," my adviser said later that week, as I sat staring blankly across her cluttered desk. "You could postpone graduation." But what was I going to do? Get a job at the local frozen yogurt store to distract myself? Sit at home with my grief, sobbing? I was halfway through my final year of medical school. I didn't know what else to do but finish.

I started making decisions really quickly because I had lost the emotional capacity to mull things over. I knew I cared deeply about women's health and enjoyed working with my hands. For the past few years, I had been leaning toward surgical specialties, particularly obstetrics and gynecology. But I had also been hoping I might fall in love with an easier field, might find a path that didn't put me at such a high risk of fulfilling my mother's lament that I was waiting too long to have a family. I felt a constant tension between living in the present and preparing for the future.

Then I considered the essential factors that my mother's profession and mine had in common: caring for people in intimate settings, communicating compassionately in difficult times, and trying not to lose ourselves in the vast abyss of human need. With newfound resolve, I traveled to San Francisco for an advanced training month in abortion techniques and family planning services. I thought back to the stories from her college days my mother had shared with my classmates in medical school. I burrowed into my long hours providing procedures and counseling at the clinic. Days and weeks passed as I lost myself in my work.

As vividly as I can remember the pale green of the hallway where I confronted the emergency medicine resident about not taking on a burn patient, as much as I can still conjure an image of the Golden Gate Bridge from a hillside near the San Francisco family planning clinic, large portions of my fourth year of medical school have completely vanished from my memory. Most of the memories that were unaffected were of things I did with Alex. He was my porthole, giving me a glimpse back into the normal world. My mother's death was like a physical trauma to me, big and dark and terrifying, casting heavy shadows across everything else in my life. Some days, Alex was the only person who could grab me by the collar and pull me out from under it.

When I started residency, my mother had been gone for less than a year. Like many of my classmates, I had moved to an unfamiliar city more than a thousand miles from anywhere I'd previously called home. Like all residents, I was starting a job that required immense responsibility but offered almost no control. Residency training is incredibly demanding in the best of circumstances, even for the most resilient and motivated person. Managing the pressure of expectations and the overwhelming insecurity that comes with being a young doctor with so little experience was nearly impossible for me. Depleted of all reserves, I was completely unable to mask frustration or displeasure. I could go to work and do my job and go home and sleep. Any finesse, any mustering of energy to be pleasant while feeling stressed or tired, was no longer within my skill set—and my evaluations showed it.

Realizing that I would need professional support to succeed in residency, I sought out a therapist. As we started off one session, we talked about what a hard week it had been, getting through another Mother's Day without my mother. When she asked what I had done that day and I told her I had spent it at the hospital, she said she was sorry I'd had to do that.

"No," I corrected her. "I scheduled myself to work. I volunteered to trade with one of the other residents because most people want to spend Mother's Day with their moms or their kids, and I don't have either."

She looked at me disapprovingly. "You're using your work to avoid your emotions."

"Yup, that's exactly right," I conceded. "It's a long, long day. I don't really know what I would do with myself if I didn't work. Every year, I trade my way into working on Mother's Day, on her birthday, and on her death day."

I had never pointed this out to her before, and she hadn't thought to ask. She started going on about how she didn't like this coping mechanism, how she would rather see me focus inward and do something kind for myself on those days. She was probably right. It was a nice theory. But I wasn't ready to confront my feelings that directly.

Alex and I got married in September during my second year of residency, almost exactly two years after my mother died. When I went looking for a gown, every other woman in the shop seemed to be there with her mother. As I watched some of them disagreeing about bridesmaid dress colors and wedding veil styles, I felt very lonely. I knew that if my mother had been there, she and I would have argued too. Alex and I weren't having our ceremony in a synagogue. Alex wasn't the nice Jewish boy she had envisioned me having babies with in my twenties. My mother was highly moral and sometimes rigid in her beliefs, and Judaism was a central part of her identity. I knew she wouldn't approve of many of my choices. Still, as I prepared for our wedding, I felt her absence in every tradition.

I was grateful she and Alex had known each other for five years before she died. While it took her more than half that time to accept him into our family, they had eventually bonded over a shared passion for art history and his ability to help recover lost computer documents in her moments of panic. On the day of our wedding, I wore a gown rewoven with the lace of my mother's dress, and I nestled a tiny photograph of us together into my bouquet of deep apricot roses and burgundy calla lilies. During our ceremony, Alex and I recalled the Sheva Brachot—the seven Jewish wedding blessings—and talked in our vows about how important it was to me to marry someone who had known my mother. We knew the relationship she and Alex had shared would carry forward into our marriage and into the family we would create.

Four years later, well into my first job out of residency, I was pregnant with Ellie. I desperately wished I could call my mother and compare our stories. When had she first felt me move? How had she chosen my name? Had she set up my room before I was born, or observed the Judaic laws of kina hora, buying no supplies until after birth, to guard her baby against the evil eye? Fortunately, from the first time I'd noticed the cesarean scar across her belly in the shower when I was a preschooler, she had answered my questions honestly, sharing details about her pregnancies that most women hear about from their mothers only once they have children themselves. As I got older, I'd heard about her obstetrician, who had decided I wouldn't fit through her pelvis for a vaginal delivery and had recommended a cesarean without labor. When I was a medical student, and just beginning to observe surgical deliveries myself, she warned me to watch out for the bladder, earnestly describing having overheard her doctor remind his assistant how important that was as I was being born.

As much as I experienced pregnancy as my mother's daughter, I also experienced pregnancy as an obstetrician. The physical stresses—standing and walking on hospital rounds, pulling back retractors during surgery, sitting on the end of a mother's bed to coach her through contractions until her baby arrived—added up to constant aches and pains in my legs and pelvis. But having witnessed the ways reproductive health could be complicated, I was continually grateful for how smoothly things were going for me. I got pregnant easily, exactly when I wanted to. I was awed by the sensation of my baby quickening inside me with her first kicks and flutters. I'd counseled so many women over the years, but having these experiences myself was humbling.

By far the hardest thing I did when I was pregnant was to take care of people who were struggling to build their own families, especially as they endured pregnancy losses and infertility. I supported families through heartbreaking deliveries, when we all knew the baby was unlikely to survive or had already died before birth. I did my best to offer compassion during the second-trimester terminations that some of my patients chose when faced with a much-loved baby's severe birth defects. I came to recognize how an early first-trimester miscarriage, even when the grainy ultrasound image revealed just a bright circle and a curved line, could bring so much anguish. As I anticipated my daughter's arrival, I felt a little closer to understanding what my patients who were experiencing losses went through. I couldn't imagine losing Ellie.

Several times during my pregnancy, I found myself telling women that I would understand if it was too hard for them to have me be their doctor right then, if they would like me to ask one of my colleagues to take over their care. I imagined I was a constant reminder of what they wanted and didn't have. I couldn't leave it unspoken. I was the elephant in the room, and I felt like an elephant some days.

None of them took me up on the offer. One colleague told me it was precisely *because* I offered. Because I acknowledged my patients' suffering and the relentless barrage of reminders in the world around them. Because I was willing to admit that their pain mattered. I hoped that was some consolation, as I thought of the emptiness I had felt in the bridal shop years ago, standing among so many other women and their mothers as they enjoyed exactly what I wished I had.

Helping manage unwanted pregnancies while I was pregnant was challenging too. I remember one patient who was courageous enough to broach this awkward topic. Preparing for her procedure on an otherwise ordinary afternoon, I felt self-conscious as she watched me maneuver my huge third-trimester bulge. She was silent while I double-checked my equipment and tested the suction on the vacuum. Then, suddenly, she said, "Is it weird for you to take care of people like me when you're pregnant?"

People like her? Were we different kinds of people? When I replied, I chose my words carefully. "This is just the right time for me to have a baby, and it's not the right time for you. So why wouldn't I want to help you? It doesn't change anything between us."

She smiled. "That's a really good answer." She told me she'd had an abortion before, twice, but never with a pregnant doctor. She said she was just asking because she'd never had the opportunity to ask. She thanked me for being willing to help.

As I reflected on our conversation later, I thought about how opportunity was exactly what it all came down to. I appreciated that I lived in a state where I was still allowed to provide abortions legally—especially as the status of women's bodily autonomy felt more and more precarious throughout much of the country. But I'd long struggled with the question of why I was able to perform them at all. The procedure itself is not one I enjoy, and I often need to distance myself and focus on the technical aspects to get through it. It was unnerving to walk into an abortion clinic at the beginning of my shift and wonder if a protester on the sidewalk would think I was headed inside to terminate my thirty-week fetus. I began to worry about how I could continue to stay safe, to be around for my family, while putting myself in the vulnerable position required to care for women in their own time of vulnerability.

But if I turned away from the opportunity to provide this crucial service because abortions were too emotionally difficult for me or too much of a risk to my own safety, women could lose the right to decide when and if they become mothers. Protecting myself could mean putting other women in danger. We could easily find ourselves again in an era of hushed phone calls, of procedures shrouded in shame and secrecy, like the time of back alleys and coat hangers that my mother had lived through. I didn't see myself as different from my patients. Maybe in a more fortunate place in my life at that moment, but not inherently different.

As I approached my due date with Ellie, I started to think less about my mother's stories of pregnancy and more about her stories surrounding my birth. I'd been born the day after my mother's birthday, so she had spent her own birthday in the hospital preparing for my arrival. In the evening, my father had stepped out to buy her a cake. Still struggling to refine his English after moving to the States from Israel less than two years earlier, and not so detail-oriented to begin with, this distracted father-to-be had been an easy mark for a shopkeeper looking to pawn off day-old desserts. My mother would laugh each time she recounted this tale over the years, the stale cake making it that much more memorable. I remember asking her if the delivery and the recovery had hurt and hearing her say yes before she added, without missing a beat, "But I didn't care because I had you."

Throughout my pregnancy, I was monitored closely for pre-eclampsia. My mother had developed this disorder of placental function and blood vessels during her pregnancy with me. Knowing how alike my mother and I were physically, and because I'd started pregnancy with the risk factor of chronic hypertension, I was relieved at every clinic check when my high blood pressure remained easily controlled on the same medication I had used for years. But at thirty-nine weeks, my obstetrician—who was also one of my trusted practice partners—and I agreed that it was time for an induction to get Ellie out safely while her placenta still seemed to be working well.

I checked in to the hospital at midnight on my scheduled date, and the nurses got me hooked up to the intravenous lines and monitors. Alex and I napped and talked as the induction medications took effect and my cervix dilated a few centimeters without much pain. When my colleague broke my bag of waters in the morning, the strangest sensation, like the core of my body being sucked down, overtook me. For years, I had told women "This is going to feel weird" before releasing their amniotic fluid because that was what I had been taught to say. But I didn't really understand what that meant until I felt it. The pain became excruciating as my daughter bore down on my cervix and I quickly progressed to seven centimeters. I asked for an epidural and fell asleep.

An hour later, I woke up sweaty and dehydrated and shivering. Ellie appeared to be faltering on the monitor. Instead of the healthy heart rate variability a baby exhibits during normal labor, her tracing showed occasional decelerations with no quick rallies afterward. The nurse took my temperature and said I was a little warm. Then she noticed the soaked sheets all around me. While I had slept, my induction medications had been delivered onto the bed from a disconnected IV line. On exam, I was still at seven centimeters.

My body had surprised me by making it this far. Knowing how much I am my mother's daughter, I had always expected I would deliver my children by cesarean just as she had. With the thought that I might have a vaginal birth after all, I had become invested in the process. Now I didn't know what to do. Should we fix the IV and restart the induction properly? Could I continue to labor with a baby who was beginning to look distressed, even though my cervix hadn't dilated in several hours? Was it time for a cesarean? Even with all my training and professional experience, all I wanted in that moment was to ask my mother's advice.

In her absence, my dad came through for our family. He had arrived that morning, flying two thousand miles to be with his granddaughter on her birthday. Not wanting to intrude, he spent much of my labor in the waiting room and had already booked a ticket to fly home the next day. When I asked the nurses to invite him to my bedside, he took in our updates of what had been happening. He looked thoughtful, like he was remembering my birth thirty-four years ago.

"Devorah," he said gently, "listen to your baby. Your baby is telling you what she wants." My dad, who had always been skeptical of mainstream medicine and critical of interventions, told me he thought it was time for a cesarean. I was immediately relieved. I wasn't scared. I was ready to be done.

A cesarean is the first surgery obstetricians learn to do in residency. After performing thousands of cesareans, I know every one of the body's landmarks intuitively. I remember picturing, from the sensations of movement that persisted even through the haze of anesthesia, what layer of my abdominal wall my colleague was separating as she worked her way through the tissue. It was a little creepy and a little comforting.

Clasp the scalpel, draw it down. Dewdrops of blood begin to crawl across the horizontal line from left to right. Smooth, firm pressure, repeat the cut, more insistently this time. The glistening yellow fat bursts through. Next comes a cut on tough fascia with heavy scissors. I push my fingers in and rake apart the abdominal muscles to expose the sheath that shields the bowel pressing up from below. I delicately separate several thinner tissue linings with tiny scissors—taking care to avoid the bladder. Finally, the uterus: bulging, squirming, ready for release. My colleague's hands have become my own hands, moving in ways so familiar but now reaching into me rather than out from me.

The pressure intensified, and the nausea became overpowering. I heard my daughter cry as she emerged. I felt lots of tugging and some sharp pain, and the anesthesiologist increased my medications. I faded out as I watched Alex standing over Ellie in the warmer. Later, in the recovery room, my colleague kept apologizing—for the failed induction, for the IV spilling all over the bed, for the twenty-two hours of labor that had ended in a surgical delivery. But I wasn't upset. I didn't care about how hard it had been. I finally understood what my mom had meant when she'd told me that the pain didn't matter, that she'd just been so happy to have me.

People ask me all the time if experiencing pregnancy and childbirth myself has changed how I practice obstetrics. It's true that now I have a deeper appreciation of what so many of my patients have been through to become mothers. I know how it feels to be faced with difficult choices during labor and to watch things unfold in ways that are not what you expected or hoped for. I understand feeling like you're trying everything in your power but there is nothing you can do to change an outcome. I feel grateful to be able to look at my patients differently now, as I stand beside them in clinic, or in labor, or in the operating room, and tell them that I truly understand what they are going through. But all of this has influenced how I take care of pregnant people much less than I expected it would.

What has changed immensely is what I can offer my patients and their families after they become parents. I've had many patients tell me that they actively sought out an obstetrician who'd been through pregnancy herself and that they really want a pediatrician or family medicine doctor who has her own kids. It's a little unfair—we don't expect an oncologist to have had cancer to be good at what she does. But I do realize now that, until I became a mother, my postpartum visits were quite useless to new families. I kept them safe and managed emergencies, but waking them up on rounds to ask about their bleeding and to request that they rate their pain on a scale of one to ten did nothing to speed their recovery or support their bonding with their new baby.

As a mother myself, I finally know the right things to say and the right questions to ask. I know how to help my patients make sense of their own stories. I think back to those bleak middle-of-the-night hours when I burst into tears for no apparent reason while trying to nurse my newborn, and I can sense whether a new mother's low mood merits an urgent mental health consult or just a few more minutes to sit talking in my office about her own concerns before she focuses again on her baby's constant stream of needs. I recall the romance of imagining that breastfeeding would require only resting my nipple on my tender newborn's lips—and the reality of latching her on with the assistance of a nurse who shoved one-third of my not-small breast deep into Ellie's mouth, convincing me I was about to suffocate her. Medical school and residency taught me nothing practical about caring for or feeding an infant. Friends and colleagues and my own family showed me the things that really mattered.

One night when Ellie was about five weeks old, Alex and I had gathered all three of her grandparents at our house for a big family dinner. As we cooked and chatted, we realized we hadn't seen my dad in a while. Thinking he had gone to settle Ellie for a nap and then fallen asleep himself, I went upstairs to her room. There, I found him sitting in the rocker holding Ellie and sobbing. The room was dark except for a sliver of light that angled in from the cracked door. He stared at two side-by-side photos on her bookshelf.

One was of me holding newborn Ellie. The other was of my mother holding newborn me. I had found the one with my mom while I was going through boxes of her things during my maternity leave and had leaned it on a shelf in Ellie's room. Alex had printed out the second one and framed them together. The similarities were eerie, especially because they were completely coincidental. We had done absolutely nothing to recreate the photo. As adults, my mom and I both have thick, wavy dark brown hair with a center part and two low ponytails. We smile down at our daughters from the upper edge of the photo, right arm cradling them from beneath. As babies, Ellie and I are both wrapped in white blankets as we look up at our mothers with huge hazel eyes.

"That picture, that picture," my father kept repeating. "I didn't know you had that picture here." We looked at it together. "I'm just so sorry you're going through this without your mother." He rocked Ellie as he whispered, "I'm trying to do it for both of us, and I don't feel like I can be enough."

He was right. As grateful as I was to have him around, it wasn't the same without her. She had been torn out of our lives, and her absence left a gaping hole. After she died, it became all too obvious that her love had played a crucial part in holding our big, close-knit family together. People stopped reaching out to each other. The reunions my mom had finally had time to plan and coordinate after her own children were grown stopped happening. I realized sadly that my connection—and therefore my children's connection—to the rest of our family would never be as strong as it might have been if she were still here.

As a grandmother, my mother would have been such an integral part of our lives. She would have flown in for visits and told Alex and me to schedule a getaway weekend while she looked after our baby. She would have sent cards and small gifts in the mail constantly. She would have invited Ellie to her house for sleepovers, carrying on the tradition she had started when I was five by sending me to stay with my grandmother every Friday night after Shabbat dinner.

In some ways that's all just a metaphor. What I really miss is her emotional support and guidance. Her presence as a witness to my days. The love she would have showered on Ellie, now in kindergarten, and Levi, who is two and a half. Being a motherless mother is the hardest thing I've ever done. Six years into motherhood, and twelve years after her death, it hasn't really gotten better. I know how much she wanted grandchildren, and it devastates me that she never got to meet them. I wonder if things would have been different if I'd chosen a different career, one that might have led me to have children sooner. When I think of questions I'd like to ask her and experiences I'd like to share with her, there's just this endless void. I feel a lot of sorrow that she doesn't know my kids.

Even when my life is filled with celebrations, I find myself reliving her loss. Graduating from medical school, getting married, finishing residency, starting a family—as wonderful as each of these days was, every milestone has been clouded with the sadness of not being able to share it with her. Each event has been something that happened to me without her, opening the wounds anew, just as the last cut had started to heal over. A mother's role is to raise her child, at every age. Even as an adult, I have longed for her at every time of transition when I was changing and growing.

I've tried to accept that losing her is part of my life. I've tried to acknowledge that grief is a natural process. I do know that losing somebody I loved so deeply has taught me how to console others who are going through loss, and I'm grateful for that. But I don't think it's changed me for the better. Since her death, it takes a lot for me to be in the moment, to get to a joyful place. Alex has grieved her loss too, for her absence from our lives, but also for the changes it brought in me. Sometimes I think he wishes I could be more like the easygoing and cheerful person I was when he met me. I don't want to cry about her anymore. But that doesn't mean I don't feel like crying. I'm just so sick of crying.

For a few years, Ellie has been old enough to understand that unexpected losses happen. One evening, when she was three, we were reading stories at bedtime. She picked up a board book with a picture of a family: mommy, daddy, sister, brother, dog. She looked up at me quizzically. "Where's *your* mommy?" she asked, scowling. I told her that my mommy wasn't here anymore. That she had died. We had opened up a chasm, huge and powerful and limitless. "Why did she die? Will I die?"

I had always wanted my daughter to know about her grandmother, but I hadn't anticipated the explanations of death I'd need to outline in such a tangible way. I wanted to be honest but not graphic. I knew she would remember what I told her, and I wanted her to trust me to tell her the truth in the kindest way possible—just as my mother had always done for me. When I couldn't answer Ellie's question about what my mother had been wearing when she'd died, she got very upset. She couldn't understand why I hadn't been there with her. Finally, we decided that she was probably wearing pajamas, since it was nighttime. That seemed to satisfy her.

Then she asked me when I was going to die.

All kids ask questions about death, but my experience has made it harder for me to prolong their innocent belief that the world is a safe and predictable place. They know I lost my mother suddenly, traumatically, and much younger than expected. Whenever we talk about something that happened before Ellie was born and she asks where she was, I tell her she was a twinkle in my eye. She asks me if she was a twinkle in my eye when my mom died.

I don't hide my sorrow from my children. I do wonder sometimes if I should shield them more. But if I did, they might think that having lost my mother doesn't bother me. Or, worse, they might realize how much it does bother me and think that I'm ashamed to share those feelings, that those kinds of feelings are something to be embarrassed about or uncomfortable with. I want my children to embrace love without hesitation, even the deepest kind of love that, when it's lost, inevitably brings great pain. I want them to understand love that can be imperfect but complete. I want them to know so much more about my mother than just the fact of her untimely death.

At bedtime, Levi and I sing the songs my mother sang to me as a child. Ellie and I curl up and read books together, and I remember days in the medical school library reading side by side with my mother, finding such peace in each other's company. On Passover, Ellie and I mix the charoset—the chutney of apples, walnuts, cinnamon, and kosher wine—that my mother and sister and I always prepared to accompany the bitter herbs that mark the holiday. We make my mother's beef and barley soup recipe to warm us on rainy weekends and use her old cookie cutters for Hanukkah treats—a dreidel, a menorah, a lion with a delicate tail that's almost impossible to get out of the mold without breaking. I tell my kids about making all these things with their grandmother, and how special it is that now we can make them together. I thank them for helping. It heals me that there are traditions I can pass down.

Alex and I have also adopted traditions in our own family that my mother may not have approved of. Christmas is a big deal for Alex's family, and it's Ellie and Levi's favorite holiday for obvious reasons. There comes a point every December when I sit alone in my home, late at night after the kids are asleep, and contemplate the hundreds of lights twinkling on our Christmas tree. It dwarfs the menorah, with its nine unassuming candles, resting on the mantel nearby. I wonder what my mom would have thought. As much as I know she would have supported me and loved the family Alex and I have made, some of my choices would have been points of contention between us. But I have faith that, even as I feel myself still seeking my mother's approval, she would have been proud to watch me becoming myself.

If she had lived, what stories would my mother be writing now? She would have looked through the boxes of old photographs and scraps of paper with me to find inspiration. She would have admitted that motherhood is difficult and wonderful and painful and complex and worthwhile. She would have cautioned me to find the balance she never found, to give selflessly to others while reserving enough energy to care for myself. She would have reminded me that, even standing beside me, she could not teach me how to be a mother. That it would be my own children who would teach me that every day.

How profound and unjust that my mother's story was much too short. I have always felt deeply connected to her, and that hasn't changed with her death. I remember her in fleeting images, with each page of her life, as I saw it through my own young eyes, falling open for just a minute or two. Maybe I appreciate these memories all the more because of their intensity and their briefness.

Can her life have told a good story, even if it didn't have a happy ending? Am I living a good story, a good enough story to honor her memory, as I spend my hours taking care of other women's daughters, other daughters' mothers, my own daughter and son? This year, on my mother's birthday, I delivered three beautiful baby girls. There are now three more people in this world who, because I witnessed their birth and was the first to touch them outside of their own mothers, will carry something forward from this woman I loved so much.

We tell our stories by who we choose to love and help and care for. We tell our stories by who we share our lives with. My mother comes back to me in the ways I spend my days in a community of women and healers and in the ways I raise my own children. In the moments between moments, when I glimpse her story woven into mine. When the joy shines through the grief.

VII:

REBUILDING

CHAPTER 13

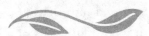

Today, more than a decade into motherhood, my memories of our early years trying to build a family are both magnified and dulled by the good fortune I've had since. I'm a little less than I would have been without my struggles, and also a little more. My children are not what make me whole. But they are part of what I needed to stop feeling broken. In their truest moments, both of them are patient and insightful beyond their years, as if they know how long we waited for them, as if they understand implicitly the value of the time between.

One night a few years ago, as we talked quietly in his room at bedtime, Zach asked me how people got scars. If I had any scars. If he had any scars. Thinking about the indelible marks that each of my five pregnancies had left behind, some visible and some invisible, I replied that we both had scars. That everyone did. I told him the story again of the night he was born, on a lucky Friday the thirteenth just like his dad, when his breathing had faltered and his lips had turned blue as the doctors had scrambled to save him. I traced circles along his rib cage where they had placed and withdrawn their needles, leaving no evidence of their work. I thought about how we are all broken but healing. How we can heal ourselves only by healing each other. How my children will keep breaking and healing and breaking again in order to grow.

Zach was quiet for a moment, then asked how he would know when his scars were gone if he couldn't see them. I told him that we can't always see our scars but that they stay with us to remind us of what we've survived. I told him our scars are our stories. I told him that scars are forever.

"I can imagine forever," he whispered in the dark.

Forever sometimes feels like how long has passed since Ian and I planted those seven kiwis outside our bedroom window. In their very first season, the shoots along the side wall withered and died, leaving the four corner plants as anchors in a square. Over the years, the enduring vines have become rough-barked and sturdy, their limbs a little farther from the beams than we'd predicted, but reaching inward to twist into a canopy of leaves and fruit that holds together, sheltering us from sun and storms.

Our family stands as four as well, and feels complete. My first three pregnancies are abstractions of grief that trail along the periphery like starts that never bore fruit, an integral part of my story but also a memory from a different life. I honestly don't think much of the three, aside from acknowledging how grateful I am that they brought us to where we are today. I can't remember who I was before them, and I can't imagine who I would be without them. But I don't lament their absence. If the three had survived, we four could not be as we are.

When I think back on building the arbor as I recovered from surgery, I see digging as so much more than putting shovel to ground. I know now that it is about finding the right angle to convince a hardened crust to yield. It is about separating unwieldy clumps of earth into pieces light enough to lift with the power we have. It is about believing that, as we remove layers of history from holes we've created, something better will come to fill the empty space. It is about being willing to break in the name of becoming something stronger.

Not so long ago, much to our children's delight, we knocked out the window overlooking the arbor to replace it with wide double doors. Sometimes we throw the doors open to invite the breeze into our room. Sometimes we forget to close them, and a little rain gets in. Sometimes Cora runs outside to pull the smooth green kiwis from their branches, then delivers them back to me. She cups her hands like tiny buckets of sweetness and promise, and I reach out to her, remembering all the years of waiting for this moment, of hoping for this fruit.

OUR THANKS

To you, for reading this book: we're grateful to each person who takes the time to learn about our stories, and we hope our words will carry forward in the conversations you have with your family, your friends, your communities, and yourself.

To my own family: Ian, for facing every complication with unwavering support and patience, for sticking with me through at least twice as many residencies as any spouse should be asked to endure, and for sharing my vision of how writing can be medicine—not to mention reading and rereading all that writing! Zach and Cora, for finding your way to us and for being such creative, adaptable, and spirited companions as we navigate the adventures of this complicated, beautiful life together. My parents, Barbara and Steve Newton, for raising me to have enough discipline to follow some rules and enough skepticism to question others, and for serving as true models of determination, kindness, and resilience. Our extended family, including Judy and Laird Thompson, Holly Thompson, Dustin Gutshall, Jennifer Thompson, Dan and Karen Salzberg, and the entire McCabe clan, for cheering us on through it all.

To our chosen family, whose love reminds us that relationships don't have to be dictated by genetics or geography: Elissa Meites, for the phone calls every Saturday, like stepping stones of comfort and companionship to hop across through the height of the pandemic. Tess, for being the kind of friend who can pick up exactly where we left off. Rob and Katrina Grant, for all the hours our families have spent exploring together, and to Rob especially, for the always-inspiring exchange of writerly ideas. The patient, compassionate teachers at Portland Montessori Collaborative—including Mitra Hasan, Sue Ann Brevig, Dena Pak, Andy Orenstein, Hilary Smith, and Mercedes Castle—for guiding our children (and us!) through the preschool years.

To so many wonderful friends, including those who've helped shape these stories: Alisa Harvey, for close and thoughtful reading of early drafts and for the coziest hand-knit shawl to brighten dreary days. Laura Moran, for all-weather walks and talks, endlessly insightful wordsmithing, and solidarity in the triumphs and fails of parenthood. Sharon Kottler-Decker, for helping me consider nuances in health and healing, inspiring a love of reading in the next generation, and being that rare educator who strives to reach children who think differently. Ilme Raudsepp and Peter Puhvel for being there in the early days.

To all the dedicated medical professionals and scientists who've cared for and collaborated with me over the years: Devorah, for saving my life and believing my story and becoming a friend, and for truly listening through it all. Those who've supported us in calm and in crisis, including Mark Nichols, Meg O'Reilly, Nancy Gordon-Zwerling, Mary Costantino, Jeff Disney, Kendra Ward, Brian Shaffer, Gwen Fraley, Dana Hargunani, and Tara Schwab. Those I've had the privilege of working with and learning from, including Annette Magner, Annette Bennion Sisk, Dixie Whetsall, Meg Hayes, Jessie Flynn, Robyn Liu, Justin Denny, John Stull, Mel Kohn, Evelyn Whitlock, Roger Garvin, John Saultz, Paul Fisher, Mike Amylon, Richard Shaw, Eric A. Weiss, Lee Frizzell, Frank Hubbell, and all my classmates and colleagues at Harvard, Stanford, OHSU, Stonehearth Open Learning Opportunities, and Northwest Primary Care.

The college and graduate school mentors who sparked my fascination with the intersection of science and the human condition, including Glenn Adelson, Dan Perlman, Ken George, and Lynne Huffman— but especially Arthur Kleinman, for encouraging me to bring my social anthropologist's mindset to medical school in order to craft the narratives of illness and healing, even if neither of us could have foreseen how profoundly that advice would shape my career.

To the booklovers and fellow storytellers who've helped me transform a yearslong vision into a published reality: Laura Gross, for your gracious good humor, your empathy and responsiveness, and your steadfast support through the evolutions of this project. Gabriella Page-Fort, for your passion for lifting up women's voices, your conviction that choice is power, and your commitment to this book from the first time we spoke. Hanna Richards, for your meticulous and thoughtful attention to the small but meaningful details, and for your willingness to engage with our stories at a level that goes deeper than grammar and syntax. Ryan Amato, for demystifying the publishing process, and for guiding me through it with such love for your work. Dana Tanamachi, for creating the most perfect cover art I could have envisioned, and for so beautifully representing everything I hope this book will offer to its readers. Yvonne Chan, for the magical interior design that brought all the pieces together. Lucile Culver, Louise Braverman, and the rest of the devoted teams at HarperCollins, for all things behind-the-scenes, including publicity and marketing efforts and keen industry sensibilities that have elevated the presentation of these printed words. The many remarkable writers and friends who've offered inspiration, advice, and support along the way, and at just the right times, including Jodi Picoult, Michelle McCann, Fonda Lee, Amber Keyser, Pauls Toutonghi, Gosia Gramstad, Meghan Paddock Farrell, Ali McCart Shaw, Robin Karr-Morse, Jen Andreson, Kelly Woods, and Sarah Tracy. The staff at the Multnomah and Washington County library systems, for creating safe spaces for people to share stories, and for feeding our family's endless appetite for books.

Finally, and above all: to all the women gathered here, for putting your trust in me and for continuing to believe in this project for more than a decade. Our collaboration is a testament to persistence, patience, and love, and I appreciate you beyond measure. I step aside to make room for your words. . . .

~ ~ ~

Shreya (*Contrasts*) lives in the Midwest with her husband, Kyle, along with their teenage son and some dogs, where she is still working as a physician. She is deeply grateful for the family and friends who carried her through all her life challenges when she couldn't do it alone, and she is in awe of their love, strength, resilience, and unwavering support. Shreya is eternally thankful for the hardworking, dedicated teams of healthcare professionals who saved her life more than twenty years ago. Her life would not be possible without her village.

Erin Russell (*Blood and Promises*). "I'd like to thank my husband, Michael, for being the best choice I've ever made. You are a remarkable partner, and I'm proud to be your wife and the mother of our son. To Cooper, from the moment I carried you, you have always been a force. I'm proud to be your mom, and it is my honor to walk the journey of hemophilia and life with you. Never stop being strong AND soft. You are my favorite kid! I'd also like to thank my brother Gavin, my uncle Joe, and my cousin Joseph for paving the way and navigating hemophilia with grace. And finally, to my mom, Nancy, for being my example of how to fiercely protect and care for my son."

Rachel Herron (*Enough for Today*) lives in the Pacific Northwest with her two daughters—who are just fifteen months apart—along with her husband and their two dogs. She owns a boutique that carries clothing in a wide range of sizes, to improve access to fashion that allows everyone to feel confident in their body. She would like to thank her husband for never missing a prenatal doctor's appointment with her (after she learned how painful it was to receive bad news alone) and for being the calm and collected one throughout their journey to parenthood. She thanks Cheri Masshardt for her counseling and for being a steady voice reminding her that she always had enough for today. She thanks her mother and her mother-in-law for sharing their family-building stories, including the struggles of multiple losses, and for being constant sounding boards and prayer warriors on her behalf. She thanks Dr. Rebecca Thompson for showing her that some doctors really do care and want the best for their patients, by listening, spending time with her, researching her medical history, developing treatment plans, and supporting her path to motherhood all while showing compassion and genuine care for her future family. Finally, Rachel is confident that her faith got her through the hard times and that God was with her every step of the way. She continues to lean on Him while parenting growing girls who happen to be quite opinionated.

Anna David (*Fairy Tales*) is an artist, a mother, and the founder and executive director of NICU Families Northwest (NFNW), a non-profit organization serving families of prematurely and medically fragile infants in Oregon and Southwest Washington. She wishes to thank her husband, Peter, for his strength, love, and partnership during the harrowing days of the NICU and the epic adventure that is parenthood. Anna would also like to thank the early champions of NFNW and all the NFNW families for the lifelong connections she's made through that work and the immeasurable impact her NICU peers have had. She is thankful for the two magical creatures that are her daughters, Miranda and Winona, whose love and curiosity are everbearing. Update: the COVID-19 pandemic forced the unfortunate closure of NFNW in late 2021.

Maya (*So Far*) would like to thank her husband for his unwavering strength and support in their partnership. The two children they are raising together have been an incredible source of joy in their lives, reminding them every day that joy can coexist with sorrow. They take care to remember Ethan and to celebrate his birthday each year, and they are still thankful for the lessons he brought into their lives during his short presence in the world. Maya would also like to thank her friends and family for continuing to be open to sharing heartfelt moments in remembering Ethan. Maya's work in clinical research and Ethan's memory propel her to better the lives of others, both professionally and personally.

Kelly Burke (*Breathe*) continues to live and breathe in the Pacific Northwest with her wife and children. "Thank you to Dr. Rebecca Thompson and Dr. Jessica Flynn for their gifted intuitive perspectives and keen medical detective skills navigating a rare disease and advocating for lifesaving treatments in protocols that allowed me to be as functional a parent as possible. You are two truly exemplary doctors and humans who always make me feel heard and seen as a whole person. To the Monday Morning circle who writes to the pulse of my oxygen tank, embodying the power of connection through the stories of our lives and holding space to archive the tender fragility, strength, and humorous ways we are human. I am forever indebted to my extended family and village of coparents who have kept me in protective arms, coached my children through physical adventures that my body could no longer perform, and invested deeply in our family's well-being. You are why E. and A. reply with a long list of names when asked about their parents. To C.D.J. and C.M.Y., my anchors in all things mothering. To E. and A., my favorite water-fight instigators, blanket-fort companions, and soccering people. You have opened my world beyond my wildest dreams and are my greatest life gifts. PS—It's your turn to make the popcorn. And finally to D.V.D., for your willingness to step into parenthood with me, for loving the many versions of myself I've been, for your generosity and dedication to community, and for your delightful ability to still surprise me after all these years."

Victoria Kukreti (*Body Of*) is a visual artist in Portland, Oregon. She would like to thank her remarkably loving and supportive husband, Rahul, and their two exceptional children, as well as the many teachers and therapists who went above and beyond to help her get to where she is today, including Albert, Thomas, Carol, Nick, Jason, and Kristine.

Marissa (*Carry*). "I would like to thank my community and village. Thank you for holding me when I needed it and for letting me do the same for you. We were never meant to do this alone. Keep advocating and fighting for the rights of all our youth. I have so much gratitude that self-forgiveness is part of my story now and that I can embrace imperfection and strive to do better as I know better. Thank you for loving me at my messiest, K. I am delighted to be a part of your story, K. and S. I will always love you, E."

Eriko (*Lines*) would like to thank her parents and sister for their unwavering support throughout her life, her husband for his strength in weathering the ups and downs in creating a family, and her children who made her biggest dream finally come true.

Stacey Kalin, LMFT, LPC, (*This One Thing*) is the mother of three young children and a licensed clinical therapist enjoying life with her family in the Pacific Northwest. She would like to thank K. for helping her become the mother she always wanted to be. Update, November 2021: Stacey passed away far too soon, taken by an aggressive form of colon cancer that she fought bravely for nearly four years. She was an incredible person: a kind and honest friend, a patient and thoughtful listener, a dedicated mental health professional, a passionate advocate for children and families, a lover of wilderness and adventure, a creative and joyous birthday-party planner, a devoted mother and partner, and a generous spirit who embraced life even in its most challenging moments. She was grateful to know that her legacy of helping others would live on by sharing her story in this project. She is deeply missed by her family and friends and fondly remembered by her community.

Lia (*Third Child*). "I wish to thank my family and friends for their love and support."

Nancy Fresco, PhD, (*Remotely*) is a faculty member at the International Arctic Research Center at the University of Alaska, Fairbanks. As the author of other books, essays, and papers (please find her at nancyfresco.com!), she chose to take a leading role in crafting her story. She would like to thank her husband for his unfailing support as coparent and partner in adventure, her twins for their resilience, open-mindedness, energy, insightfulness, and humor, and her family doctor for being a conscientious and generous role model. She would also like to thank her parents, in fond memory, for always allowing her to be herself.

Tina Lamers, PhD, (*Solving for Unknowns*) is an engineering executive based out of Fort Collins, Colorado, with career-driven stints in many other locations across the globe. She hopes her story will inspire others to find a new life path when the one they planned is no longer an option. She wishes to thank her son, Justin, for his inner strength on his journey, from resilience in the face of loss to fully embracing life; her parents for their emotional support and for disrupting their lives to spend copious amounts of time away from their home to help her; her sister, Trisha, for moving to Colorado for a year; and her husband, Josh, for his quiet, steadfast support in her life's evolution over the past eighteen years.

Eileen Andersen (*Doing the Math*) is a postpartum doula in Minnesota. "I'd like to acknowledge my outstanding, kind, and smart medical cheerleaders: David Lee, MD; Leonardo Pereira, MD; Daniel Herzig,

MD; Sarah Wylie, ND; Melissa Kuser, ND; Jelena Stefanovic, LAc; Paula Acker, LCSW; Liliana Barzola, Intuitive; Clare Katner, LMT; and Antoinette Newman, MFT. You are the best and I cannot thank you enough. To my dog, Lily, who was always there to lick my tears of sadness and frustration. To my three living children: Sam, for choosing me to be your mom, Max, my rainbow baby, and Claire, my bright star. And to Spirit Max, for being oh so brave and paving the way for your siblings. Finally, to my husband, Paul, for always knowing it would all work out."

Lydia (*Given*) would like to thank her teachers, healers, and friends who have been guides in overcoming her childhood trauma, in particular Chad Angotta, Sister Paula Modaff, Colleen Taylor, and her best friend and husband, Nathaniel.

Carolyn (*Anyone Else's Family*). "I have always relied on my friends to fill the void I felt in my own family, so thanks to all of them, past and present, who have supported me during the challenges life has presented. You know who you are. I am so grateful to them all but most importantly to my loving husband, Bryan, who for almost thirty years has shown me kindness and love when in the beginning I didn't even know what that meant. I also want to acknowledge the love and support my Al-Anon friends have given me in my journey of healing and self-discovery. I've learned so much and continue to grow because of this program. And to my beloved daughter who had the courage to seek me out and put it all on the line to find me after more than thirty years apart. To finally hold her in my arms helped heal the hole in my heart I had endured for all those years."

Mitra Hasan (*Other Women's Children*). "I want to give thanks to the Creator, not only for the blessings but also for the trials. I would not be who I am or where I am without having followed this path. Along the way, I have met my amazing husband, Elijah, have been loved by him and his family, have been supported by him, and have grown with him. The journey with my own family has not always been easy but we continue to show up and support each other. To my circle of women, I am forever grateful to you for accepting me and for loving me. To all the mothers who have trusted me with their tiny babies, I thank you. Your precious gift has allowed me to love and care for many children. There is love, trust, and community that can be built outside one's family. My work as an assistant to infancy has given me the opportunity to be one of the first people that can show this to the tiny humans that I have cared for."

Dafna Lohr, MD, (Devorah (*A Good Story*)) is an OB/GYN in Portland, Oregon. "I would like to thank my husband, Andy, who has been right there with me through so much joy and pain. I am so lucky we found each other in the right place and time. You make me a better person and support and protect me like no one else. I am grateful for my two wonderful children, Zandy and Reuben, who are my whole heart and, no doubt, my greatest accomplishment. Thank you to my mom, Sue Ellen Schwartz, who modeled unconditional love and shared so much about herself with me when I was young that, even after she died too soon, I could keep her stories alive for my own children. And finally, I wish to thank Becca Thompson for writing this book, including me in it, and trusting me from the day we met. You have a true gift for making lemonade from lemons."

ABOUT THE AUTHOR

Rebecca N. Thompson, MD, is a family medicine and public health physician who specializes in women's and children's health. She trained at Harvard, Stanford, and Oregon Health and Science University and will always be learning from her most influential teachers—her patients, colleagues, family, and friends. She lives in Portland, Oregon, where she spends her free time wandering through green spaces, reading in cozy nooks, playing unreasonably complicated board games, repurposing found objects, and accompanying her husband and children on all-weather adventures near and far.